**Handb**
**Pediat**

**Second Edition**

QM
24

D1331221

# Handbook of Pediatric Urology

## Second Edition

## EDITORS

**Laurence S. Baskin, M.D.**
Chief, Pediatric Urology
Professor Urology and Pediatrics
University of California, San Francisco
University of California, San Francisco Children's Medical Center
San Francisco, California

**Barry A. Kogan, M.D.**
Falk Chair in Urology
Chief, Division of Urology
Albany Medical College
Albany, New York

## FOREWORD BY

Sam Hagwood, M.D.
W. H. and Marie Wattis Distinguished Professor
Chairman, Department of Pediatrics
University of California, San Francisco School of Medicine
San Francisco, California

## LIPPINCOTT WILLIAMS & WILKINS
### A **Wolters Kluwer** Company
Philadelphia • Baltimore • New York • London
Buenos Aires • Hong Kong • Sydney • Tokyo

*Acquisitions Editor*: Brian Brown
*Managing Editor*: Michelle M. LaPlante
*Project Manager*: David Murphy
*Manufacturing Manager*: Benjamin Rivera
*Marketing Manager*: Adam Glazer
*Compositor*: TechBooks
*Printer*: R.R. Donnelley

**© 2005 by LIPPINCOTT WILLIAMS & WILKINS**
**530 Walnut Street**
**Philadelphia, PA 19106 USA**
**LWW.com**

Printed in the USA

**Library of Congress Cataloging-in-Publication Data**

Handbook of pediatric urology / editors, Laurence S. Baskin, Barry A. Kogan;
foreword by Sam Hagwood.—2nd ed.
        p. ; cm.
    Includes bibliographical references and index.
    ISBN 0-7817-5162-4 (alk. paper)
        1. Pediatric urology—Handbooks, manuals, etc.   I. Baskin, Laurence S.
II. Kogan, Barry A.
    [DNLM: 1. Urinary Tract—abnormalities—Child—Handbooks.
2. Urinary Tract—abnormalities—Infant—Handbooks.
3. Urologic Diseases—Child—Handbooks.   4. Urologic Diseases—Infant—
Handbooks.   5. Urogenital Diseases—Child—Handbooks.
6. Urogenital Diseases—Infant—Handbooks.   WS 39 H2364 2005]
RJ466.H36 2005
618.92'6—dc22                                                          2004029980

                                                        10  9  8  7  6  5  4  3  2  1

# Dedication

We all have heroes that we look to for guidance and help. Mine was Dr. John Duckett, Jr., senior editor of the first edition of the *Handbook of Pediatric Urology*. Dr. Duckett was my role model and teacher for pediatric urology. He taught me the intricacies of patient care and the nuances of pediatric urologic surgery. Most importantly, his vibrant personality was reflected in the hope and spirit that he was able to give to his patients and colleagues. Dr. Duckett is greatly missed by all. This edition is dedicated to his memory. His spirit lives on in all who have learned from this great teacher, leader, mentor and friend.

*Laurence S. Baskin, M.D.*

I would like to dedicate this book first to the children whose care will be enhanced by the knowledge gleaned from these pages. Second, and no less important, to my wife Cheryl and my daughters Rebecca and Sarah, who have consistently provided both the balance and the love needed to make my life whole and productive.

*Barry A. Kogan, M.D.*

# Contributor List

**Ahmet R. Aslan, M.D.,** *Attending Physician, Department of Urology, Haydarpasa Numune Research and Education Hospital, Tibbiye Caddesi, Üsküdar, Istanbul, Turkey*

**Laurence S. Baskin, M.D.,** *Chief Pediatric Urology, Professor Urology and Pediatrics, University of California, San Francisco, University of California, San Francisco Children's Medical Center, San Francisco, California*

**James M. Betts, M.D.,** *Clinical Professor of Surgery, University of California, San Francisco, Department of Surgery, San Francisco, California; Surgeon-in-Chief, Department of Surgery, Children's Hospital Oakland, Oakland, California*

**Guy A. Bogaert, M.D., PH.D.,** *Professor in Urology, Faculty of Medicine, Katholieke Universiteit Leuven; Associate Professor, Department of Urology-Pediatric Urology, UZ Leuven-Gasthuisberg, Leuven, Belgium*

**Pamela A. Bogan, M.S., F.N.P.,** *Nurse Practitioner, The Urological Institute of Northeastern New York, Division of Urology, Department of Surgery, Albany Medical College, Albany, New York*

**Paul R. Brakeman, M.D., PH.D.,** *Adjunct Instructor, Department of Pediatrics, University of California, San Francisco, San Francisco, California*

**Michael DiSandro, M.D.,** *Voluntary Assistant Professor, Department of Urologic Surgery, University of Miami School of Medicine; Staff Physician, Department of Urologic Surgery, Miami Children's Hospital, Miami, Florida*

**Michele Brophy Ebbers, M.D.,** *Fellow, Pediatric Urology, Department of Urology, University of California, San Francisco, San Francisco, California*

**Melissa A. Ehlers, M.D.,** *Assistant Professor of Anesthesia, Director of Pediatric Anesthesia, Albany Medical Center, Albany, New York*

**Jack S. Elder, M.D.,** *Carter Kissell Professor of Urology and Pediatrics, Case School of Medicine; Director of Pediatric Urology, Rainbow Babies and Children's Hospital, Cleveland, Ohio*

**Karla M. Giramonti, R.N., M.S., F.N.P.,** *Instructor, Division of Urology, Department of Surgery, Albany Medical College, Nurse Practitioner, The Urological Institute of Northeastern New York, Albany, New York*

**Angelique C. Hinds, R.N., M.N., C.P.N.P.,**   *Pediatric Urology Nurse Practitioner, Department of Urology, University of California San Francisco Children's Hospital, San Francisco, California*

**Nicholas M. Holmes, M.D.,**   *Assistant Professor of Surgery, Department of Surgery, F. Edward Hébert School of Medicine, Uniformed Services University of Health Sciences, Bethesda, Maryland; Head, Pediatric Urology, Department of Urology, Naval Medical Center San Diego, San Diego, California*

**George W. Kaplan, M.D., F.A.C.S., F.A.A.P.,**   *Clinical Professor, Surgery and Pediatrics, University of California at San Diego; Chief, Department of Surgery, Children's Hospital, San Diego, California*

**Barry A. Kogan, M.D.,**   *Chief, Division of Urology, Professor, Surgery and Pediatrics, Department of Surgery, Albany Medical College, Albany, New York*

**Martin A. Koyle, M.D., F.A.C.S., F.A.A.P.,**   *Professor of Surgery and Pediatrics, Vice-Chief, Division of Urology, The University of Colorado; Chairman, Department of Pediatric Urology, The Children's Hospital, Denver, Colorado*

**Eric A. Kurzrock, M.D., F.A.A.P.,**   *Assistant Professor, Department of Urology, U. C. Davis School of Medicine; Chief, Pediatric Urology, U.C. Davis Childrens Hospital, Sacramento, California*

**Robert S. Mathias, M.D.,**   *Professor, Department of Pediatrics, University of California San Francisco Medical Center, San Francisco, California*

**Gerald C. Mingin, M.D.,**   *Assistant Professor, Department of Surgery, The University of Colorado; Attending Physician, Department of Urology, Denver Children's Hospital, Denver, Colorado*

**Hiep Thieu Nguyen, M.D., F.A.A.P.,**   *Assistant Professor, Surgery (Urology), Harvard Medical School; Assistant in Urology, Pediatric Urology, Children's Hospital, Boston, Massachusetts*

**Anthony Portale, M.D.,**   *Professor Pediatrics, University of California San Francisco Children's Hospital, San Francisco, California*

**Michael Ritchey, M.D.,**   *Professor, Surgery and Pediatrics, University of Texas Houston Medical School, Houston, Texas*

**Jeffrey A. Stock, M.D.,**   *Clinical Associate Professor of Surgery, University Medicine and Denistry, New Jersey Medical School; Director, Division of Pediatric Urology, Children's Hospital of New Jersey, Newark, New Jersey*

**Ronald S. Sutherland, M.D.,**   *Associate Clinical Professor, Department of Surgery, University of Hawaii; Chairman, Urology Service and Urology Residency Program, Tripler Army Medical Center, Honolulu, Hawaii*

**Hubert S. Swana, M.D.,**   *Clinical Instructor, Department of Urology, University of California San Francisco, San Francisco, California*

# Preface

A thousand new books are published every day. Why a pediatric urology handbook? We asked this question many times before writing the first edition, and the answer has been reinforced by the subsequent feedback we have received. There simply is no other resource that covers the breadth of pediatric urology in one highly readable, easy-to-use, and accessible source.

Extensively illustrated for the benefit of both patients and health care professionals, the second edition of the *Handbook of Pediatric Urology* is a comprehensive resource to answer your pediatric urology questions. An excellent complement for your office, clinic, emergency room, or classroom, the second edition has been expanded to include new chapters on laparoscopy in pediatric urology, sports recommendations for patients with solitary kidneys and other genitourinary anomalies, preparing your patient for pediatric anesthesia, and the treatment of urinary incontinence and constipation. The chapters on the classic pediatric urology problems such as hypospadias, hydronephrosis, reflux, urinary tract infection, undescended testes, hernia and hydroceles, and congenital anomalies have all been updated. We have included a new appendix of online recommendations because so many of our patients are computer savvy. Finally, the Pediatric Urology Facts and Figures: Data Useful in the Management of Pediatric Urologic Patients has been updated for a quick reference on important pediatric urology medication issues.

We hope you find the second edition of the *Handbook of Pediatric Urology* an excellent resource.

*Laurence S. Baskin, M.D.*
*Barry A. Kogan, M.D.*

# Foreword

Urinary tract malformations and anomalies as well as urinary tract infections are among the most common problems with which neonatologists, pediatricians, and primary care physicians must deal. Chronic renal failure with an attendant need for hemodialysis and/or transplantation, although somewhat less common, extracts a substantial toll on the ever more constrained financial resources of our health care system, and is the precipitant of major life adjustments for children and families who are affected by these conditions. Renal trauma and primary kidney cancer are also frequently encountered in pediatric practice. It is for these reasons that the publication of this concise and well-organized text is particularly welcome and should meet the needs of the busy practitioner in conveying important information about pediatric urologic disease, methods of evaluation, and therapeutic modalities.

*Sam Hagwood, M.D.*
*W. H. and Marie Wattis Distinguished Professor*
*Chairman, Department of Pediatrics*
*University of California,*
*San Francisco School of Medicine*
*San Francisco, California*

# Credits

The editors thank the following who gave educational grants in support of the publication of this handbook: Albany Medical College, Division of Urology; University of California–San Francisco, Department of Urology; Q–MED; and Braintree Laboratories.

# Contents

# Circumcision

Laurence S. Baskin

## I. THE ORIGINS OF CIRCUMCISION

**A.** Egyptian artifacts date circumcision to 6,000 years ago.

**B.** Four thousand years ago, the Old Testament references ritual circumcisions to be performed on the eighth day after birth with a flint knife.

**C.** Both the Old and New Testaments make numerous references to circumcision without any relationship to health benefits.

**D.** Widespread practice of circumcision originated in the 19th century, allegedly as a prophylaxis against disease.

**E.** The present incidence of circumcision in the United States is estimated to be between 60% and 90% of newborn boys, with a much lower incidence in Europe. Geographic variations exist, with the Midwest having a higher incidence of circumcision compared to the East and West coasts.

**F.** Circumcision is the most common operation performed in the United States.

## II. AMERICAN ACADEMY OF PEDIATRICS RECOMMENDATIONS

In 1975 and 1983, the American Academy of Pediatrics stated that "there is no absolute medical indication for circumcision in the neonatal period." This statement was reiterated and endorsed by the College of Obstetrics and Gynecology. In 1989, the American Academy of Pediatrics task force on circumcision concluded that newborn circumcision has potential medical benefits and advantages as well as disadvantages and risks. When circumcision is being considered, the benefits and risks should be explained to the parents and informed consent obtained.

## III. POTENTIAL MEDICAL ADVANTAGES

**A.** Prevent phimosis

**B.** Repair phimosis

**C.** Prevent balanoposthitis [superficial infection of the glans penis (*balano-*) and foreskin (*-posthitis*)]

**D.** Eliminate the risk of penile cancer

**E.** Potentially decrease the incidence of sexually transmitted diseases, cervical cancer, and human immunodeficiency virus infection

**F.** Reduce the incidence of urinary tract infection in male neonates (newborns to 3 months of age) by approximately tenfold

## IV. DISADVANTAGES

**A.** Transient behavioral and physiologic changes that the infant experiences

        **B.**  Pain

        **C.**  Potential complications of circumcision

        **D.**  Irreversible removal of the prepuce

**V.**  **CONTRAINDICATIONS**

All boys born with penile anomalies (hypospadias, epispadias, megalourethra)

**VI.**  **RELATIVE CONTRAINDICATIONS**

        **A.**  Bleeding diathesis

        **B.**  Prematurity

        **C.**  Severe medical problems

**VII.**  **OTHER FACTORS**

        **A.**  Emotional

        **B.**  Cultural

        **C.**  Religious

        **D.**  Father's foreskin status

**VIII.**  **NORMAL FORESKIN**

        **A.**  **Development**

            **1.**  The foreskin begins to develop in the third month of intrauterine life with normal completion by 4 to $4^1/_2$ months.

            **2.**  It is normal for the newborn's foreskin to be adhered to the glans.

            **3.**  Separation of the foreskin from the glans penis occurs late in gestation with only 4% of newborn boys having a completely retractable foreskin. In 50% of newborn boys, the foreskin can not be retracted far enough to visualize the urethral meatus.

            **4.**  By the age of 6 months, 20% of boys will have a completely retractable foreskin, and by 3 years that number increases to 90%. By the teenage years, complete separation of the foreskin has occurred in virtually all boys.

        **B.**  **Foreskin Care**

            **1.**  The uncircumcised penis needs no special care other than the same attention given to the rest of the body.

            **2.**  Genital hygiene in little boys does not require retraction of the foreskin.

            **3.**  For undetermined reasons, possibly folklore or tradition, many physicians, parents, and grandparents remain convinced that the foreskin must be retracted at an early age.

            **4.**  Painful early foreskin manipulation can lead to bleeding, scarring, phimosis, and psychological trauma for the child and parent.

**IX.**  **PHIMOSIS PENILE ADHESIONS AND PARAPHIMOSIS**

        **A.**  *Phimosis* is a narrowing of the opening of the prepuce, preventing it from being drawn back over the glans penis (typically from scarring and/or recurrent infection). Treatment in severe cases is surgical release of the scarred tissue, which may be referred to as a *cicatrix*. In less severe cases, the phimosis responds to local treatment with topical steroids. Betamethasone

0.05% ointment applied to the tip of the penis at the area of the phimosis for 6 to 8 weeks twice a day has a 50% to 90% success rate. After 1 week the patient (if old enough) or parent should gently pull back the foreskin to facilitate release of the phimosis.

**B.** Penile adhesions in children with and without circumcision typically resolve over time without formal treatment. If concerning to parents they may also be treated with topical steroids in the same fashion as described for phimosis. Recalcitrant adhesions after circumcision may require surgical release. Simple adhesions can be lysed with the use of EMLA cream and a sharp iris scissors in the office. More dense adhesions or multiple adhesions may require general anesthesia.

**C.** *Paraphimosis* is a painful constriction of the glans penis by the foreskin, which has been retracted behind the corona of the glans penis. Prolonged retraction of the foreskin leads to a relative obstruction of the lymphatics. This may cause lymphedema distally. Treatment requires reducing the foreskin after manual compression of the edematous glans penis. In severe cases, the constricting foreskin may need to be surgically released via a dorsal slit (see below).

**X.  METHODS**
The goal of circumcision is to remove an adequate amount of shaft skin along with inner-preputial skin so as to obtain an acceptable cosmetic result and prevent future development of phimosis and paraphimosis. There are four major techniques, which are described below.

**A. Dorsal Slit:** The dorsal slit is performed by incising the dorsal aspect of the foreskin, exposing the glans and thereby preventing phimosis and paraphimosis, but is usually cosmetically unacceptable. The dorsal slit is reserved for acute cases of phimosis or paraphimosis.

**B. Shield Technique (Mogen Clamp):** The Shield technique requires separation of the adhesions between the foreskin and the glans (Fig. 1–1A–C). The shield protects the glans by forcing it away from the stretched penis. The excess skin is excised and hemostasis achieved by manual compression.

**C. Gomco Clamp (Fig. 1–2) or Plastibell Clamp** (modifications of the Shield technique): When using a Gomco clamp, after freeing the inner preputial adhesions, the prepuce is drawn through a ring and hemostasis achieved by pressure between the ring and the Gomco clamp. If any separation occurs between the opposed skin edges after removal of the foreskin, the healing occurs either by secondary intention or primary suture. In the Plastibell technique, excess prepuce is allowed to necrose off (typically within 3 to 7 days) by placing a tight suture across the excess foreskin. A more common practice is to cut the prepuce off just distal to the absorbable suture.

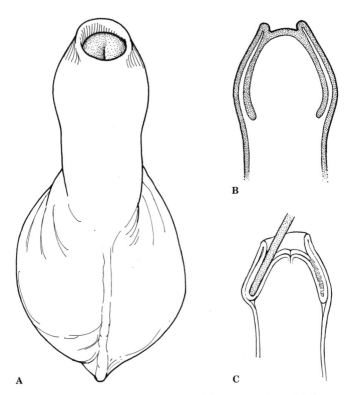

**A**                                                      **C**

**B**

Fig. 1–1A–C.   Schematic of separation of the prepuce from the glans, the critical step in a successful circumcision.

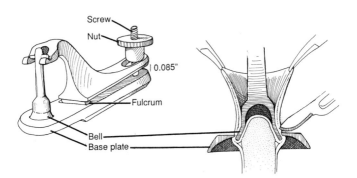

Fig. 1–2.   Schematic of Gomco clamp and application to penis.

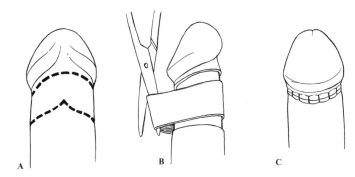

**Fig. 1–3A–C.   Schematic of freehand circumcision technique.**

In both the Gomco and the Plastibell techniques, the glans is protected by the respective clamps.

**D.   Freehand Surgical Excision** (Fig. 1–3A–C): This is done by a combination dorsal slit or Sleeve technique. The wound is primarily closed by approximating the skin with small absorbable sutures.

Most complications of circumcision can be avoided by careful attention to complete separation of the glans from the inner preputial epithelium (Fig. 1–1A–C), careful symmetric removal of the inner and outer preputial skin collar, and attention to hemostasis.

**XI.   COMPLICATIONS**

Complications are listed in Table 1–1.

**A.   Acute**

**1.**   Bleeding is probably the most common acute complication, and is typically controlled by direct pressure (the rare case will require placement of a suture).

**Table 1–1.   Circumcision complications**

| Acute | Nonacute |
| --- | --- |
| Bleeding | Skin loss |
| Infection | Skin excess |
| Amputation | Skin asymmetry |
| Urinary retention | Skin bridges |
| | Skin chordee |
| | Epidermal inclusion cyst |
| | Concealed penis |
| | Phimosis |
| | Meatal stenosis |
| | Urethrocutaneous fistula |

Incidence of circumcision complications has been estimated to range from 0.2% to 5.0%.

2. Partial penile amputation (glans or corporal injury) is a very rare complication of circumcision. If a serious amputation injury occurs, the patient should be immediately transported to the care of a pediatric urologic surgeon for an attempt at immediate penile reconstruction. Injury to the glans penis is typified by excess bleeding at the time of circumcision, or bleeding that is difficult to control with direct pressure.

3. Infections after circumcision are usually self-limiting and respond to local dressing changes. Serious necrotizing soft tissue infections have been reported, but are quite rare.

4. *Skin issues:* If during the course of routine circumcision an excessive amount of skin is inadvertently removed, such as the penile shaft skin, this should be treated by local wound care with a barrier cream such as petroleum jelly (Vaseline) and the penile skin allowed to heal by secondary intention. Rarely, if ever, is immediate penile skin grafting necessary. More common is too little skin being removed in asymmetric fashion, which can be treated electively. Caution must be used with electrocautery as a means for hemostasis during circumcision because the current may ground through the penile blood supply, resulting in thrombosis and necrosis of the glans penis.

**B. Nonacute**

1. Meatal stenosis is essentially unheard of in uncircumcised boys and is most likely a result of meatitis and meatal ulcers, which presumably occur because the meatus is no longer protected by the prepuce. The mechanism of meatitis is most likely an irritant reaction to ammonia produced by bacteria in a urine-soaked diaper. The meatus may also be subjected to mechanical trauma from rubbing against the diaper. Diagnosis of meatal stenosis is not based on visual inspection of the urethral meatus, but on visualization of the urinary stream. If the stream is deviated significantly, usually more than 30 degrees in an upward direction, a functional impairment with respect to hitting the toilet with the urinary stream is present and a meatotomy indicated. Meatotomy in an older cooperative child can be performed with the use of EMLA cream in the office. Younger children require a quick general anesthetic.

2. *Skin issues:* Late complications that may require repeat circumcision include inadequate foreskin removal; asymmetric skin removal; skin bridges, which occur from the raw surface of the glans healing to the cut edge of the foreskin; epidermal inclusion cysts, which occur when an island

of skin is left to heal underneath the skin that is primarily closed; and penile curvature, which can occur from skin tethering secondary to scar tissue from a circumcision that was performed at the time of acute inflammation.

3. Urethral cutaneous fistulas are known complications secondary to aggressive removal of the foreskin with entrapment of the penile urethra and subsequent ischemia from a crush injury.

XII. **LOCAL ANESTHESIA FOR NEONATAL CIRCUMCISION**

The dorsal penile nerve block and circumferential block at the base of the penis both have potential complications including local hematoma and bleeding. Techniques include the following.

A. **Dorsal Penile Nerve Block:** Lidocaine (0.02 to 0.4 cc of 1% lidocaine) is injected with a 27-gauge needle at the base of the penis at both the 10 o'clock and 2 o'clock positions dorsal laterally to infiltrate the neurovascular bundle.

B. **Circumferential Block at the Base of the Penis:** This is done with a 25 or 27 tuberculin syringe using 0.6 to 1.0 cc of 1% lidocaine without epinephrine using a single injection site ventrally at the penoscrotal junction. Care is taken to angle the needle laterally to avoid the urethra and a bilateral subcutaneous infiltration is achieved. The circumcision is performed 3 to 5 minutes after injection, allowing time for the anesthetic to take effect.

C. **EMLA Local Anesthetic Circumcision Technique:** EMLA is a eutectic mixture of local anesthetics which has not been approved for use in infants younger than 1 month or infants under the age of 12 months who are treated with methemoglobin-inducing agents. EMLA can be applied directly to the foreskin and has been useful as an anesthetic for meatal stenosis and may possibly have a role in pediatric circumcision.

D. **Oral Agents**
   1. Tylenol
   2. Sucrose
   3. Pacifier
   4. Manischewitz wine

XIII. **POSTOPERATIVE CARE OF NEWBORN CIRCUMCISION**

A. Proper postoperative care has the objective of minimizing postoperative bleeding; avoiding the formation of adhesions, skin bridges, and buried penis; and preventing infection.
   1. Postoperative care begins with a proper bandage. Recommended is either a petroleum jelly or petrolatum (Xeroform) bandage.
   2. An approximate 1- × 10-in. strip is cut from the prepackaged dressing and gently wrapped around the coronal sulcus.

3. The bandage is left for 24 hours if it does not fall off with the first diaper change. A lubricating (e.g., KY jelly) or antibiotic ointment may be applied to the exposed penis and petroleum jelly to the diaper.

4. If the petrolatum gauze has not fallen off in 24 hours, it is gently soaked off with cotton balls and tepid water. At that time the skin at the head of the penis is pushed back so the groove can be seen under the glans penis (the coronal sulcus), thus preventing penile adhesions. A wet cotton swab can aid in this process.

5. Parents are counseled that a few drops of blood or ooze may be seen on the diaper. Typically the baby may bathe at the time that the umbilical cord has fallen off. A soft yellow scab should not be confused with infection or pus; it is normally present, will fall off in time, and should not be removed.

**B.** The major complication that occurs and can be prevented at a 1-week follow-up visit is adhesions of the mucosal skin to the glans penis.

This can be corrected at this 1-week visit by gently pushing the skin at the head of the penis back so the groove under the glans penis is visible, thereby breaking up any adhesions that have formed.

## RECOMMENDED READING

Baskin L, Canning DA, Snyder HM, et al. Treating complications of circumcision. *Pediatr Emerg Care* 1996;12:62–68.

Goldman R. The psychological impact of circumcision. *BJU Int* 1999;83[Suppl 1]:93–102.

Moses S, Bailey RC, Ronald AR. Male circumcision: assessment of health benefits and risks. *Sex Transm Infect* 1998;74:368–373.

Schoen EJ, Anderson G, Bohon C, et al. American Academy of Pediatrics: Report of the Task Force on Circumcision. *Pediatrics* 1989;84:388–391.

Wiswell TE. John K. Lattimer Lecture. Prepuce presence portends prevalence of potentially perilous periurethral pathogens. *J Urol* 1992;148:739–742.

Wiswell TE, Geschke DW. Risks from circumcision during the first month of life compared with those for uncircumcised boys [see comments]. *Pediatrics* 1989;83:1011–1015.

# Hypospadias

Laurence S. Baskin

I. **INTRODUCTION**
   A. *Hypospadias* is a congenital defect of the penis, resulting in incomplete development of the anterior urethra, corpora cavernosa, and prepuce (foreskin).
   B. Clinically, the hypospadiac urethral meatus does not cause significant symptoms other than a urinary stream, which may be deflected downward.
   C. Hypospadias is also associated with penile curvature and may result in infertility secondary to difficulty in semen delivery.
   D. Hypospadias is not associated with an increased risk of urinary tract infection.

II. **EMBRYOLOGY**
   A. At 1 month gestation the male and female genitalia are essentially indistinguishable.
   B. Under the influence of testosterone, the male external genitalia become masculinized.
   C. By the end of the first trimester (at approximately 16 to 18 weeks), the penile urethra and accompanying prepuce are completely formed.
   D. Abnormalities in this development can lead to hypospadias and associated penile anomalies.
   E. In hypospadias, incomplete development of the glandular urethra does not allow the preputial folds to fuse.
   F. Consequently, in hypospadias the foreskin is absent on the ventrum and there is excessive foreskin on the dorsal surface (dorsal preputial hood).

III. **CLASSIFICATION**
   A. Hypospadias can be classified as to the location of the urethral meatus without taking into account penile curvature. Penile curvature or chordee is germane in that a distal hypospadias with severe curvature will require extensive reconstruction to correct both the curvature and urethra, as the abnormal meatus, which may now be at the penoscrotal junction.
   B. A more useful surgical classification is the location of the meatus after penile straightening or chordee correction at the time of reconstructive surgery, where
      1. Fifty percent of patients have anterior hypospadias with the meatus on the glans or subcoronal (Fig. 2–1A).
      2. Twenty percent have the urethral meatus on the penile shaft (Fig. 2–1B).
      3. Thirty percent have the meatus between the perineum and the penoscrotal junction (Fig. 2–1C).

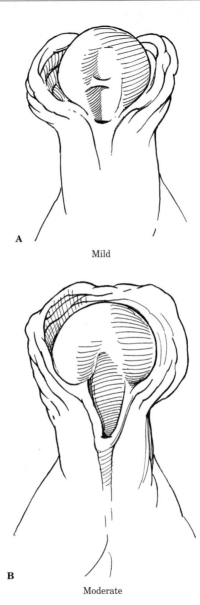

Mild

Moderate

Fig. 2–1.   Classification of hypospadias. A: Anterior hypospadias.
B: Penile shaft hypospadias.

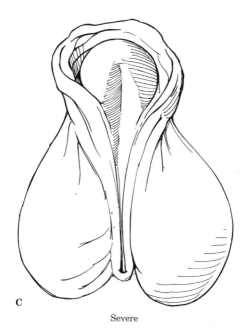

C

Severe

**Fig. 2–1.** (*Continued*) C: Scrotal hypospadias.

## IV.  INCIDENCE, GENETICS, AND ETIOLOGY

**A.**  Hypospadias occurs in 1 per 250 live male births.

**B.**  There is a 14% incidence in male siblings and an 8% incidence in offspring.

**C.**  The majority of cases of hypospadias have no known etiology. Extensive research into abnormal androgen metabolism or the levels of the androgen precursors, testosterone, or the more potent dihydrotestosterone has revealed only a small percentage of patients with any abnormalities.

**D.**  Environmental pollutants or endocrine disruptors have been suggested to cause hypospadias by maternal exposure that is carried to the developing fetus. Case reports human data and experimental animal data are cause for concern and further investigation is warranted.

## V.  ASSOCIATED ANOMALIES

**A.**  Undescended testes occur in approximately 9% of patients with hypospadias.

**B.**  There is increased incidence of up to 30% in patients with penoscrotal or more severe hypospadias.

**C.**  Inguinal hernias also occur in approximately 9% of patients with hypospadias.

**D.**  A utricle or Müllerian remnant in the posterior urethra is found in a high percentage of patients with severe hypospadias.

E. Associated urinary tract anomalies are uncommon in patients with isolated hypospadias because the external genitalia are formed much later than the kidneys, ureter, and bladder.

F. Patients with hypospadias and an undescended testicle or an inguinal hernia do not need further urinary tract evaluation.

G. Patients who have hypospadias in association with other organ system anomalies such as a cardiac murmur, imperforate anus, limb malformations, cleft lip, or pyloric stenosis require renal and bladder imaging with an abdominal ultrasound.

H. Patients with severe hypospadias and undescended testes should be karyotyped and undergo a further endocrinologic workup (see Chapter 4).

VI. **TREATMENT**

A. There are five basic phases for the successful reconstruction of the hypospadiac penis:
1. Creation of a normal urethral meatus and glans penis
2. A straight penis
3. A normal urethra
4. Skin covering
5. Normal position of the scrotum in relationship to the penis

VII. **TIMING OF SURGERY**

A. Hypospadias surgery is best performed between the ages of 6 and 18 months, prior to toilet teaching and during the psychological window when genital awareness has not been recognized by the patient.

B. Outpatient surgery is now the standard of care. The majority of hypospadiac defects can be repaired in a single-stage operation; severe cases often require a staged procedure. Early hypospadias repair with minimal hospitalization helps to avoid separation anxiety and fears related to genital surgery.

VIII. **ANESTHESIA**

A. Hypospadias surgery is performed under general anesthesia.

B. A penile nerve block or a caudal supplementation is standard to minimize postoperative discomfort.

IX. **HYPOSPADIAS OPERATIONS**

A. **Primary tubularization** (GAP, Thiersch-Duplay, King, Pyramid) (Fig. 2–2)

B. **Meatal advancement and glanuloplasty procedure** (MAGPI) (Fig. 2–3)

C. **Primary tubularization** with incision of the urethral plate (Snodgrass) (Fig. 2–4)

D. **Onlay island flap procedure** (Fig. 2–5)

E. **Staged repairs:** In patients with severe hypospadias, two planned operations performed about 6 months apart yield a controlled outcome with fewer complications. The first stage consists of penile straightening and the transfer of vascularized skin from the excess prepuce from the dorsal to the ventral

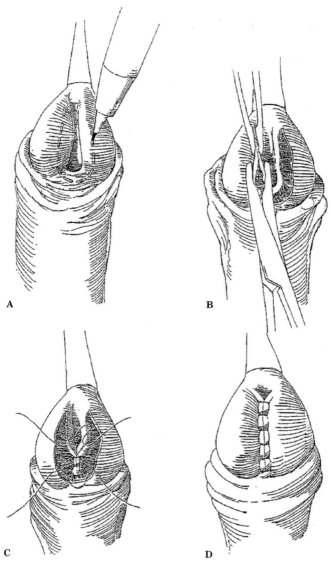

Fig. 2-2.   A–D: GAP hypospadias repair.

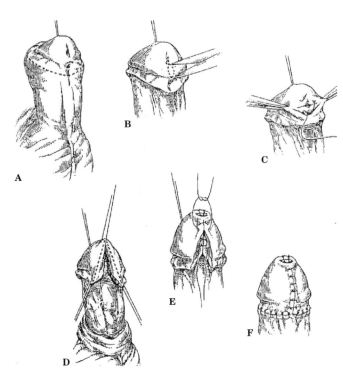

**Fig. 2–3.** A–F: MAGPI hypospadias repair.

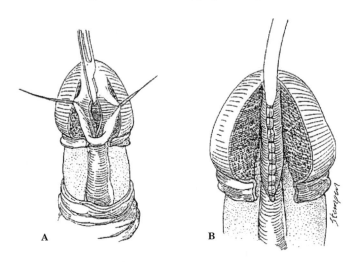

**Fig. 2–4.** A–B: Snodgrass hypospadias repair.

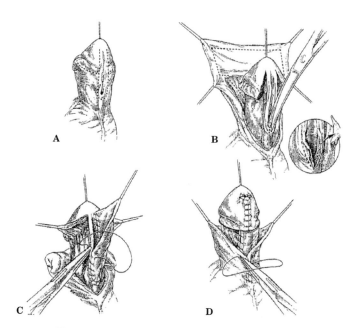

**Fig. 2–5.  A–D: Onlay island flap hypospadias repair.**

aspect of the penis. The second stage consists of the reconstruction of the new urethra, glans penis, and skin.

**F. Salvage repairs** with buccal mucosa grafts (taken from the inside of the cheek) can be used for urethral replacement, typically in a secondary procedure when local vascular flaps have failed (Fig. 2–6).

**G. Straightening the penis** can be performed with a midline dorsal tunica plication procedure that does not violate the nerve supply, thereby preserving normal erectile function (Fig. 2–7).

## X. SURGICAL COMPLICATIONS

**A. Urethno-cutaneous Fistula:** A communication between the new urethra and the penile skin, which typically allows urine to come out through two separate holes. Fistulas require operative closure approximately 6 months after the initial operation, when tissue swelling has subsided.

**B. Meatal Stenosis:** Stricturing of the new urethra, which can occur anywhere along the urethroplasty, but most commonly occurs in the glans penis.

**C. Urethral Diverticulum:**  A large outpouching or ballooning of the urethra secondary to too large of a urethroplasty or an obstruction distally (i.e., meatal stenosis).

**D. Superficial Skin Loss:** A relatively common complication after hypospadias surgery that typically heals

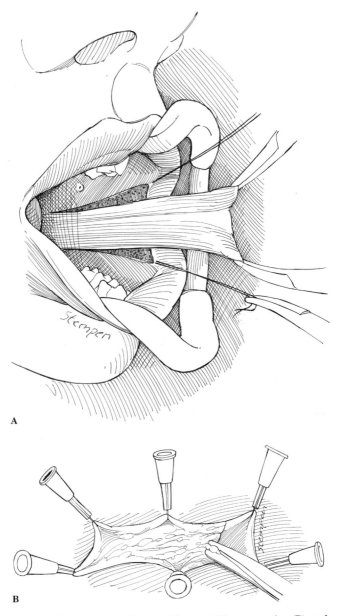

A

B

**Fig. 2–6.** Buccal mucosa free graft harvest (A), preparation (B), and tubularization

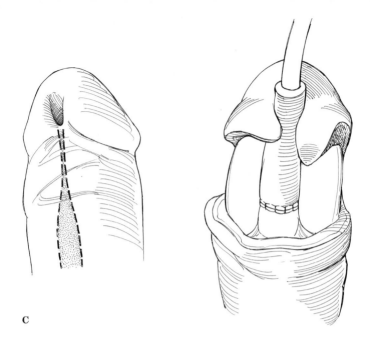

C

Fig. 2–6. (*Continued*) (C) into new urethra for secondary hypospadias procedures.

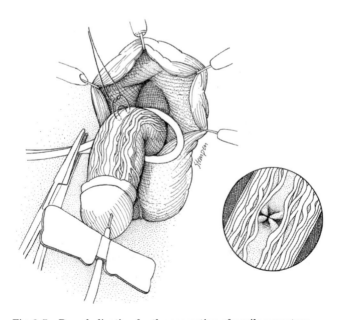

Fig. 2–7. Dorsal plication for the correction of penile curvature.

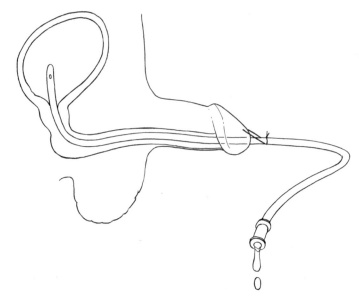

**Fig. 2–8. Urinary diversion drippy stent for hypospadias repair.**

spontaneously without the need for further surgical intervention by secondary penile skin granulation. This can be treated with local wound care and daily bathing.

   **E. Residual Penile Curvature:** If severe, reoperation with penile straightening is required.

**XI. POSTOPERATIVE CARE**

(See pediatric patient handout Web site Chapter 31.)

   **A.** Anterior hypospadias repair such as the MAGPI and GAP are often done without the use of a drippy stent and require no special treatment.

   **B.** More severe hypospadias requires the use of an indwelling drippy stent, which is typically removed 7 to 14 days after surgery by cutting a stitch that secures the urethral catheter to the glans penis (Fig. 2–8).

   **C.** Prophylactic doses of antibiotics (see Chapter 32) such as cotrimoxazole (Bactrim) or nitrofurantoin are typically prescribed while the stent is in place to keep the urine sterile.

   **D.** Postoperative symptoms include

      **1.** Bladder spasms, which can be treated with oxybutynin (Ditropan)

      **2.** Urinary retention (uncommon); secondary to a stent malfunction such as blockage or kinking

      **3.** Postoperative pain, controlled with acetaminophen (Tylenol), acetaminophen with codeine elixir, and antiinflammatory agents such as ibuprofen (Motrin)

E.  Dressings
    The most common dressing used after hypospadias is a plastic dressing such as Tegaderm, which is used with gauze to sandwich the penis onto the abdomen and is typically removed at home 2 to 3 days after surgery.

## XII. POSTOPERATIVE CARE

A.  The majority of patients with hypospadias can expect excellent outcomes with one operation. The reconstruction tends to grow with the child and results in a normal phallus for voiding, appearance, and sexual function after puberty.

B.  To ensure patient satisfaction and an understanding of their congenital anomaly, my practice is to see patients who have had hypospadias reconstruction 1 year after the repair, after toilet teaching, and after puberty.

C.  Patients with complications are seen as needed. With better primary surgical techniques, the goal is to eliminate the need for salvage surgery.

## RECOMMENDED READING

Baskin LS. Hypospadias. In: *Pediatric surgery,* 4th ed. O'Neill, 2002.
Baskin LS. Hypospadias. In: O'Neill JA Jr, Rowe MI, Grosfield JL, et al, eds. *Pediatric surgery,* 5th ed. New York: Elsevier, 2004.

# Undescended Testes

Guy A. Bogaert

I. **DEFINITION**

The testis is *undescended* if it is not in the scrotum or cannot be brought there during physical examination.

  **A.** From a clinical point of view, the testis may be palpable or nonpalpable.

  **B.** A palpable testis may be found along the normal descending pathway (exiting the abdomen at the internal inguinal ring in the direction of the external inguinal ring).

  **C.** *Cryptorchidism* means hidden or obscure testis in Greek and is often used interchangeably with *undescended testis*. Therefore, a cryptorchid testis maybe atrophic or ectopic as opposed to truly undescended.

  **D.** A testis that is not in the scrotum on physical examination is either palpable elsewhere or nonpalpable.

  **E.** A testis outside the scrotum, but palpable, can be either *retractile* (not truly undescended), *incompletely descended* (within the inguinal canal or just outside), or *ectopic* (following a different pathway, e.g., perineal or femoral).

  **F.** The inability to palpate a testis (nonpalpable) means the testis is either beneath the external oblique fascia (unusual), in the abdomen, or atrophic/absent.

  **G.** A boy with a unilateral normal descended testis has the same paternity chance as a boy with bilateral normal descended testes (90%). Paternity rate in bilateral undescended testes is 62%.

  **H.** The incidence of bilateral undescended testes is 5% to 15% of all boys with undescended testes.

II. **CLASSIFICATION**

  **A.** A *retractile testis* is not truly undescended and is generally palpated in the inguinal area. A retractile testis has an extrascrotal position intermittently because of an active cremasteric reflex. By definition retractile testes function normally.

  **B.** An ectopic testis (Fig. 3–1) (fewer than 5% of cases) descends properly until misdirected outside the external inguinal ring, presumably by an abnormal gubernaculum. These testes may be found in the perineum, prepenile, or femoral areas. These testes are thought to be more normal than incompletely descended testes.

  **C.** An incompletely descended testis (Fig. 3–1) (95% of cases) can be intraabdominal, in the inguinal canal, or just exiting the external ring (prescrotal).

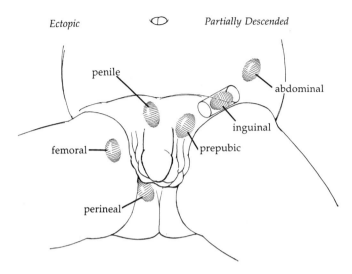

*Ectopic*    *Partially Descended*

penile

abdominal

inguinal

femoral    prepubic

perineal

**Fig. 3–1.   Patient's left side depicts normal pathway for testicular descent illustrating possible locations of undescended testes. Patient's right side shows possible location of normal testes that descend into an ectopic position.**

**D.** An absent or atrophic testis is uncommon (3.3% of all cryptorchid testis, likely the result of perinatal torsion).

**III.   INCIDENCE**

A unilateral cryptorchid testis is the most common disorder of sexual differentiation in boys and the most common surgical condition in pediatric urology.

**A.** The undescended palpable testis
   1. Newborns have an incidence of 3% to 5% of cryptorchidism (of those, 15% are bilateral).
   2. Serial studies at 3 and 9 months of age have shown that most of these cryptorchid testes descend spontaneously.
   3. By the age of 1 year, only 0.7% to 1.0% of these children will still have a cryptorchid testis (palpable along the expected descending pathway).
   4. The same incidence of 0.7% has been found in young adults (military recruits), suggesting that no spontaneous descent occurs after 9 months of age.

**B.** The nonpalpable testis
   1. In 20% of all children with a cryptorchid testis, the testis will be nonpalpable; however, only 25% of those will ultimately prove to be absent at surgical exploration.
   2. A nonpalpable testis is generally found intraabdominally, or, depending on the examiner,

sometimes inguinally (75% of all patients with an originally nonpalpable testis).

3. The information that a testis might be found even if nonpalpable is useful in reassuring concerned parents.

C. Risk factors for a higher incidence of an undescended testis

1. Newborn children who are premature, have a low birth weight, are small for gestational age, and twins have a significantly higher incidence of cryptorchidism.

2. Although it has been suggested that boys born after in vitro fertilization or intracytoplasmic sperm injection would present more frequently with cryptorchidism, it has not been demonstrated in large epidemiologic studies.

## IV. EMBRYOLOGY

A. Until the 6th week of gestation, gonads remain indifferent. During weeks 6 and 7, the effects of the testis-determining SRY gene (on the Y chromosome) result in differentiation into a testis. Also, during weeks 6 and 7, Sertoli cells develop and secrete müllerian-inhibiting substance, causing müllerian duct regression. From the 9th week of gestation, Leydig cells produce testosterone, which stimulates Wolffian duct development.

B. Testicular descent usually occurs during the third trimester (this can now be documented by prenatal ultrasound, in that no descent is seen before 28 weeks gestation).

## V. ETIOLOGY

Many theories have been proposed to explain the etiology of cryptorchid testes.

A. Abnormality of the gubernaculum testis

1. The gubernaculum is a cordlike structure that extends from the lower pole of the epididymis and the testis to the scrotum.

2. It appears that the gubernaculum does not pull the testis into the scrotum, but rather guides it by providing a space into which it can descend.

3. Absence or abnormality of the gubernaculum may be a cause of maldescent.

4. An ectopic testis is likely to be secondary to an abnormally positioned distal extension of the gubernaculum, leading the testis to an abnormal position.

B. Reduced intraabdominal pressure

1. Overall, it is doubtful that diminished intraabdominal pressure is an etiologic factor in most cases of cryptorchidism.

2. All patients born with the prune-belly syndrome have intraabdominal testes.

3. These may be due to reduced intraabdominal pressure, but may also relate to a mass effect from bladder distension.

   **4.** Similarly, patients with gastroschisis have a
   higher incidence of cryptorchidism. However,
   these patients also have central nervous system
   abnormalities, suggesting the possibility of pituitary or other endocrine dysfunction that may
   lead to incomplete descent.

**C.** Abnormal testis (inborn error)
   **1.** This hypothesis originates from the observation
   that a lower fertility rate is common even after
   successful orchiopexy (fertility rate does not equal
   paternity rate).
   **2.** Therefore, congenitally abnormal testes from otherwise healthy newborns might not descend normally.
   **3.** However, it has been shown in animal studies
   that a normal testis is not even a prerequisite
   for testicular descent: a testicular prosthesis will
   descend in place of a testis.

**D.** Endocrine abnormality (at the testicular level)
   Most likely an endocrine abnormality is the primary cause of cryptorchidism in the majority of
   healthy newborns. Human chorionic gonadotropin
   (hCG), testosterone, dihydrotestosterone, calcitonin
   gene–related peptide, epidermal growth factor, in-
   hibin, and luteinizing hormone (LH) all may influence directly or indirectly the process of testicular
   descent. Hence, an abnormality in one of these may
   result in cryptorchidism. In fact, several studies have
   shown reduced testosterone and LH during the first
   6 months of life in children with unilateral undescended testes. However, it is unclear how a generalized endocrinologic problem causes cryptorchidism
   on only one side. It is therefore suggested that the
   situation of hypogonadotropic hypogonadism is at the
   testicular level.

**VI. SIGNIFICANCE**
   **A. Cancer**
      **1.** Of all testis cancers, 11% originate in cryptorchid
      testes; there is a 25 to 30 times increased risk of
      testis cancer in cryptorchid patients.
      **2.** Looked at another way, some studies have shown
      that 1 in 100 patients with undescended testes
      develop testis cancer.
      **3.** Surgical orchiopexy does not alter the incidence of
      cancer.
      **4.** However, there are no long-term data on children
      treated with modern techniques, who have under-
      gone surgery around the age of 1 year.
   **B. Fertility and Paternity**
      **1.** The incidence of clinical infertility after treat-
      ment is hard to judge scientifically, owing to
      the variability in the cause of the anomaly,
      the difficulty in diagnosis and in quantifying
      testicular position, the variability in treatment
      and the lengthy follow-up necessary, as well as

disagreement about the best measure of fertility. Per definition, *fertility* consists of histologic evaluation or sperm analysis of the ejaculate. However, *paternity* is the most relevant and important aspect for the patient, but paternity consists of a combination of male and female fertility factors.

2. In general, the following information is useful.
   a. The histologic appearance of testes brought down in older children is less favorable.
   b. Studies of semen analysis in an attempt to measure fertility in patients with unilateral undescended testes show that 50% are abnormal. However, the paternity rate in these patients is almost normal (89%) and therefore the results of semen analysis are of no clinical importance.
   c. In patients with bilateral undescended testes, the semen analysis is abnormal in 75%.
   d. Studies of paternity by questionnaire have shown that patients with unilateral cryptorchidism have normal paternity rates, but those with a bilateral problem have markedly reduced paternity rates.
   e. Because current treatment recommendations (surgical repair at about 1 year of age) have not been in effect for long enough, there are no adequate studies of the effect of early treatment on fertility or paternity.

C. **Associated Findings**
   1. A cryptorchid testis is more prone to torsion and probably more susceptible to trauma.
   2. The psychological effects of the undescended testis are not well known, but are probably not as important as those from penile abnormalities.
   3. Also, the majority of children with a cryptorchid testis will have a patent processus vaginalis (indirect inguinal hernia).

VII. **DIAGNOSIS**
   The diagnosis of cryptorchidism is made by physical examination. If a child has no testis in the scrotum, the most important task for the examining physician is to determine whether the testis is palpable [retractile (not truly undescended), inguinal, or ectopic] or nonpalpable (abdominal/inguinal/absent-atrophic). There is no role for radiographic imaging in the diagnosis of cryptorchidism.

A. **Clinical Examination**
   1. Although dependent on the experience of the examiner, the clinical examination is the most reliable, accurate, least invasive, and least expensive test for a child with a cryptorchid testis.
   2. The best time to make the initial diagnosis of cryptorchidism is before 6 months of age. This is because the cremasteric reflex is weak in the

newborn period and overlying body fat is minimal. Of note is that a patient seen for an undescended testis, who had a normal testis for the first 6 months of life, is likely to have a retractile and not a truly undescended testis.

3. The shape of the scrotum on the side of the cryptorchid testis can be an indication of whether the testis was ever present. A normal hemiscrotum suggests that the testis will be found below the internal ring.

4. The inspection of the inguinal, suprapubic, scrotal, and perineal region will find an ectopic testis.

5. Palpation should start well above the scrotum, usually in the region of the superior anterior iliac crest. Then, a firm downward pressure (toward the sacrum) is applied as the examiner's hand moves obliquely toward the symphysis. While the examiner maintains this downward pressure (toward the sacrum, not the feet), the opposite hand is used to palpate the ipsilateral scrotum.

6. Another helpful maneuver to differentiate a retractile testis from a cryptorchid testis is to place the child in a frog-leg position and have him press the soles of his feet together. Having an older child squat often makes it possible to palpate a retractile testis.

7. It is unreliable to have the family check for the testis in the bath or other circumstances.

8. Repetitive examination or referral to an experienced examiner can avoid additional and invasive diagnostic procedures as well as reduce confusion or differentiation between an undescended (and in some cases, nonpalpable) testis with a retractile testis.

**B. Localization Studies**

In essence, if the testis is found by an imaging study, surgery is needed; if it is not found, surgery is needed to be definitive.

1. Imaging studies are popular, but should only be considered for nonpalpable testes. Even so, radiologic evaluation of the nonpalpable testis is not generally helpful because surgery will still be necessary.

2. Although ultrasonography is noninvasive, this technique commonly produces false-negative and false-positive results, which preclude its clinical usefulness.

3. Gonadal arteriography, contrast peritoneography, and gonadal venography have all been advocated but have fallen into disuse because they are invasive and have significant false-negative and false-positive rates.

4. Computed tomographic scanning has been utilized, but despite technical refinements, there is

radiation exposure and failure to find a testis does not preclude surgery.

5. Magnetic resonance imaging does not use ionizing radiation but requires sedation or anesthesia in young children. It is the most accurate radiographic test available, yet it is expensive and not reliable enough to preclude surgery.

6. Laparoscopy is the most reliable technique of localizing a nonpalpable testis or proving its absence. Although it requires general anesthesia, it is a safe, accurate, and fast procedure in the hands of an experienced examiner. In addition, the laparoscopic findings will define the next operative step, which can be a standard inguinal incision, or the placement of additional ports to mobilize the testis and its vessels and perform a laparoscopic orchiopexy (one stage or a two-staged Fowler-Stephens orchiopexy). This means that laparoscopy as a diagnostic tool is essentially the first step of treatment.

C. **Hormonal Evaluation**

1. Hormonal evaluation is of debatable usefulness. It is definitely of no clinical value when the undescended testis is palpable.

2. In the situation of bilateral undescended testes, a chromosome and hormonal analysis is essential. Girls with congenital adrenal hyperplasia may be fully virilized and present as boys with an empty scrotum. To prove anorchia, there must be a high baseline LH and follicle-stimulating hormone as well as a low testosterone and no testosterone response to a prolonged trial of hCG. If these criteria are completely met, anorchia is most likely and laparoscopic confirmation may be postponed until puberty, when testicular prostheses are likely to be placed. Otherwise, early surgical exploration of anorchia is necessary.

3. Vanishing testis syndrome is noted in a boy (XY) with a normal penis and scrotum and bilateral anorchia. If penile and scrotal development is normal, testes must have been present until the 12th to 14th week of gestation, when masculinization is completed. Most likely this syndrome is the result of neonatal torsion. Surgical exploration confirms the presence of bilateral vas deferens and blind-ending vessels.

VIII. **THERAPY**

The rationale for treatment of patients with cryptorchidism is based on limiting complications. Fertility and malignancy are the main considerations, although the chance of torsion, trauma, and the psychological aspect of missing a testis also play a role. Furthermore, there is the common association of a patent processus vaginalis that requires surgical correction when the processus is patent after the age of 1 year.

A. **Hormonal Therapy** (before or after surgery, or none)

In a large metaanalysis of published data using hCG or luteinizing hormone-releasing hormone (LHRH) in an attempt to treat undescended testes, the success descent rate was 12%. Early studies suggest that LHRH in a long-term low-pulsatile dosage after successful scrotal orchiopexy can increase germ cell counts. However, there are no data available to support the benefit or the clinical relevance, if the aim is to improve fertility or paternity. There are no known side effects to long-term low-dose LHRH treatment.

1. Hormonal therapy should not be considered in cases with an obvious patent processus vaginalis (hernia), in ectopic testes, or where these testes are mechanically prevented from entering the scrotum (previous unsuccessful surgery).

2. hCG and LHRH can be used individually or in combination. hCG acts on the Leydig cells, whereas LHRH acts indirectly through the pituitary, and may be more efficient than LHRH at increasing testosterone, but neither agent is clinically superior to the other.

3. hCG (preferred in the United States) is administered intramuscularly and the dosage depends on the age and weight of the child. One dosage schedule is 1,000 IU weekly for a child up to 10 kg, 1,500 IU weekly for those between 10 and 20 kg, and 2,500 IU weekly for children weighing more than 20 kg for 4 consecutive weeks.

4. LHRH, which is preferred in Europe, is administered as a nasal spray. If used in an attempt to treat before surgery, the success rate is about the same as that seen with hCG, namely 10% to 15%. The dosage suggested to improve the number of germ cells after surgery is 0.2 mg biweekly for a period of 6 to 24 months (studies ongoing).

B. **Surgery**

1. Operative treatment should be undertaken early, between 9 and 18 months of age. This is after the time where most spontaneous descent would have occurred (between 0 and 9 months) and before elevated intraabdominal temperature has a chance to damage testicular germ cells. Also, from a psychological point of view, it is well accepted that children do better with genital surgery before the age of 18 months. There is less separation anxiety and fewer castration concerns.

2. Standard inguinal exploration and orchiopexy: Surgery for a palpable cryptorchid testis consists of a 3-cm inguinal incision (usually hidden in an inguinal skin crease), mobilization of the spermatic cord and testis, and ligation of the associated patent processus vaginalis. The testis is mobilized into a subdartos pouch in the scrotum.

The procedure can nearly always be performed as an outpatient with minimal morbidity (young children will be essentially normal within 2 days). The success rate is 99%. An adjunctive caudal or ilioinguinal nerve block allows the patient to awaken without pain and greatly reduces stress for all concerned.

3. Surgery for intraabdominal testes: Surgery for intraabdominal testes is technically challenging. Numerous options have been suggested, including orchiectomy when the condition is unilateral. Because a nonpalpable testes is unlikely to descend into the scrotum after 6 months of age, surgery can be performed at 6 months of age.

   a. A standard inguinal orchiopexy will only succeed in rare cases.

   b. Acceptable results have been achieved with a planned two-stage inguinal operation, with or without a Silastic sheath around the spermatic cord to facilitate the dissection. Nonetheless, this can cause a fair amount of morbidity and the second stage can be quite difficult, often resulting in damage to cord structures.

   c. Alternatively, modifications have allowed good success in highly skilled hands with additional dissection underneath the skin incision or by the Fowler-Stephens (see below) approach through an inguinal incision.

   d. Microvascular transfer of an intraabdominal testis has a high success rate (88%), but requires the availability of a microvascular surgeon and equipment and the procedure is time intensive (the last is particularly relevant as the necessity for the procedure cannot be determined preoperatively). In addition, this approach has required 8 to 11 days of postoperative hospitalization and immobilization. Hence it has fallen out of favor at most centers.

   e. In recent years, however, laparoscopy has become the treatment of choice in the approach of abdominal testes. In many centers, laparoscopy is performed to visualize the testis and plan the approach. In skilled hands, the testis may be mobilized laparoscopically and brought into the scrotum this way (with a minimum of morbidity and as an outpatient procedure). In some cases, the testis is too high and the spermatic vessels must be divided to provide sufficient length. In these cases, the collateral blood flow from the vas deferens must be carefully preserved and keeps the testis alive in most instances (two-stage Fowler-Stephens procedure).

     **f.**  Removal of the testis is recommended currently if an abdominal testis is found in a boy older than 10 years who has a normal contralateral descended testis. In these cases, the chance of the testis contributing to fertility is minimal and the testis is still prone to malignancy; therefore, orchiectomy is advised.

  **4.**  There is presently no indication for routinely performing a testicular biopsy in every child undergoing surgery for cryptorchidism.

  **5.**  A suture in the testis can cause damage. Recent studies have shown that the relative risk of fertility problems increases 7.6 times after a suture through the tunica albuginea of the testis, 5.5 times if bilateral cryptorchidism is found.

**C.** **Combination** **of** **Hormonal** **Therapy** **and** **Surgery**

As mentioned, there is ongoing, highly innovative work on long-term hormonal stimulation after surgical orchiopexy. In theory, if these patients have reduced LH and testosterone levels (perhaps the cause of the failure to descend), their testes, even if brought into the scrotum, would not function normally. Therefore, a 6-month course of biweekly stimulation with an LHRH agonist (0.2 mg) has been suggested. However, this approach is still unproven in the long term and should be considered experimental.

## RECOMMENDED READING

Cortes D. Cryptorchidism—aspects of pathogenesis, histology and treatment. *Scand J Urol Nephrol Suppl* 1998;196:1–54.

Hadziselimovic F, Herzog B, eds. Cryptorchidism, its impact on male fertility. *Horm Research* 2001;55(1):1–56.

Hadziselimovic F, Herzog B. Treatment with a luteinizing hormone-releasing hormone analogue after successful orchiopexy markedly improves the chance of fertility later in life. *J Urol* 1997;158:1193–1195.

Heyns CF, Hutson JM. Historical review of theories on testicular descent. *J Urol* 1995;153:754–767.

Nistal M, Paniagua R, Diez-Pardo JA. Histological classification of undescended testes. *Hum Pathol* 1980;11:666–674.

# Abnormalities of Sexual Differentiation

Hiep T. Nguyen

Sexuality is defined by a complex interaction between our genetic makeup, environmental stimulus, and cultural influences. The origins of our sexuality occur at the time of conception when the genetic material from two sources of the opposite sex coalesce into a new individual. From that moment sexual differentiation occurs by a highly organized process. Sex chromosomes and autosomes dictate the development of gonads; the gonads in turn produce hormones, which then direct the development of the internal and external genitalia. Disorders of sexual differentiation arise from abnormalities in chromosomes, gonadal development, or hormonal production/activity.

Patients with disorders of sexual differentiation may present (a) as a newborn with ambiguous genitalia or if chromosomal sex of amniocentesis differs from that of the infant's phenotype; (b) with inappropriate pubertal development; (c) with delayed pubertal development; or (d) later in life with infertility.

## I. NORMAL SEXUAL DIFFERENTIATION
### A. Chromosomes
1. Male: The genetic materials necessary for the development of the male phenotype are located on the short arm of the Y chromosome [the sex-determining region of the Y chromosome (SRY)]. The SRY region or testis-determining factor (TDF) gene codes for proteins that have the ability to bind to DNA and RNA. These proteins in turn regulate the expression of other genes on the X chromosome and on autosomes that subsequently direct the development of the testis.
2. Female: The genetic information for the development of the female phenotype is located on the X chromosome and on autosomes. However, the molecular processes involved remain unknown.

### B. Gonads:
The gonads develop from the genital ridges, which are formed during the 4th week of gestation. The germ cells located in the endoderm of the yolk sac migrate to the genital ridges where the cells are compartmentalized and differentiated into specific components of the gonads.
1. Male: At approximately the 6th to 7th week of gestation, the development of the testis begins under the influence of TDF and its downstream protein products. Some of the primordial germ cells differentiate into Sertoli cells, providing early endocrine function in the fetal testis. Others differentiate

into Leydig cells, which are responsible for the production of testosterone. The remaining primordial germ cells differentiate into spermatogonias. Loose mesenchymal tissue condenses into a thick layer, the tunica albuginea, that surrounds the testis and separates their connection with the coelomic epithelium and prevents further migration of mesonephric cells into the testis.

2. Female: Without TDF gene products, the primitive gonads begin to differentiate into the ovaries at approximately the 15th week of gestation. The primordial germ cells differentiate and are arrested in the last phase of meiotic prophase to form the oocytes. The cells in the genital ridges develop into granulosa cells, which surround the oocytes. The fetal ovaries produce estradiol; however, the exact site of estradiol synthesis in the fetal ovaries is currently not known.

C. **Hormones:** At 3.5 weeks of gestation, the wolffian system (Fig. 4–1) appears as longitudinal ducts, cranially connecting to the substance of the mesonephros and caudally draining into the urogenital sinus. At approximately the 6th week of gestation, the Müllerian duct develops as an evagination in the coelomic epithelium just lateral to the wolffian duct.

1. Male: At the 8th to 9th week of gestation, the Sertoli cells of the fetal testis secrete müllerian-inhibiting factor (MIF; also known as müllerian inhibiting substance or anti-müllerian hormone). This glycoprotein induces the regression of the müllerian ducts. Because MIF acts locally, müllerian duct regression only occurs on the ipsilateral side of the fetal testis producing this hormone. MIF also induces the formation of seminiferous tubules and further differentiation of the testis. At the 9th or 10th week of gestation, the Leydig cells appear in the testis and begin to synthesize testosterone. This hormone transforms the wolffian duct into the male genital tract, which is completed by the end of the 11th week of gestation. Beginning in the 9th week of gestation, testosterone also induces the development of the external genitalia from the genital tubercle, urogenital sinus, and genital swellings. In these tissues, testosterone is converted by 5-$\alpha$ reductase into dihydrotestosterone (DHT), which regulates the transformation of these tissues into the glans penis, penile and cavernous urethra, Cowper's glands, prostate, and scrotum. At the 28th to 37th week of gestation, testicular descent into the scrotum begins. Although the mechanisms of this process are not completely understood, they are thought to be androgen dependent.

2. Female: The female internal genitalia develop from the müllerian ducts. Without testosterone,

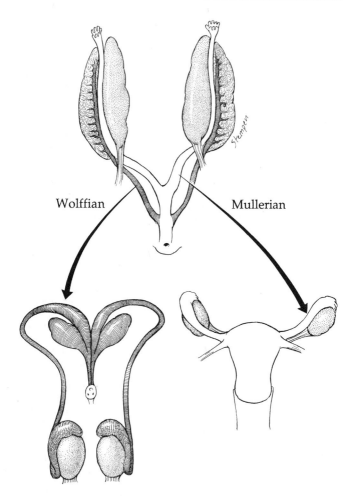

**Fig. 4–1.** Embryologic development of both the male and female reproductive tracts from a common origin.

the wolffian ducts regress at the 9th week of gestation. At this time, the müllerian ducts begin to differentiate; the cranial portion forms the fallopian tube, and the caudal portion from both ducts fuses to form the uterus, cervix, and upper portion of the vagina. Concurrently, the external genitalia (the lower portion of the vagina, vestibule, Bartholin and Skene glands, clitoris, and labia minora and majora) develop from the urogenital sinus and genital tubercles. Like the testis, the ovary undergoes a partial transabdominal descent. However, transinguinal descent of the ovary does not occur, leaving the ovaries just below the rim of the true pelvis. The role of estrogen in the differentiation of the female phenotype is unclear.

## II. DISORDERS OF SEXUAL DIFFERENTIATION

Abnormal sexual differentiation may be divided into three categories.

**A. Disorders of chromosomal sex** result from abnormalities in the number or structure of the sex chromosomes. These abnormalities may arise from nondisjunction, deletion, breakage, rearrangement, or translocation of genetic material on these chromosomes. These disorders are summarized in Table 4–1.

**B. Disorders of gonadal sex** result from abnormalities in gonadal development. In these disorders, the karyotype is normal (i.e., 46XX or 46XY). However, mutations in the sex chromosomes or autosomes, teratogen, or trauma to the gonads interfere with their normal development. These disorders are summarized on Table 4–2.

**C. Disorders of phenotypic sex** result from abnormalities in hormonal production or activity. Etiologies include defective synthesis by the gonads, abnormal production by the adrenal glands, presence of exogenous sources, or abnormalities in receptor activity. These disorders are summarized in Table 4–3. Figure 4–2 illustrates the pathway of hormone synthesis by the adrenal glands.

## III. EVALUATION AND DIAGNOSIS OF INTERSEX

The accurate diagnosis of a patient with intersex is a challenging process. Based on the diagnosis, decisions will be made for gender assignment, which will have a great impact not only on the patient but also the patient's family. Furthermore, in cases such as severe salt-wasting congenital adrenal hyperplasia, accurate diagnosis is often life-saving.

**A. History**

1. A detailed history is of great importance. Because many of the disorders such as XX male syndrome and true hermaphrodite are hereditary, a family history should carefully be examined not only for similarly affected individuals but also for variant forms, unexplained death during infancy, infertility, amenorrhea, and hirsutism.

2. Drugs ingested during pregnancy such as progesterone and virilizing signs in the mother during pregnancy should be ascertained.

**B. Physical Examination**

1. **General:** The abdomen and perineum should be carefully palpated for midline structures as a uterus. Other helpful physical findings include dehydration, failure to thrive (in patients with salt-wasting congenital adrenal hyperplasia), and the presence of other associated anomalies (in patients with Turner or Klinefelter syndrome).

**Table 4-1. Disorders of chromosomal sex**

| Disorder | Pathology | Chromosomes | Incidence | Gonads | Internal Genitalia | External Genitalia | Other Features | Risk of Cancer | Treatment |
|---|---|---|---|---|---|---|---|---|---|
| Klinefelter syndrome | Extra X and/or Y chromosome | 47XXY 46XY/47XXY | 1 in 500 | Hyalinized testis no spermatogenesis | Wolffian | Male | Gynecomastia Tall stature Mild mental retardation Elevated FSH/LH Low testosterone Elevated estradiol Infertility | Breast Extragonadal germ cell | Supplemental androgens Surgery for severe gynecomastia |
| Klinefelter variant | Extra X and/or Y chromosome | 48XXYY 48XXXY/ 49XXXYY 49XXXXY | Rare | Hyalinized testis No spermatogenesis | Wolffian | Male | As in Klinefelter More severe mental retardation | Similar to Klinefelter | Same as Klinefelter |
| XX male | No Y chromosome Translocation of SRY/TDF Activation of downstream TDF genes | 46XX | 1 in 20,000 to 24,000 | Hyalinized testis no spermatogenesis | Wolffian | Male | Gynecomastia Short stature Increased incidence of hypospadias Normal mental status May be familial | Rare germ cell | Same as Klinefelter |

| Disorder | Pathology | Chromosomes | Incidence | Gonads | Internal Genitalia | External Genitalia | Other Features | Risk of Cancer | Treatment |
|---|---|---|---|---|---|---|---|---|---|
| Turner syndrome | Absence of X chromosome | 45X | 1 in 2700 | Streak gonads -no germ cells | Müllerian | Immature female | Short stature Little breast development Webbed neck and other somatic abnormalities Cardiovascular abnormalities (i.e., coarctation) Renal abnormalities (horshoe or malrotation) Autoimmune disease (hypothyroid, diabetes) Infertility Amenorrhea | Germ cell in Y-chromosome mosaic | Supplemental estrogen Removal of streak gonads in Y-chromosome mosaic |
| Turner variant (X-chromatin–positive gonadal dysgenesis) | Partial X chromosome deletion or addition | 45X/46XX 45X/47XXX 45X/46XX/ 47XXX 46XXqi or 45X/46XXqi 46XXpi 46XXr or 45X/46XXr 46XXp- or 45X/46XXp- 46XXq- or 45X/46XXq- | Rare | Streak gonads | Müllerian | Immature female | Similar to Turner | Similar to Turner | Same as Turner |

(Continued)

**Table 4-1. (Continued)**

| Disorder | Pathology | Chromosomes | Incidence | Gonads | Internal Genitalia | External Genitalia | Other Features | Risk of Cancer | Treatment |
|---|---|---|---|---|---|---|---|---|---|
| Mixed Gonadal Dysgenesis (X-chromatin Negative Gonadal Dysgenesis) | Incomplete virilization and müllerian regression | 45X/46XY (70%) undetected mosaic- 46XY 45X/47XYY 45X/46XY/ 47XYY | | One testis (usually undescended) and streak gonad | Wolffian and Müllerian | Usually ambiguous 60%; reared female | Somatic features like 45X | Germ cell | Female Prophylatic gonadectomy Male Streak gonads removed -Intraabdominal testis excised unless can be relocated and no ipsilateral Müllerian structure present Reconstructive surgery |
| True hermaphrodite | Unknown | 46XX (70%) 46XY (10%) mosaic | Unknown | Bilateral ovitestis (20%) Ovitestis and ovary or testis (40%) One ovary and testis (40%) | Wolffian and Müllerian | Usually ambiguous; 70% reared male | Gynecomastia at puberty Menstruation at puberty May be familial | Rare germ cell | Reconstructive surgery Possible remove gonads |

Abbreviations: −, deletion; FSH, follicle-stimulating hormone; i, insertion; LH, luteinizing hormone; P, short arm of the chromosome; q, long arm of the chromosome; r, ring chromosome.

**Table 4-2. Disorders of gonadal sex**

| Disorder | Pathology | Chromosomes | Incidence | Gonads | Internal Genitalia | External Genitalia | Other Features | Risk of Cancer | Treatment |
|---|---|---|---|---|---|---|---|---|---|
| Pure gonadal dysgenesis | Unknown mutation prevents normal differentiation of gonads | 46XX 46XY | 1 in 8,000 | Bilateral streak gonads | Müllerian | Immature female | Normal to tall stature Miminal somatic abnormalities Female: Estrogen deficiency Male: Testosterone deficiency May be familial | Germ cell in 46XY | Estrogen supplement Remove gonads in 46XY |
| Absent testes syndrome | Mutation, teratogen or trauma to testis | 46XY | Unknown | Absent/rudiment testis No streak gonads | Wolffian | Variable virilization | Normal | Usually none | Female Estrogen supplement -Reconstructive surgery Male -Androgen supplement |

**Table 4–3. Disorders of phenotypic sex**

| Disorder | Pathology | Chromosomes | Incidence | Gonads | Internal Genitalia | External Genitalia | Other Features | Urinary Steroids | Risk of Cancer | Treatment |
|---|---|---|---|---|---|---|---|---|---|---|
| **Female Pseudohermaphrodite** | | | | | | | | | | |
| 3-β-Hydroxysteroid dehydrogenase deficiency | Excess androgens | 46XX | Second most common of CAH | Ovary | Müllerian | Mild ambiguous | Severe salt wasting No cortisol No aldosterone | DEAS | None | Replacement mineralocorticoids and glucocorticoids Reconstruction as needed |
| 11-β-Hydroxylase deficiency | Excess androgens | 46XX | Rare | Ovary | Müllerian | Ambiguous | Hypertension Decreased cortisol Decreased aldosterone | 11-DCS 11-DOC | None | Replacement glucocorticoids |
| 21-Hydroxylase deficiency Partial | Excess androgens | 46XX | 1 in 5,000 to 15,000 | Ovary | Müllerian | Ambiguous | Normal cortisol Increased aldosterone | 17-OH-P | None | Reconstruction as needed |
| Severe | Excess androgens | 46XX | | Ovary | Müllerian | Ambiguous | Severe salt wasting Decreased cortisol Decreased aldosterone | 17-OH-P | None | Replacement mineralocorticoids and glucocorticoids Reconstruction as needed |
| Excess maternal androgens | Excess androgens | 46XX | — | Ovary | Müllerian | Ambiguous | Drugs such as progestational agents Virilizing ovarian adrenal tumors | None | None | None |

## Male Pseudohermaphrodite

| Disorder | Pathology | Chromosomes | Incidence | Gonads | Internal Genitalia | External Genitalia | Other Features | Urinary Steroids | Risk of Cancer | Treatment |
|---|---|---|---|---|---|---|---|---|---|---|
| 20,22 Desmolase deficiency | Defect in testosterone synthesis | 46XY | | Testis | Wolffian | Ambiguous | Severe salt wasting No cortisol No aldosterone | None | None | Replace mineralocorticoids and glucocorticoids |
| 3-β-Hydroxy-steroid dehydro-genase deficiency | Defect in testosterone synthesis | 46XY | Second most common of CAH | Testis | Wolffian | Ambiguous | Severe salt wasting No cortisol No aldosterone | DEAS | None | Replace mineralocorticoids and glucocorticoids Reconstruction as needed |
| 17-α-Hydroxylase deficiency | Defect in testosterone synthesis | 46XY | | Testis | Wolffian | Ambiguous | Hypokalemic alkalosis Hypertension Decreased cortisol Decreased aldosterone Gynecomastia | CS 11-DCS | None | Replacement glucocorticoids |
| 17,20-Desmolase deficiency | Defect in testosterone synthesis | 46XY | Rare | Testis | Wolffian | Ambiguous | Normal cortisol and aldosterone | ASD | None | Supplemental testosterone |
| 17-β-Hydroxy-steroid dehydrogenase deficiency | Defect in testosterone synthesis | 46XY | Most common | Testis | Wolffian | Ambiguous | Virilization at puberty | ASD | None | Decision reared as female or male |
| 5-α-Reductase deficiency | Defect in androgen action | 46XY, autosomal recessive | Testis with spermato-genesis | Wolffian | Female | No gynecomastia Normal testosterone Normal virilization | None | None | None |

(*Continued*)

**Table 4-3.** *(Continued)*

| Disorder | Pathology | Chromosomes | Incidence | Gonads | Internal Genitalia | External Genitalia | Other Features | Urinary Steroids | Risk of Cancer | Treatment |
|---|---|---|---|---|---|---|---|---|---|---|
| Complete testicular feminization | Androgen receptor defect | 46XY X-linked | 1 in 20,000 to 64,000 | Testis Not fertile | Absent | Female reared as female | Increased testosterone Increased estrogen | None | Germ cells | Remove gonads after puberty Estrogen replacement |
| Incomplete testicular feminization | Androgen receptor defect | 46XY X-linked recessive | 1/10th of complete | Testis Not fertile | Wolffian | Female | Increased testosterone Increased estrogen | None | Germ cells | Remove gonads prior to puberty Estrogen replacement |
| Reifenstein syndrome | Androgen receptor defect | 46XY X-linked recessive | | Testis Not fertile | Wolffian | Hypospadias male | Gynecomastia Increased testosterone Increased estrogen | None | None | Reconstruction as needed |
| Infertile male syndrome | Androgen receptor defect | 46XY ? X-linked recessive | | Testis Not fertile | Wolffian | Male | Infertility Normal or increased testosterone Normal or increased estrogen | None | None | None |
| Receptor + resistance | Androgen receptor defect | Unknown | | Testis Not fertile | Wolffian | Ambiguous | Normal or increased testosterone Normal or increased estrogen | None | None | None |
| Persistent müllerian duct | Persistent müllerian duct syndrome | Unknown | | Testis | Wolffian with rudimentary uterus and tubes | Male usually cryptorchid | Normal testosterone Normal estrogen | None | None | Orchipexy Leave uterus and tubes |

   **2.** **Genitalia:** It is important to palpate for a gonad in the labioscrotal fold or the scrotum. Because ovaries do not descend, it is likely to be a testis. It is important to document the size of the phallus (Table 4–4) and the location of the urethral meatus. Any patients with bilateral cryptorchidism or with unilateral cryptorchidism with hypospadias should be suspected of having abnormalities in sexual differentiation. Other helpful physical findings include hyperpigmentation of the areola and labioscrotal fold, common in patients with congenital adrenal hyperplasia.

**C.** **Chromosomal Evaluation**

   **Chromosomal analysis:** The most accurate assessment of chromosomes is from cultured peripheral blood leukocytes. This method provides the exact chromosomal complements, presence of mosaicism, and structural features of the chromosomes. In the case of mosaicism, several different tissue samples may be required to accurately determine the presence of mosaicism. Table 4–5 summarizes the chromosomal abnormalities found in most intersex disorders.

**D.** **Hormonal Evaluation**

   In evaluating patients with intersex due to hormonal abnormalities, biochemical tests are often crucial.

   **1.** Urinary steroids: In the case of congenital adrenal hyperplasia, the specific enzyme defect can be differentiated based upon the presence or absence and the type of steroid excreted in the urine. These findings are illustrated in Table 4–3 and Figure 4–3.

   **2.** Human chorionic gonadotropin (hCG) stimulation test: In other disorders caused by hormonal abnormalities (such as $5\alpha$-reductase deficiency and androgen resistance), direct measurement of plasma testosterone is often not helpful because abnormalities in testosterone levels in these pathologic states have not been consistently characterized. A more useful test is the testosterone response following stimulation by hCG (2000 IU per day for 4 days). If plasma testosterone levels rise greater than 2 ng/mL from baseline, the abnormality is due to androgen resistance rather than defective testosterone synthesis. In addition, this test is also used to diagnose $5\alpha$-reductase deficiency. A post-hCG stimulation ratio of testosterone to DHT greater than 30 establishes this diagnosis.

**E.** **Other Evaluation**

   **1.** Ultrasound (US): Examining the abdomen by US may help to identify the presence of Müllerian-derived structures such as the uterus and fallopian tubes. On US, the uterus appears as a solid organ behind the bladder with a white streak through the center. The adrenal glands can also be

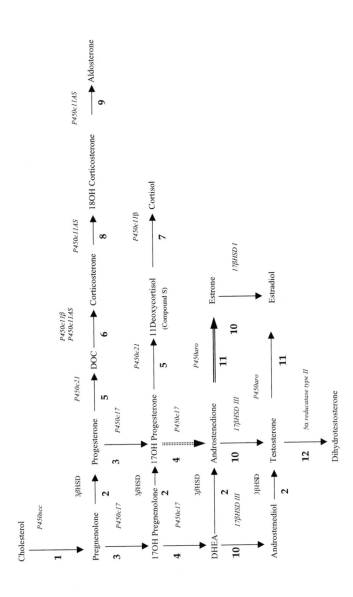

**Table 4–4.    Stretched penile length**

| Age | Range (cm) |
|---|---|
| Newborn (30 wk) | 1.7–3.2 |
| Newborn (34 wk) | 2.2–3.8 |
| Newborn (term) | 2.7–4.3 |
| <1 y | 2.3–5.9 |
| 1–3 y | 3.1–6.9 |
| 3–11 y | 3.7–8.6 |
| Adults | 10.1–16.5 |

examined for enlargement by US. Although this finding is not diagnostic for congenital adrenal hypoplasia, it is suggestive and directs further evaluation.

2.  Genitography: When US findings are not clear, injecting radiographic contrast through the opening of the urogenital sinus is helpful in delineating the urogenital sinus and internal duct structures. This helps to determine the presence of wolffian versus müllerian ductal structures.

3.  Exploratory laparotomy/laparoscopy: Occasionally, exploratory laparotomy or laparoscopy with gonadal biopsy is required for diagnosis. This is indicated for patients in whom the biopsy will influence the sex assignment, which is based on several

←

**Fig. 4–2.    Principal pathways of steroid hormone synthesis.** *Reaction 1:* Mitochondrial cytochrome P450scc catalyzes 20α-hydroxylation, 22-hydroxylation, and scission of the C20-22 carbon bond resulting in the conversion of cholesterol to pregnenolone. *Reaction 2:* 3βHSD type II, a short-chain dehydrogenase in the endoplasmic reticulum, catalyzes 3β-hydroxysteroid dehydrogenase and isomerase activities. *Reaction 3:* P450c17 catalyzes the 17α-hydroxylation of pregnenolone to 17OH-pregnenolone and of progesterone to 17OH-progesterone. *Reaction 4:* The 17,20-lyase activity of P450c17 converts 17OH-pregnenolone to dehydroepiandrosterone (DHEA), but very little 17OH-progesterone is converted to Δ4 androstenedione. *Reaction 5:* P450c21 catalyzes the 21-hydroxylation of progesterone to deoxycorticosterone (DOC) and of 17OH-progesterone to 11-deoxycortisol. *Reaction 7:* P450c11β converts 11-deoxycortisol to cortisol. *Reactions 6, 8, and 9:* In the adrenal zona glomerulosa, DOC is converted to corticosterone and then to 18OH-corticosterone by P450c11β in the zona fasciculata. Reactions 10 and 11 are found in the testes, ovaries, and in some peripheral, nonglandular tissues. *Reaction 10:* Several forms of 17β-HSD, a reversible non-P450 enzyme of the endoplasmic reticulum, mediate 17β-hydroxysteroid dehydrogenase activities, converting DHEA to androstenediol (type III), androstenedione to testosterone (type III), and estrone to estradiol (type I). The reverse 17-ketosteroid reductase activities are catalyzed by the type II and IV enzymes. *Reaction 11:* Testosterone is converted to estradiol by P450aro (aromatase). *Reaction 12:* Testosterone is converted to dihydrotestosterone by 5α-reductase type II. (Modified from Miller WL: Molecular biology. *Endocr Rev* 1988;9:295–318, with permission.)

**Table 4–5.  Chromosomal abnormalities in intersex disorders**

| Genital Appearance | Karyotype | Gonads | Diagnosis |
|---|---|---|---|
| Ambiguous | 46XX | Ovaries | $21\beta$-hydroxylase deficiency |
| Ambiguous | 46XX | Ovaries | $11\beta$-hydroxylase deficiency |
| Ambiguous | 46XX | Ovaries | $3\beta$-hydroxylase deficiency |
| Ambiguous | 46XX | Ovaries | Maternal virilization |
| Ambiguous | 46XY | Testis | $17\beta$-hydroxysteroid dehydrogenase deficiency |
| Ambiguous | 46XY | Testis | 20,22 desmolase deficiency |
| Ambiguous | 46XY | Testis | $3\beta$-hydroxysteroid dehydrogenase deficiency |
| Ambiguous | 46XY | Testis | 17,20 desmolase deficiency |
| Ambiguous | 46XY | Testis | $5\alpha$-reductase deficiency |
| Ambiguous | 46XY | Testis | Relfenstein syndrome |
| Ambiguous | 46XY | Testis | Receptor + androgen resistance |
| Ambiguous | 46XX; 46XY; 46XX/46XY | Ovary, testis, ovotestis | True hermaphrodite |
| Ambiguous | 45X/46XY; 46XY; 45X/47XYY; 45X/46XY/ 47XYY | Testis and streak | Mixed gonadal dysgenesis |
| Male | 46XX | Testis | XX Male |
| Male | 47XXY; 46XY/47XXY; Klinefelter variant | Testis | Klinefelter syndrome |
| Male | 46XY | Testis | Persistent müllerian duct syndrome |
| Male | 46XY | Testis | Infertile male syndrome |
| Female | 46XY | Testis | Testicular feminization |
| Female | 46XY | Testis | $17\alpha$-hydroxylase deficiency |

(*Continued*)

**Table 4–5.** *(Continued)*

| Genital Appearance | Karyotype | Gonads | Diagnosis |
|---|---|---|---|
| Female | 46XY; 46XX | Streak | Pure gonadal dysgenesis |
| Female | 45X and Turner variant | Streak | Turner syndrome |

Turner variant:
    45X/46XX
    45X/47XXX
    45X/46XX/47XXX
    46XXqi
    45X/46Xxqi
    46Xxpi
    46XXr
    45X/46XXr
    46 XXp-
    45X/46XXp-
    46XXq-
    45X/46XXq-
Klinefelter variant:
    48XXYY
    48XXXY/49XXXYY
    49XXXXY

factors including laboratory results, functional external genitalia, fetal/neonatal exposure to androgen and its effect on the brain, and parental opinion. Furthermore, in cases such as incomplete testicular feminization, Turner syndrome (Y variant), and mixed gonadal dysgenesis, removal of streak gonads may be required at the time of exploratory laparotomy/laparoscopy because of the risk of cancer in the gonads.

**IV. AN APPROACH TO THE DIAGNOSIS OF INTERSEX**
Figures 4–3A–C illustrate a clinical approach to differentiating the disorders of intersex. It is based on grouping these disorders by their common manifestations: (a) ambiguous genitalia or discordant chromosomal findings in the newborn, (b) inappropriate pubertal development, (c) impaired pubertal development, and (d) infertility.

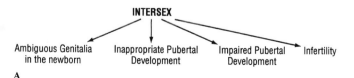

Fig. 4–3. A: Four types on intersex.

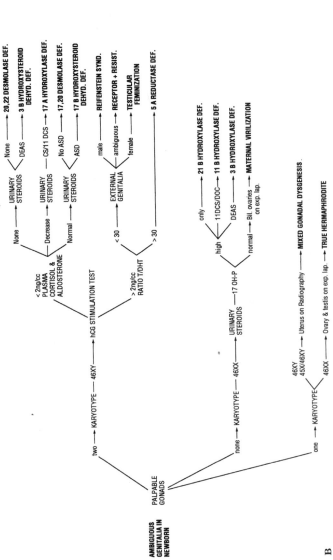

**Fig. 4-3.** *(Continued)* B: Algorithm for the investigation of ambiguous genitalia in the newborn.

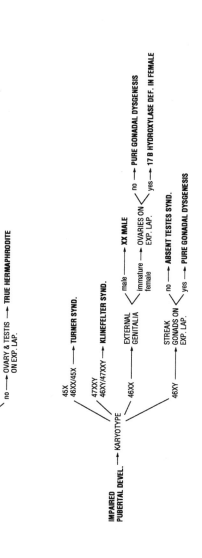

**Fig. 4-3. C** *(Continued)* C: The specific enzyme defect can be differentiated based upon the presence or absence and the type of steroid excreted in the urine.

## V. SEX ASSIGNMENT

In the past, the baby born with ambiguous genitalia was considered incomplete until either a male or female sex was assigned. Unfortunately, a prompt (but inappropriate) assignment, although timely and comforting for family, physicians, nurses, and staff, can lead to more complex problems in the future. We advocate an immediate attempt to make a definitive and accurate determination. Fortunately, for the majority of patients with ambiguous genitalia (congenital adrenal hyperplasia) this can be accomplished. In patients where ambiguity remains after initial testing and the diagnosis cannot be made or the diagnosis is clear but sex assignment remains difficult, we advocate for a more cautious approach, with a reversible or nonbinding sex assignment.

It is clear that both social (the nurturing hypothesis) and biologic (the genetic and hormonal hypothesis) factors all play a role in determining our sexual identity. The parents' perception of their child's genitalia influences interactions such as naming, clothes, play orientation, and social organization, and is, therefore, critical to the child's identity. In addition, sexual identity is predetermined by the genetic and hormonal make up. Animal experimentation and human data suggest a role of steroid or androgen imprinting of the brain and subsequent sexual identity. The process of sexual identity is not an all-or-none process; male and female characteristics exist as a continuum. Clinical experience has shown that the patients, themselves, will reassign their sex. In cases where the genotype does not match the phenotype, it is clear that surgical reconstruction from male to female does not guarantee a successful sexual identity. Consequently, genital surgery in patients with intersex should be considered carefully and tailored for each individual patient.

## VI. TREATMENT OF COMMON INTERSEX CONDITIONS

### A. Congenital Adrenal Hyperplasia (Female Pseudohermaphrodite)

1. Treatment of CAH requires accurate diagnosis of the enzymatic defect that led to the excess production of androgens.
2. Sex assignment is usually female.
3. Replacement therapy with glucocorticoid (hydrocortisone) with or without mineralocorticoid ($9\alpha$-fluorohydrocortisone) is needed to prevent salt wasting. Serial measurements of plasma renin activity (PRA), $17\alpha$-hydroxyprogesterone, and androgens can be used to monitor the therapy.
4. Antihypertensive medication may be needed for those with $11\beta$-hydroxylase deficiency.
5. Surgical therapy may include clitoral reduction, feminizing genitoplasty, and vaginoplasty. Adequate hormonal replacement often normalizes clitoral appearance and clitoral reduction is not necessary.

6. Timing of feminizing genitoplasty and vaginoplasty remains controversial, with some advocating early repair and others suggesting delaying surgery until puberty or early adulthood.

7. Because congenital adrenal hyperplasia is hereditary, prenatal counseling is required, and prenatal therapy with dexamethasone is of some benefit.

B. **Congenital Adrenal Hyperplasia (Male Pseudohermaphrodite)**

1. Medical therapy with glucocorticoid, mineralocorticoid, and antihypertensives are indicated for specific enzymatic defects.

2. Sex assignment should be carefully made based on considerations mentioned previously, and irreversible surgery such as orchiectomy should be delayed until appropriate counseling has been given.

3. Bilateral orchiectomy is usually performed at the time of hernia repair, after workup for delayed puberty, or following female sex assignment.

4. Hypospadias repair and scrotoplasty in phenotypically male patients can be undertaken after 6 months of age. Preoperative treatment with testosterone may be of benefit in specific patients to increase the size of the phallus and improve local tissue vascularity.

C. **Mixed Gonadal Dysgenesis**

1. The streak gonad should be removed at time of diagnosis because of a higher risk of malignancy.

2. The undescended testis should be brought down into the scrotum or removed depending on gender assignment.

3. In patients with male gender assignment, the descended testes or undescended testes that have been brought down into scrotum should be carefully followed for the development of malignancy.

4. Genital reconstruction should be performed in accordance with gender assignment.

5. Hormone replacement is often required during adolescence.

D. **True Hermaphrodite**

1. This condition is quite rare and can only be made after histologic evaluation demonstrating the presence of both ovarian and testicular tissues in the same individual. It should not be used in cases of dysgenetic gonads in which scattered primordial follicles may be present.

2. Excision of the discordant gonadal tissue should only be done after gender assignment is firmly established. When this tissue cannot be completely excised, gonadectomy may be necessary.

3. Adequate excision of testicular tissue can be confirmed postoperatively by measurement of hCG-stimulated androgen levels. However, the presence of ovarian tissue cannot be similarly evaluated in

prepubertal patients. Residual ovarian tissue may manifest as gynecomastia at puberty.

**VII.  KEY POINTS**

**A.**   Newborns with ambiguous genitalia and evidence of dehydration are likely to have severe salt-wasting congenital adrenal hyperplasia and require immediate replacement therapy.

**B.**   Gender identity is strongly influenced by prenatal androgen exposure. In the newborn period, the family should be counseled by a team of health care professionals with experience in the area of intersex. When gender identity is not clear cut, irreversible genital surgery is not recommended.

**C.**   Specific disorders of sexual differentiation are associated with an increased risk of cancer. An accurate diagnosis is required to identify these individuals.

**RECOMMENDED READING**

Diamond DA. Sexual differentiation: normal and abnormal. In: Walsh PC, Retik AB, Vaughan Jr D, et al. *Campbell's urology*, volume 3, 8th ed. Philadelphia: WB Saunders, 2002.

Forest MG. Ambiguous genitalia/intersex: endocrine aspects. In: Gearhart JP, Rink RC, Mouriquand PDE, eds. *Pediatric urology*. Philadelphia: WB Saunders, 2001.

Grumbach MM, Conte FA. Disorders of sex differentiation. In: Larson PR, Kroneneberg HM, Melmed S, et al, eds. *Williams textbook of endocrinology*, 10th ed. Philadelphia: WB Saunders, 2002.

Park JM. Normal and anomalous development of the urogenital tract. In: Walsh PC, Retik AB, Vaughan Jr D, et al, eds. *Campbell's urology*, volume 3, 8th ed. Philadelphia: WB Saunders, 2002.

# Hydrocele, Hernia, Neonatal Torsion, and Scrotal Masses

Barry A. Kogan

**HYDROCELE/HERNIA**

I. **DEFINITION**
   A. **Hydrocele:** An accumulation of fluid around the testicle.
      Types: Communicating or noncommunicating (Fig. 5–1A–B).
      1. Communicating: persistence of a patent processus vaginalis with the same pathophysiology as an indirect hernia (see below) but a smaller opening, preventing bowel from entering. The fluid around the testis is peritoneal fluid. This is a congenital defect.
      2. Noncommunicating: no connection to the peritoneum; rare in children, occurs mostly in adolescents and adults. The fluid comes from the mesothelial lining of the tunica vaginalis and is often the result of inflammation of the testis or epididymis. This is an acquired lesion.
   B. **Hernia:** A protrusion of an organ or tissue through an abnormal opening (Fig. 5–2).
      Types: Indirect inguinal, direct inguinal, or femoral.
      1. Inguinal, indirect: persistence of a patent processus vaginalis. This defect is congenital and allows protrusion of peritoneal contents (usually small intestine) through the internal inguinal ring along the spermatic cord for a variable distance, in some cases, as far as the scrotum. This may become incarcerated if it cannot be reduced back into the peritoneum. If so, the pressure of the hernia may alter blood flow to the testis, which can be damaged from ischemia. In addition, the blood flow to the bowel may be affected and, in this circumstance, it is called a *strangulated hernia*.
      2. Inguinal, direct: weakness in the floor of the inguinal canal. This is an acquired condition and is uncommon in children.
      3. Femoral: rare in children.

II. **EMBRYOLOGY OF INDIRECT INGUINAL HERNIAS AND HYDROCELES**
   A. During the 3rd month of gestation, the peritoneal lining of the abdominal cavity protrudes out of the internal inguinal ring following the gubernaculums, which attaches to the base of the scrotum (or, in girls, to the labia majora). This is the processus vaginalis. Late in gestation, the testis descends along the same path from the retroperitoneal space through the inguinal canal just

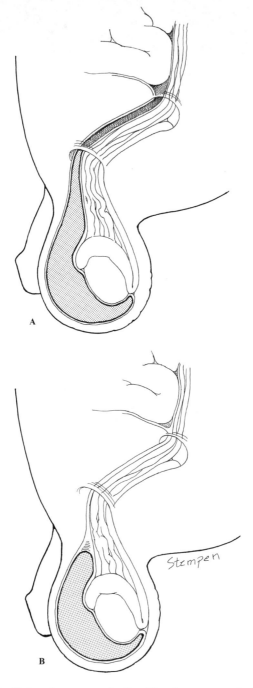

Fig. 5–1.   Hydroceles: communicating (A) and noncommunicating (B).

Hernia

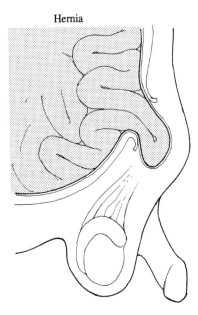

**Fig. 5–2. Anatomic diagram depicting a hernia.**

    posterior to the processus vaginalis and into the scrotum.

**B.** At approximately the time of birth, the portion of the processus vaginalis between the peritoneum and the scrotum obliterates, separating the residual tunica vaginalis in the scrotum from the peritoneum. If the processus fails to obliterate, it is said to remain *patent.*

**C.** For obvious embryologic reasons, premature infants have a much higher rate of patency of the processus vaginalis. If the patent processus is large enough to allow the bowel to enter, there is an indirect inguinal hernia. If the processus is patent, but the connection is small, a communicating hydrocele is likely to result when peritoneal fluid enters the inguinal canal. If the processus does obliterate, a noncommunicating hydrocele may result by secretion of fluid into the residual tunica vaginalis. This is usually associated with inflammation in the scrotum.

**III.  INCIDENCE**

    **A.**  Approximately 1% to 3% of children have a hernia.

    **B.**  In premature babies, the rate is approximately 3 times as high depending on the degree of prematurity.

    **C.**  About 10% of children with hernias have a family history of hernia, although there is no known inheritance pattern or gene identified.

    **D.**  At least one-third are diagnosed before 6 months of age.

     **E.**  The male/female ratio is 8/1. The right/left ratio is 2/1; about 16% are bilateral.

**IV. DIAGNOSIS**

     **A.**  The diagnosis is made, in most cases, by observation, often by the parents. A lump or bulge is present in the groin, scrotum, or labia. The lesion is noted particularly at times of increased intraabdominal pressure (e.g., crying or straining). Generally, the lump disappears soon after the intraabdominal pressure returns to normal. In older children, the enlargement may be progressive during the day and recede during naps or at night. When present, the diagnosis is clear. On occasion, the lesion is reported by the parents but cannot be demonstrated in the office, even when the child is crying or straining. Sometimes, the examiner can elicit a "silk glove" sign, in which the layers of the processus vaginalis can be felt around the spermatic cord feeling like "silk rubbing on silk" in the absence of a lump. Alternatively, the parents can bring in a photograph to document it or, if the parents are good historians, repair can be based on history alone.

     **B.**  Because hydroceles in the first year of life do not require surgical intervention, it is important to differentiate them from hernias. Most often the physical examination is clear, with the bowel clearly palpable as distinct from fluid. Sometimes, bowel sounds can be heard in the sac. Transillumination is of no value in that both hydrocele fluid and bowel fluid/air transmit light. Needle aspiration is dangerous for obvious reasons. In rare circumstances, a plain abdominal x-ray or an ultrasound can be useful.

     **C.**  When the diagnosis of a hernia is unclear, some surgeons have recommended herniography. A 60% iothalamate solution is injected blindly into the peritoneum using a small needle. The child is placed upright for 10 minutes and an x-ray is taken to determine if the contrast outlines the patent processus vaginalis. The diagnostic accuracy is high. Complications include the obvious potential for bowel injury, contrast reactions, and peritoneal irritation from the hyperosmolar contrast. In practice, this procedure is useful only rarely.

     **D.**  An attempt should be made to reduce the hernia/hydrocele by keeping the child calm and applying gentle pressure on the lump. The bowel is most often reduced easily. When the sac is filled with fluid, this may also reduce easily. An interesting circumstance occurs when there is a large hydrocele noted in the scrotum that does not reduce easily. Although there is some pressure to repair this because of its obvious appearance, the fact that it does not easily reduce suggests that the connection with the peritoneum is small. In infants, these may well resolve spontaneously.

     **E.**  A special circumstance is the incarcerated hernia. Any child with symptoms of a bowel obstruction (e.g., vomiting and abdominal distention) should be examined carefully for a hernia. In these cases, the mass is usually tender and sometimes there is skin erythema. The hernia may be palpable on rectal examination or confirmed by plain x-ray or ultrasound. An attempt to reduce the hernia should be made as described. If it cannot be reduced, emergent operative intervention is needed. If it can be reduced, the child should be observed closely for signs of bowel injury. Operative repair should be performed soon after.

## V.  TREATMENT

**A.**  There is no medical management for hernias/hydroceles and the use of trusses is of historical interest only. Hernias will persist indefinitely and will almost always need to be repaired at some time. Hydroceles may resolve during the first or second year of life and, hence, in most circumstances, a period of observation is justified in most infants.

Hernias in premature infants are often repaired prior to hospital discharge, but the majority of hernias and communicating hydroceles in children can be repaired as an outpatient surgical procedure with minimal discomfort and morbidity. Surgical repair is performed by ligating the processus vaginalis at the internal inguinal ring, thereby separating the peritoneum from the distal tunica vaginalis. The success rate approaches 99% and the major risk is from the anesthetic. There is some danger of damage to spermatic cord structures because the processus vaginalis is intimately attached to them. In normal circumstances, the risk is about 1%. If surgery on an incarcerated hernia is necessary, the risk is significantly higher, as high as 6% to 10%, although it is unclear if the damage is related to the repair or the prolonged incarceration, which reduces testicular blood flow.

**B.**  In infants, at the time of the inguinal hernia repair, it is appropriate to explore the contralateral groin; approximately 60% have a contralateral patent processus vaginalis. In older children, the rate of positive exploration is much lower and, hence, in most circumstances, contralateral surgery is not indicated. To be more certain, some authors have recommended intraoperative herniography. Recently, laparoscopy has been used to evaluate the contralateral internal ring. One popular technique has been to insufflate the peritoneum via the processus vaginalis prior to ligation. Crepitus in the contralateral groin indicates a patent processus vaginalis. In addition, a 70-degree lens can be inserted into the processus vaginalis and maneuvered to provide a visual inspection of the contralateral internal ring. If the contralateral ring is open, it is repaired. This procedure is somewhat controversial in that there are no controlled studies to determine if an open ring is associated with a clinically significant hernia/hydrocele in the future. On the other hand, without laparoscopy, at least 2% to 3% of children will present with a contralateral problem that requires surgical intervention.

## VI. SPECIAL CIRCUMSTANCES

### A. Testicular Feminization

1. Approximately 2% to 3% of girls with hernias will be found to have a testis within the hernia sac. These girls have testicular feminization syndrome. They have completely normal external genitalia, a shallow vaginal cavity, and should still be raised as girls.
2. Depending on the philosophy of the local pediatric endocrine group, the testes may be left in place until after puberty (after which they should be removed due to the risk of gonadoblastoma) or removed at the time of hernia repair because of the risk of virilization if the syndrome is incomplete.
3. These girls will be normal except for infertility and the need for hormone replacement.

### B. Increased Intraabdominal Pressure

1. Communicating hydroceles are unlikely to resolve spontaneously in children with increased intraabdominal fluid.
2. This is seen in children on peritoneal dialysis and those with ventriculoperitoneal shunts.
3. Early surgical repair is indicated. In these cases, there is a high recurrence rate and repair should be performed with particular caution.

### C. Hernia Uterae Inguinale

1. A rare syndrome resulting from the persistence of müllerian structures secondary to the failure of paracrine secretion of anti-müllerian hormone (AMH) or to an AMH receptor defect.
2. Affected boys are not ambiguous at birth and generally present later with undescended testes for orchiopexy, or with inguinal hernias.
3. Although not absolutely essential, most recommend removing the residual müllerian remnants.

### D. Connective Tissue Disorders

Hernias are more common in children with connective tissue disorders. In particular, children with Ehlers-Danlos and Hurler-Hunter syndromes are prone to hernias. Sometimes, the children develop the hernias before the diagnosis of the syndrome.

## NEONATAL SCROTAL MASSES

### I. NEONATAL TORSION

A. Neonatal torsion is the most common scrotal mass among infants.
B. Most often an incidentally discovered mass is found on physical examination.
C. The mass is generally nontender, and there is no scrotal edema.

**D.** Torsion usually begins before birth and only rarely is it possible to salvage the testis.

**E.** Ultrasound is usually diagnostic if there is a question about the diagnosis.

**F.** Although controversy exists, many will explore through the scrotum, remove the testis if necrotic, and perform a scrotal orchiopexy on the contralateral side, as there have been increasing numbers of cases of bilateral asynchronous torsion.

## II. TESTICULAR TUMORS

**A.** Testicular tumors are rare among children. If present in neonates, they are most likely teratomas.

**B.** These are usually also asymptomatic and discovered on routine physical examination.

**C.** They are of mixed embryological origin and usually have calcified areas on ultrasound. In addition, they generally do not occupy the entire testis (differentiating them from torsion on ultrasound).

**D.** In children, they are virtually always benign and excision is generally curative. Partial orchiectomy is adequate treatment when feasible based on the anatomy.

**E.** An endodermal sinus tumor (yolk sac) is a more serious lesion, in that it may metastasize. It tends to occur in older children. These tumors make $\alpha$-fetoprotein (AFP); however, in newborns, the levels of AFP are already elevated, so measuring levels may not be useful, except for comparisons with later measurement. These tumors are amenable to retroperitoneal lymph node dissection, chemotherapy, and radiation therapy when needed, but in most cases, radical orchiectomy and confirmation that the tumor has not spread (by computed tomography for staging) is all that is needed.

## RECOMMENDED READING

Husmman, D. Intersex. In: Gillenwater JY, Grayhack JT, Howards SS, et al, eds. *Adult and Pediatric Urology,* 4th ed. Philadelphia: Lippincott Williams and Wilkins; 2002:2533–2564.

Weber TR, Tracy TF. Groin hernias and hydroceles. In: Ashcraft KW, Holder TM, eds. *Pediatric surgery,* 2nd ed. Philadelphia: WB Saunders; 1993.

# Urinary Tract Infections in Children

Angelique C. Hinds and Nicholas M. Holmes

I. **INTRODUCTION**

Controversy exists in the diagnosis, treatment, and management of children with urinary tract infections, from method of collection of the urine specimen to who gets a voiding cystourethrogram (VCUG). Practice patterns vary extensively, and depend on region, specialty, and practitioner age. Historically, the focus in patients diagnosed with urinary tract infection has been to demonstrate vesicoureteral reflux, which in itself is not the cause of recurrent infection and the potential subsequent renal scarring or renal insufficiency. Recent efforts have focused on the more likely causes of urinary tract infections: bacteria, genetics (bad luck), and abnormal bladder function. Evidence-based medicine shows that there is a general consensus with respect to some aspects of treatment of urinary tract infections in the pediatric population, whereas other areas remain controversial.

II. **EPIDEMIOLOGY**

A. Urinary tract infections account for as many as 8 million office visits and 1.5 million hospitalizations in the United States.

B. The prevalence of urinary tract infection varies with age and sex.

1. Symptomatic infections occur in 1.4 per 1000 neonates and are more common in uncircumcised males. Thereafter, infections are more common in girls, with a prevalence of 1.2% to 1.9%.

2. Young girls have a high incidence of cystitis or nonfebrile first-time urinary tract infection between the ages of 2 and 6 years.

3. Febrile urinary tract infections or symptomatic pyelonephritis have a higher rate in young girls of 4.1% to 7.5%. The recurrence rate in girls has been reported to be as high as 30% within 1 year of the initial infection, and as high as 50% within 5 years.

C. Urinary tract infections are caused by bacteria, with *Escherichia coli* accounting for more than 75% of all infections. *Klebsiella* and *Proteus* are the next most common bacteria with Staphylococcus and Enterococcus, also known to cause urinary tract infection.

III. **RISK FACTORS** (Table 6–1)

A. **Female Gender**

1. In girls, bacteria can gain access to the urinary tract more easily than in boys because of the

**Table 6–1.   Gender ratio of urinary tract infections by age**

|            | Girls | Boys |
|------------|-------|------|
| Neonate    | 0.4   | 1.0  |
| 1–6 mo     | 1.5   | 1.0  |
| 6–12 mo    | 4.0   | 1.0  |
| 1–3 y      | 10.0  | 1.0  |
| 3–11 y     | 9.0   | 1.0  |
| 1–16 y     | 2.0   | 1.0  |

perineal location of the urethral orifice and the shorter urethra.

   **a.**  The normal perineal bacterial flora may enter the urethra. These bacteria are normally washed out with voiding without consequence. However, if there is a disruption of this normal flora (due to vaginitis, illness, stress, medications) the growth can increase and potentially allow access of enough bacteria to the bladder to cause infection.

   **b.**  In the sexually active adolescent, the mechanics of vaginal penetration can predispose them to infection.

   **2.**  Vaginal voiding (see Chapter 8) can lead to increased moisture in the perineum allowing for bacterial overgrowth. These children often complain of smelly urine and/or underpants.

**B.  Male Gender**

   **1.**  Foreskin

   **a.**  In the neonate (younger than 6 months), an intact foreskin increases the incidence of urinary tract infection 10 times compared to boys who have been circumcised.

   **b.**  Phimosis

   **(1)**  *Phimosis* is the inability to retract the foreskin, and is a normal physiologic occurrence in *newborn* boys. At birth, only 4% of boys have a completely retractable foreskin. By 6 months of age, 20% have a retractable foreskin. By 3 years, 90%, and 100% of teenagers will have a retractable foreskin.

   **(2)**  The prepuce can serve as a reservoir for potentially uropathogenic bacteria. Studies have demonstrated the P-fimbriated *E. coli* is more adherent to the inner preputial skin.

**C.  Abnormal Bladder or Voiding With or Without Incontinence** (see Chapter 8)

   **1.**  High pressures in the bladder (poor bladder compliance)

The low-pressure storage ability of the bladder can be described as bladder compliance. This allows the bladder to fill and store urine at low pressures (approximately 10-20cm/$H_2O$). Abnormal bladder compliance reduces one of the bladder defense mechanisms against bacterial invasion. Poor compliance may be secondary to a neurogenic bladder, dysfunctional voiding, or an uninhibited bladder.

2. Incomplete bladder emptying or infrequent voiding

Normally, any bacteria that enter the bladder are flushed out of the bladder with complete and frequent voiding. Infrequent voiding and residual urine in the bladder (stasis) allows bacteria that enter the bladder to grow and multiply enough to cause infection.

3. Difficulty relaxing the pelvic floor during voiding

Incomplete relaxation of the pelvic floor during voiding can cause poor compliance and/or incomplete emptying, both of which can lead to urinary tract infection.

D. **Constipation/Encopresis** (see Chapter 10)

E. **Congenital Genitourinary Tract Anomalies:** vesicoureteral reflux, ureteropelvic junction obstruction, megaureter, ureteroceles, posterior urethral valves, hydronephrosis, ureterovesical junction obstruction and ureteropelvic junction obstruction, prune-belly syndrome, bladder extrophy, and neurogenic bladder abnormalities

1. Kidney transplant registries throughout the world show that one of the most common causes of end-stage renal disease is congenital structural anomalies and reflux nephropathy. Clearly the implication is that urinary tract infection with anatomic abnormalities (Fig. 6–1) puts the patient at the greatest risk for renal failure.

2. Reflux nephropathy has been shown to cause chronic renal insufficiency and is reported to occur in 5% to 10% of patients presenting for renal transplantation. Most patients with hypertension and scarred kidneys have a history of vesicoureteral reflux. What is unclear is whether these patients were born with dysplastic kidneys, with the natural history being renal failure, or whether recurrent urinary tract infections causes progressive renal damage.

Reflux does not necessarily increase the risk of urinary tract infection; however, it may increase the *morbidity* of a urinary tract infection. For example, if reflux is present at the same time bacteria gain access into the bladder, this bacteria is allowed to ascend into the

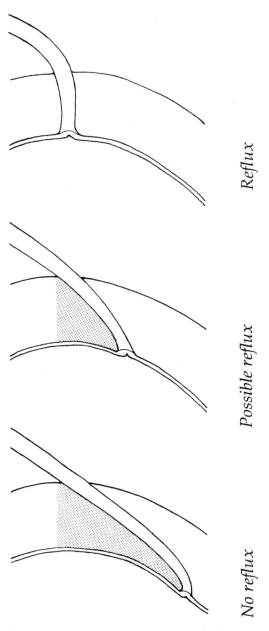

*No reflux*          *Possible reflux*          *Reflux*

Fig. 6–1.   Ureterovesical junction. Inadequate length of the submucosal muscular backing can lead to vesicoureteral reflux.

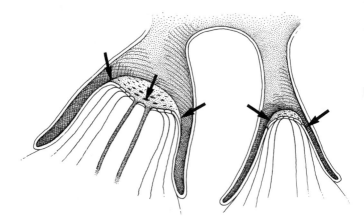

**Fig. 6–2.   Anatomy of concave and convex renal papillae.**

  kidneys (due to the reflux) and cause a true
  *upper tract infection* (pyelonephritis) instead
  of a lower urinary tract (bladder) infection.

**3.** The renal papillary configuration and the location of the renal papillae can also predispose to
  urinary tract infection. Renal papillae in the upper and lower poles are in direct line for possible
  refluxing urine, thus accounting for renal scarring in either portion of the kidney. The renal
  papillary configuration can be either convex or
  concave. Convex papilla are typically nonrefluxing and concave papilla are at more risk for reflux
  and therefore increase in scarring (Fig. 6–2).

**F.** **Neurogenic Bladder:** caused by spina bifida, spinal
  lesions, or spinal injury (see Chapter 11)

**G.** **Catheterization/Drainage Tubes**
  **1.** Children who have been "in and out" catheterized or have had any indwelling urinary drainage
   catheter in place
  **2.** Patients on clean intermittent catheterization
   (see Special Circumstances)

**H.** **Predisposition or Colonization**
  Children who have recurrent urinary tract infections and have no other anatomic causes have
  been found to have increased adherence of specific
  bacteria to the cells of the perineum, including
  the vaginal introitus and the urethra. These children are found to be colonized with *E. coli.* Often
  these *E. coli* are P-fimbriated (an extra bacterial
  adherence mechanism), which are more virulent
  *E. coli* and have greater affinity for urothelium.
  These children may also have a decrease in cellular immunity with lower levels of the antibodies immunoglobulin A and G. In summary, these

patients have susceptible urothelium that allows an increase in bacterial colonization.

IV. **PRESENTATION**

  A.  The presenting symptoms of urinary tract infection depend on the anatomic site of the infection and the age of the patient.

  1.  Anatomic site of infection

  a.  An upper tract infection (kidney infection or pyelo-nephritis) typically cause general malaise-type symptoms such as fever, nausea/vomiting, or flank pain.

  b.  A lower tract infection (bladder infection) most often presents with symptoms such as dysuria, frequency/urgency, or incontinence.

  c.  It is important to note that, although an upper tract infection is assumed when there is a positive urine culture and a fever, children may have fever with lower tract infections as well. The only way to truly differentiate would be a dimercapto-succinic acid (DMSA) scan at the time of the infection, which is not warranted in most cases.

  2.  Age

  a.  Younger children (infants) will have nonspecific symptoms such as fever, irritability, poor feeding, vomiting, diarrhea, failure to thrive, and jaundice. A certain level of suspicion is therefore required.

  b.  Older children most often complain of dysuria, suprapubic discomfort, frequency, urgency, and change in urine odor or color if they have a lower tract infection and fever and flank pain if they have an upper tract infection.

  B.  **Asymptomatic Bacteriuria**

  It is certainly possible to have bacteria within the urinary tract and be asymptomatic without having clinical infection or renal scarring. The prevalence of asymptomatic bacteriuria has been documented to be approximately 0.9% among young schoolgirls. Of these patients, 10% were found to have vesicoureteral reflux without any renal scarring.

V. **DIAGNOSIS**

  A.  Once a urinary tract infection is suspected diagnosis is based on examination of the urine.

  1.  Method of collection

  a.  We recommend an accurate diagnosis of all patients with suspected urinary tract infections. In neonates and young children, this translates into a catheterized urine specimen to reduce ambiguous diagnosis.

  b.  In toilet-trained children a clean-catch, midstream urine specimen can be obtained after carefully retracting the foreskin and cleaning the glans penis in boys and spreading the labia and cleaning the periurethral area in girls.

    **c.** It is critical to accurately predict who has a urinary tract infection. For example, the contamination rate and difficulty in interpreting bagged urine collection specimens may lead to unwanted invasive and expensive further investigations. A bagged specimen is only useful if it is negative. If a bag specimen is positive then a catheterized specimen should be obtained.

**2.** Urinalysis

    **a.** The urine specimen should be checked at minimum for leukocyte esterase and nitrite urine dipstick plus microscopic analysis. In patients who have a negative dipstick and/or microscopic analysis, further urine culture is unwarranted and an alternative source of the fever should be sought. A positive leukocyte esterase or nitrite test with 5 or more white blood cells per high power field or a microscopic with bacteria in an unspun specimen is highly predictive of a urinary tract infection.

    **b.** Specimens for urine culture should be refrigerated if they cannot be sent to the laboratory within 30 minutes.

**3.** Urine culture

    **a.** Simply stated, results of urine cultures that are greater than $10^5$ colony-forming units constitute a urinary tract infection and less than $10^5$ does not. However, if the urine is collected in a sterile fashion (catheterized specimen and a single organism is documented by culture, even though the colony-forming units are less than $10^5$), the patient should be considered to have a urinary tract infection. In addition, if the symptoms are consistent with urinary tract infection and antibiotics improved those symptoms, a diagnosis of a urinary tract infection must be entertained despite a less than $10^5$ colony count. Conversely, multiple different organisms or mixed genital flora obtained from a voided specimen should be considered suspicious for contamination even if the greater than $10^5$ colony forming units are documented. Strict reliance on colony forming units is unwarranted.

    **b.** Urine cultures in infants and young children without a clear focus of infection show an incidence of urinary tract infection in 7.5% with a temperature of greater than 38.3°C. This incidence increases up to 17% in white girls with a temperature higher than 39.0°C. In contrast, patients with lower tract infection or cystitis typically have a temperature of 38°C or less.

## VI.  IMAGING (Fig. 6–3)

A.  Present recommendations are that all neonates and children (boys and girls) that have their first culture proven documented urinary tract infection with a fever greater than 38.5°C have follow-up imaging studies consisting of a renal and bladder ultrasound and a contrast VCUG to determine any anatomic abnormalities.

1.  Pyelonephritis (kidney infection) and renal scarring have been associated with renal insufficiency, hypertension, and end-stage renal disease.

2.  Pyelonephritis scarring is the most common cause of unilateral renal disease, as well as hypertension in young children and young adults.

3.  It has been shown that the incidence of renal scarring is less if worked up after the first infection and much greater if workup is done after multiple infections.

4.  The natural history of recurrent infection and reflux is renal scarring. Historically, untreated high-grade (IV and V) vesicoureteral reflux leads to poor renal outcomes.

5.  Older children who present with lower tract infection or cystitis, defined as a fever less than 38°C with lower tract symptoms, do not necessarily need to be imaged after the first infection. "Older" children who can verbalize or otherwise express lower tract symptoms generally translate to children during or after toilet teaching.

B.  **Renal/Bladder Ultrasound**

1.  The renal/bladder ultrasound may be obtained at any time after infection.

2.  The ultrasound should always include evaluation of the kidneys and bladder.

3.  Ultrasound alone is not sufficient to rule out vesicoureteral reflux. A child may have a normal ultrasound and still have severe reflux.

C.  **VCUG**

1.  The VCUG should be obtained after urine sterility has been documented.

2.  The initial VCUG should always be a contrast VCUG and not a nuclear VCUG.

A nuclear VCUG, although the better test for demonstrating reflux, only diagnoses the presence or absence of vesicoureteral reflux and does not reveal any other congenital anomalies such as ureterocele or posterior urethral valves. If reflux is identified, subsequent VCUGs should be nuclear VCUGs; the nuclear study exposes the child to much less radiation. Newer techniques with "pulsed" fluoroscopy may obviate this difference in radiation exposure.

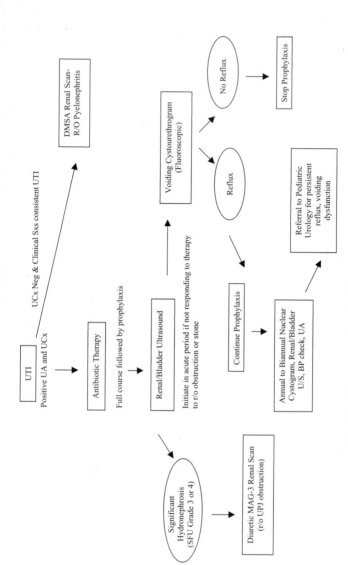

**Fig. 6–3. Treatment algorithm for urinary tract infections.**

**D. DMSA Scan**
1. The DMSA scan is becoming more and more popular and useful in the management of children with urinary tract infections.
2. The DMSA scan can be used to differentiate a true pyelonephritis.
3. It can help the urologist to assess the severity of an individual's recurrent infections.
4. Although further data are needed, newer studies suggest that the DMSA scan may help to predict children who will have more trouble long term than other children. In addition, the DMSA scan may help to predict which children's reflux will and will not resolve.

**VII. TREATMENT**
**A. Antibiotics**
1. It has been shown in a number of prospective studies that treating urinary tract infections is effective in preventing recurrent infections.
2. Empiric therapy should be initiated if an infection is suspected. Intensity and mode of therapy are based on the clinical appearance of the child.
   a. If the child appears toxic with signs of dehydration, inability to tolerate oral intake, or signs of sepsis, intravenous antibiotics should be administered. Typically, gentamicin and ampicillin are administered as first-line therapy.
   b. Those patients who have a fever, but appear clinically well otherwise, may be started on ceftriaxone given intramuscularly and continued treatment with oral antibiotics. Trimethoprim-sulfamethoxazole (TMP-SMX) or nitrofurantoin can be used pending the culture results.
3. Antibiotic therapy should continue for at least 7 days because of the risk of recurrent infection.
4. Antibiotic prophylaxis (with TMP-SMX or nitrofurantoin) should be instituted following full-dose therapy until radiologic imaging can be obtained to verify an anatomically normal urinary tract. Follow-up urine culture should be attained to document sterilization of urine.

**B. Prevention**
1. As with many ailments, including urinary tract infections, prevention is the best medicine.
2. Prevent and treat constipation (see Chapter 10)
3. Prevent and treat voiding dysfunction (see Chapter 8)
4. Antibiotic prophylaxis
   a. Prophylaxis for young children with vesicoureteral reflux continues to be the standard of care. Current studies are looking at whether older refluxing children without other risk factors and with lower grades of

reflux could be followed safely without prophylactic antibiotics.

   **b.** In children with recurrent infections without congenital anomalies (reflux) in whom constipation and voiding dysfunction have been addressed, prophylaxis may also be warranted (rare).

5. Some patients benefit from prophylaxis only with certain behaviors (sexual activity, change in routine).

6. Although there is an increase of urinary tract infections in neonates who are uncircumcised, justification of circumcision to prevent urinary tract infections still seems unwarranted.

7. Although controversial, boys with identified urinary tract anomalies (posterior urethral valves, ureteropelvic junction obstruction, vesicoureteral reflux) may benefit from neonatal circumcision, thereby decreasing the incidence of urinary tract infection.

8. Breastfeeding may confer protection against urinary tract infections in the newborn period with secretory immunoglobulin A antibodies and lactoferrin.

## VIII.   SPECIAL CIRCUMSTANCES

   **A.** There are many urologic conditions (prune-belly syndrome, posterior urethral valves, neurogenic bladders, bladder extrophy) where clean intermittent catheterization is used as an intervention to either preserve renal function or allow for urinary continence. These children may be at further risk for urinary tract infection owing to their conditions. Interestingly, if these children follow basic guidelines of frequent and complete emptying (no different than for the child who does not catheterize), then this technique can prevent infections.

   **B.** If the child has had bladder augmentation surgery (see Chapter 11) and is suffering from recurrent infections, then he or she should be instructed on more frequent catheterization and more frequent and efficient bladder irrigation.

## RECOMMENDED READING

Riccabona M. Urinary tract infection in children. *Curr Opin Urol* 2003;13:59–62.

Rushton HG, Pohl HG. Urinary tract infection in children. In: Bellman AB, Lowell R, King SA, et al, eds. *Clinical pediatric urology,* 4th ed. London: Martin Dunitz; 2002.

# Vesicoureteral Reflux

Laurence S. Baskin

## I. INTRODUCTION

*Vesicoureteral reflux* is the abnormal retrograde flow of bladder urine into the upper urinary tract through an incompetent ureterovesical junction. Reflux in itself that is without bacterial contamination and low in pressure has not been documented to be deleterious. Reflux in the presence of bacteria is a risk factor for upper urinary tract infections or pyelonephritis. Untreated upper urinary tract infections have been shown to lead to acquired renal scarring or reflux nephropathy in children. Congenital abnormalities of renal development may have associated vesicoureteral reflux, resulting in a clinical picture of reflux nephropathy but without a history of urinary tract infection.

A. **Reflux Nephropathy** is defined as the following clinical triad.
   1. Renal scarring
   2. Hypertension
   3. Vesicoureteral reflux

## II. EPIDEMIOLOGY

The prevalence of reflux varies with several demographic factors of the patient population. Reflux may occur as an isolated entity or with other associated anomalies of the genitourinary tract.

A. **History of Urinary Tract Infection**
   In children without urologic symptoms or history of infection, the incidence of reflux is likely less than 1%. In children with a history of symptomatic urinary tract infection, the incidence of reflux has been estimated to range from 20% to 50%.

B. **Age**
   The prevalence of reflux correlates inversely with the age of the study population. With linear growth, spontaneous resolution of reflux occurs in many patients.

C. **Race**
   Reflux is more commonly a disease of fair-skinned children. The prevalence of reflux appears to be significantly lower among black children and children of Mediterranean origin when compared to white children. The prevalence of reflux in black children with a history of urinary tract infection is estimated to be approximately 25% of the incidence in the population of white children.

D. **Sibling Predisposition**
   Siblings of patients with known reflux have approximately a 30% prevalence of reflux, with younger siblings being at greatest risk. In many of these children,

there may be no documented history of symptomatic infections. For this reason, routine screening of the siblings of children with reflux grade 3 or higher has been advocated by most pediatric urologists and nephrologists.

E. **Gender**

Because of the epidemiology of urinary tract infection in children, boys and girls may present with reflux at different ages. Because urinary tract infections are more common in uncircumcised boys than girls during the neonatal period, many boys are diagnosed with reflux in the neonatal period. However, after the first year of life, the incidence of urinary infections is much higher among girls than boys. Therefore, most school-aged children diagnosed with reflux are girls.

F. **Associated Anomalies**

Although vesicoureteral reflux may occur as an isolated entity, reflux may also occur with other genitourinary abnormalities.

1. Posterior urethral valves: Congenital bladder outlet obstruction has been associated with reflux in up to 50% of patients.
2. Duplicated collecting system: Reflux is commonly associated with the lower pole moiety of a duplicated system.
3. Prune-belly (Eagle-Barrett) syndrome
4. Bladder exstrophy
5. Severe voiding dysfunction

III. **CLASSIFICATION OF REFLUX**

A. **Primary Reflux**

Primary reflux occurs as a result of a congenital deficiency in the formation of the ureterovesical junction in the absence of any other predisposing pathology. Accordingly, these patients may have a laterally ectopic ureteral orifice consistent with a deficient submucosal ureteral tunnel. The majority of otherwise healthy children who present with symptomatic urinary tract infection have primary reflux. It should be noted that the majority of the current guidelines, which have been developed to treat children with reflux, apply mainly to those patients with primary reflux.

B. **Secondary Reflux**

Secondary reflux occurs as a result of other urinary tract dysfunction, which leads to a decompensation of a normally formed ureterovesical junction. Although secondary reflux may have many different underlying etiologies, the key to the treatment of these patients depends on the identification of these underlying etiologies. Successful treatment of these patients ultimately depends on the management of the underlying causes.

1. Neurogenic bladder
   a. Myelomeningocele
   b. Spinal cord injury

**Table 7–1.  Grading of vesicoureteral reflux**

**Grade 1:** Appearance of contrast in the ureter only
**Grade 2:** Appearance of contrast in the ureter and renal pelvis without associated dilation or blunting of calyces
**Grade 3:** Mild calyceal dilation without ureteral tortuosity
**Grade 4:** Moderate calyceal dilation and blunting without ureteral tortuosity
**Grade 5:** Severe calyceal dilation with ureteral tortuosity

  2. Obstruction
    a. Voiding dysfunction
    b. Posterior urethral valves
    c. Ectopic ureteroceles
  3. Infection: Cystitis may also predispose an otherwise marginally competent ureterovesical junction to demonstrate reflux.

IV. **GRADING OF REFLUX**
Grading of the degree of reflux is important to the management and ultimate prognosis of the patients. More severe grades of reflux are associated with lower rates of spontaneous resolution and a higher incidence of renal scarring. According to the international system, reflux is graded by the severity of calyceal changes, ureteral dilation, and redundancy that occur secondary to reflux (Table 7–1, Fig. 7–1).

V. **CLINICAL PRESENTATION**
A. **Urinary Tract Infection**
Most children with reflux initially present with an episode of urinary tract infection. Pyelonephritis is the initial presentation in most cases.

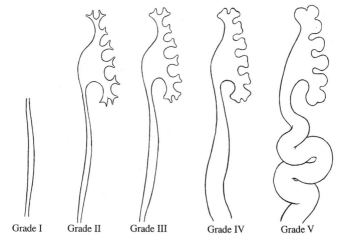

Grade I     Grade II     Grade III     Grade IV     Grade V

**Fig. 7–1.  International reflux classification.**

**B. Unexplained Febrile Illness**

Other patients may have no documented history of urinary tract infection, but may instead have a history of frequent recurrent illness with unexplained fevers. Some children with reflux and pyelonephritis are mistakenly treated for presumed recurrent otitis. It is, therefore, of utmost importance to evaluate all children with unexplained fever with a urinalysis and urine culture.

**C. Associated Genitourinary Anomalies**

As mentioned, reflux commonly occurs in conjunction with other urologic abnormalities. The finding of any of the previously mentioned conditions should prompt an investigation for reflux.

**D. Prenatal Diagnosis**

Because of the recent advent and popularity of prenatal ultrasound screening, fetal hydronephrosis can often be detected in utero. Although fetal hydronephrosis can be due to any number of pathologic or physiologic causes (see Chapter 12), all children with prenatally diagnosed hydronephrosis should be placed on antibiotic prophylaxis until a cystographic examination can be done to either confirm or exclude reflux.

## VI. DIAGNOSIS

Once the acute illness is resolved, the diagnosis of reflux can be entertained. A voiding cystourethrogram (VCUG) should never be performed in the presence of infected urine. However, the likelihood of detecting reflux is highest if the child is evaluated soon after the acute infection episode. It is believed that the presence of recent infection in the bladder predisposes a marginally competent ureterovesical junction to reflux. The presence of reflux in these marginally competent ureterovesical junctions may be missed if the evaluation is conducted several weeks following the acute episode. Because the real danger is vesicoureteral reflux in the presence of infection, many authorities have advocated early radiographic evaluation at 1 to 2 weeks following the acute episode.

**A. VCUG**

Vesicoureteral reflux is a radiographic diagnosis. The gold standard study is contrast VCUG. VCUG allows accurate diagnosis and grading of the severity of reflux. In a small number of cases, more than one cystographic examination may be needed to make the diagnosis of reflux.

**B. Urodynamic Evaluation**

Many children with reflux also have voiding dysfunction. Often the diagnosis is suspected by a history of incontinence, frequency, or urgency. If indicated, urodynamic evaluation with monitoring of intravesical compliance can be done at the same time as the VCUG. This information is important in the management of patients with reflux and other abnormalities of the lower urinary tract (e.g., neurogenic bladder).

Appropriate management of the voiding dysfunction often results in resolution of reflux.

C.  **Renal Ultrasound**

Renal ultrasound is relatively insensitive in the detection of mild and moderate reflux. As an adjunctive technique, ultrasound can be useful in the grading of hydronephrosis (see Chapters 12 and 13), and as a baseline for follow-up studies to monitor renal growth.

D.  **Nuclear Medicine Renal Scan**

Renal scan using DMSA is useful in the detection of renal cortical scars. Some centers have employed renal scans to confirm the diagnosis of acute pyelonephritis.

E.  **Nuclear Medicine Cystogram**

Nuclear cystogram is useful as a follow-up study in patients with known reflux. It has the advantage of high sensitivity and lower radiation exposure than the standard VCUG. However, because of its inability to accurately grade reflux and detect associated anomalies (spina bifida, ureteroceles, duplicated systems), nuclear cystograms should not be used for the initial evaluation of reflux.

VII.  **MANAGEMENT**

The primary goal in both medical and surgical management of reflux is to prevent development of pyelonephritis, recurrent urinary tract infections, and the formation of renal cortical scarring.

A.  **Medical Management of Reflux**

Once the diagnosis of reflux is suspected, low-dose continuous antibiotic prophylaxis should be initiated. The patient should continue antibiotic prophylaxis until the reflux resolves spontaneously or is corrected surgically. Each patient should have periodic follow-up (yearly to 18 months) to check for the resolution of reflux.

1.  Antibiotic prophylaxis

There are relatively few effective antibiotic agents available for use in urinary tract prophylaxis in children. Prophylactic antibiotics are generally given in a dosage that is approximately one-half to one-third of the normal therapeutic dose. Table 7–2 lists the commonly used agents and potential serious-but-rare side effects.

2.  Anticholinergic therapy

For patients with uninhibited bladder contractions (dysfunctional voiding; see Chapter 8) and secondary reflux, treatment with anticholinergic medications (e.g., oxybutynin) in addition to antibiotics may allow spontaneous resolution to occur.

3.  Office visits and follow-up testing

Patients on medical management should be under surveillance for urinary tract infections. However, routine monitoring of urine is not

**Table 7–2. Commonly used agents for urinary tract prophylaxis in children**

| Agent | Oral Dosage | Precautions |
|---|---|---|
| Trimethoprim/ sulfamethoxazole | 2 mg/kg PO qhs (Trimethoprim) | Avoid use in the first 2 months due to kernicterus, megaloblastic anemia. |
| Nitrofurantoin | 2 mg/kg qd | Pulmonary fibrosis, hemolytic anemia in G6PD deficiency. |
| Amoxicillin | 20 mg/kg PO qd | Good choice for first 2 months. Development of resistance common thereafter. |
| Cephalexin | 20 mg/kg PO qd | Good choice for first 2 months. Development of resistance common thereafter. |

recommended unless the patient has signs and symptoms of a urinary tract infection. Urine should periodically be monitored for protein and the patient checked for hypertension, although in most cases proteinuria and hypertension will not be an issue until well into adulthood. Kidney growth as well as scarring should be monitored with ultrasound (every 1 to 2 years). The critical issue is to keep the urine sterile while reflux is present, thereby decreasing the chance of pyelonephritis and new renal scarring.

**B. Surgical Correction**

Although many patients with reflux can be managed successfully with antibiotic prophylaxis, surgical correction of reflux is often indicated when medical therapy is unsuccessful.

1. Indications
   a. Recurrent episodes of pyelonephritis on antibiotic prophylaxis
   b. Medical noncompliance
   c. Breakthrough infections by resistant organisms
   d. Persistence of reflux into puberty

2. Results

   In experienced hands, antireflux surgery is highly safe and effective. In the American section of the International Reflux Study Group, ureteral reimplantation successfully corrected reflux in 99% of cases with complication rates less than 2%.

**3.** Techniques

    **a.** Open surgery: The goal of surgery is to create a functional value at the vesi-coureteral junction. This is accomplished by mobilization of the ureter and reimplantation using stronger muscular backing. Two general approaches are used intravesical (Fig. 7–2) and extravesical (Fig. 7–3). As noted, surgical repair has an extremely high success rate.

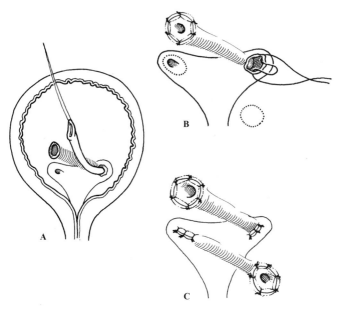

Fig. 7–2.  A–C: Intravesical ureteral reimplantation technique.

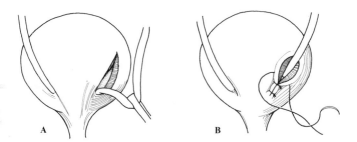

Fig. 7–3.  A–B: Extravesical ureteral reimplantation technique. Posterior aspect of the bladder (Lich-Gregor procedure).

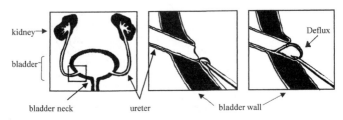

**Fig. 7–4. Endoscopic injection of dextranomer/hyaluronic acid copolymer for the correction of vesicoureteral reflux.**

   **b.** Endoscopic treatment
      **(1)** Injectable agents
         The endoscopic treatment of vesicoureteral reflux has become accepted in the United States with the FDA approval in 2001 of injectable dextranomer/hyaluronic acid copolymer (Deflux). The procedure is performed by inserting a cystoscope, through the urethra to access the inside the bladder (Fig. 7–4). A small amount of the injectable copolymer is introduced into the wall of the bladder near the opening of one or both ureter(s). Although the exact mechanism of reflux correction is unknown, the copolymer seems to fix the ureterovesical junction in place and recreate the natural intravesical tunnel between the ureter and bladder. There are no incisions made in the abdomen for this procedure. Including the administration of general anesthesia in children, the procedure takes 15 to 30 minutes.
      **(2)** Risks
         The use of this injectable substance has minimal risks. These include mild bleeding, infection, and dysuria after the procedure. The theoretical risk of ureteral obstruction and kidney blockage has been reported only rarely. Nevertheless, follow-up upper tract imaging with an ultrasound 4 to 6 weeks after the procedure is prudent.
      **(3)** Outcomes
         Using the dextranomer/hyaluronic acid copolymer, there is a higher success rate with this procedure for those with lower grades of reflux. Capozza and Caione (2002) reported a 95% success rate for grade II, 71% success rate for grade III,

and 43% success rate for grade IV reflux. Similarly, in their study Capozza et al. (2001) reported an 87% success rate for grade II, 75% success rate for grade III, and 41% success rate for grade IV reflux. In another study, Lackgren et al. (2001) reported a 78% success rate for both grades II and III reflux, and 66% success rate for grade IV reflux. The treatment can be performed more than once and does not impede open surgical correction if not successful.

**(4)** Candidates for This Procedure
Based on the success rates, this procedure is recommended for use in children with grade II, grade III, and possibly grade IV reflux.

**(5)** Contraindications
  **(a)** A large bladder diverticulum
  **(b)** An extra ureter (tube that carries urine from the kidney to the bladder)
  **(c)** Active urinary tract infection
  **(d)** Active voiding dysfunction (abnormal emptying of the bladder)

## VIII. SUMMARY

Vesicoureteral reflux is one of the most common urologic abnormalities treated by pediatric urologists. An increased understanding of the pathologic mechanisms, bladder dysfunction, and natural history of reflux has led to improvements in both medical and surgical approaches to treating this disease. The effective treatment of patients with reflux depends on early detection of reflux and institution of antibiotic prophylaxis. Close followup and periodic reevaluation are necessary for all patients. When indicated, surgical correction of reflux has been shown to be safe and effective. Endoscopic treatment with agents such as the dextranomer/hyaluronic acid copolymer has proven to be safe and effective alternative treatment.

## RECOMMENDED READING

Capozza N, Caione P. Dextranomer/hyaluronic acid copolymer implantation for vesico-ureteral reflux: a randomized comparison with antibiotic prophylaxis. *J Pediatr* 2002;140:230–234.

Capozza N, Patricolo M, Lais A, et al. Endoscopic treatment of vesico-ureteral reflux: twelve years' experience. *Urol Int* 2001;67:228–231.

Lackgren G, Wahlin N, Skoldenberg E, et al. Long-term followup of children treated with dextranomer/hyaluronic acid copolymer for vesicoureteral reflux. *J Urol* 2001;166:1887–1892.

U.S. Food and Drug Administration. *New device approval: Deflux injectable gel.* 2001. Accessed March 20, 2003. Available from: URL: http://www.fda.gov/CDRH/PDF/P000029.HTML

Walker RD, Atala A. Vesicoureteral reflux and urinary tract infection in children. In: *Adult and pediatric urology,* volume 3, 4th ed. Philadelphia: Lippincott Williams and Wilkins; 2002:2671–2718.

# Daytime Urinary Incontinence (in the Otherwise Healthy Child)

Angelique C. Hinds

## I. INTRODUCTION

To understand childhood urinary incontinence one must first understand the development of normal bladder control.

- **A.** The neurophysiologic mechanism of normal urinary bladder is controlled by a complex integration of sympathetic, parasympathetic, and somatic innervation that involves the lower urinary tract, the micturation center in the sacral spinal cord, the midbrain, and higher cortical centers. Successful development of normal bladder function requires bladder storage of urine at low pressures with a closed sphincter and complete emptying of the bladder with a voluntary bladder contraction and an involuntary sphincteric relaxation.
- **B.** Starting in the fetus, micturation occurs mainly by reflex voiding at frequent intervals without voluntary control. Bladder filling triggers afferent nerves that, through spinal reflexes, cause both relaxation of the external urinary sphincter and detrusor contraction and result in complete emptying of the bladder.
- **C.** By 6 months of age, the bladder capacity increases and the frequency of micturation decreases.
- **D.** Between the ages of 1 and 2 years, conscious sensation develops.
- **E.** By 2 to 3 years of age, the ability to initiate and inhibit voiding from the cerebral cortex develops. It is at this point that the lower urinary tract is most susceptible to abnormal learned cortical input (this may be as simple as a child who is told not to wet his or her pants).
- **F.** A school-aged child will normally void four to nine times per day.
- **G.** Normal bladder capacity of a child is age related and can be calculated as the age in years plus 2 (in fluid ounces).

## II. DEFINITION

- **A.** *Urinary incontinence* is the involuntary leakage of urine in a child older than 5 years of age (the age at which a healthy child in our society should have acquired daytime continence). This particular age, however, depends on the culture of the family. Some cultures expect continence at much younger ages, often because of socioeconomic reasons (lack of availability of diapers and laundering facilities).

**B.** Causes of urinary incontinence in children can be thought of as acquired (dysfunctional, secondary) or nonacquired (familial, primary). Interestingly, the nonacquired causes of incontinence can lead to acquired (dysfunctional) problems.

### III. CLASSIFICATION

#### A. Voiding Dysfunction

1. *Voiding dysfunction* in childhood is a dysfunction or discoordination of the lower urinary tract without a recognized organic cause (neurologic disease, injury, or congenital malformation).

2. Voiding dysfunction, in general terms, is a discoordination between the bladder muscle and the external sphincter activity (Fig. 8–1) and can take many forms, including inability to voluntarily start or to stop voiding, poor bladder emptying, increased bladder capacity, incontinence, and high pressures in the bladder.

3. Because older children can control their external sphincter more easily than their bladder muscle, it is easier for them to stop urination than to start it. The contraction of the external sphincter is subconscious and normal during bladder filling, but is pathologic during bladder contraction. Although this may be a normal response to an inappropriate bladder contraction, if this continues, it leads to lower and, less often, upper urinary tract deterioration.

4. The contraction of the external sphincter at the time of a bladder contraction has been referred to as *detrusor-sphincter-dyssynergia* (DSD). With voiding dysfunction, the DSD is a learned response; unfortunately, the same term is used for

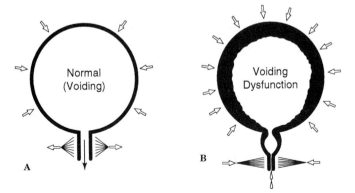

**Fig. 8–1.  Schematic of normal coordinating voiding (A) and dysfunctional voiding (B).**

children with a neurogenic cause for the DSD (spina bifida). To avoid confusion, we prefer to use *voiding dysfunction* for the learned response and *DSD* for those with a neurogenic cause.

**B. Dysfunctional Elimination Syndrome**

When voiding dysfunction has progressed to include not only urinary incontinence but also constipation, stool incontinence, and/or recurrent urinary tract infections, we classify this as *dysfunctional elimination syndrome.*

**C. Nonneurogenic Neurogenic Bladder** (NNNB or Hinman syndrome)

Current thinking is that the NNNB (Hinman syndrome) is the final clinical result of prolonged and severe voiding dysfunction in children without an identifiable neurologic lesion. In this most severe form, the abnormal learned voiding pattern can lead to residual urine, vesicoureteral reflux, recurrent pyelonephritis, and ultimately to renal insufficiency. This is most often thought of as an acquired problem, but has also been seen in small children prior to the accepted age of normal continence, so there may be a primary problem not yet identified. NNNB is very rare.

**D. Vesicovaginal Voiding**

Vesicovaginal voiding can be acquired or nonacquired. The acquired form is common and thought to be caused by children voiding with their legs in complete adduction and results in a portion of voided urine deflecting off the labia and pooling in the vagina. This urine slowly dribbles out when the girl stands or walks after voiding. This problem is often found in obese children, but can be seen with any body habitus. Children with congenital anomalies such as common urogenital sinus anomalies (congenital adrenal hyperplasia) often have primary vaginal voiding.

**E. Transient Wetting**

Transient wetting can occur in association with a bladder infection, illness, or stress (birth or death of family member, sexual abuse).

**F. Uninhibited Bladder**

The uninhibited bladder can be primary or acquired. A primary uninhibited bladder is also known as a *hyper bladder* or *spastic bladder* and is manifested by incontinence, urgency, and frequency. It occurs when the bladder involuntarily contracts (usually prior to age-appropriate capacity). The cause of this is unknown, but it tends to run in families and is often chronic. The hyper bladder often becomes more hyper in response to stress or other triggers, not unlike asthma. The younger child may have incontinence at the time of this unexpected contraction, and the older child may remain dry but void more frequently than normal. Often, to remain continent, children contract their pelvic floor at the time of the contraction, which can lead to voiding dysfunction, thereby exacerbating the original problem. In its acquired form, a child with severe voiding dysfunction can have such high pressures in the bladder that the bladder muscle hypertrophies, which subsequently may cause the bladder to exhibit uninhibited contractions, again exacerbating the original problem.

G. **Voiding Frequency Disorders**
   1. Voiding frequency disorders come in two forms, either voiding too frequently or voiding too infrequently. These problems are often self-limited, but can be quite frustrating for the child and family. Both may be associated with a psychosocial trigger, but not in all cases can one be identified.
   2. Lazy bladder: The lazy bladder is a bladder with a large capacity and manifests itself with very infrequent voiding. The bladder may have poor contractility. It is usually a result of prolonged voiding dysfunction, but can also be seen in very young children who void with normal relaxation of the external sphincter (infrequent). Children may void as few as one to three times in 24 hours.
   3. Benign urinary frequency: Children with severe urinary frequency syndrome experience an acute onset of extraordinary urinary frequency. They can feel the need to void as often as every 5 to 15 minutes during the day; however, most sleep through the night and remain dry. Children usually experience spontaneous remission, although temporary recurrence is common.

H. **Giggle Incontinence**
   *Giggle incontinence* occurs when a normally continent girl is incontinent only when she laughs. Interestingly, this same child will not become incontinent with other Valsalva maneuvers such as coughing, sneezing, or jumping. True giggle incontinence is rare.

IV. **EPIDEMIOLOGY**
   A. Most otherwise healthy children can manage to stay dry during the day by the age of 4 years.
   B. Of all children with a wetting problem, 10% will only have symptoms by day, 75% only by night, and 15% by both day and night.
   C. Studies in children just starting school (6 to 7 years of age) have shown that 3.1% of the girls and 2.1% of the boys had an episode of daytime wetting at least once a week. Most of these children had urinary urgency (82% of the girls and 74% of the boys). For reasons that are not understood, there is also a difference in prevalence depending if the child lives in colder (2.5%) or hotter areas (1.0%).

**D.** Spontaneous Cure Rate

The spontaneous cure rate for daytime wetting is similar to that for nocturnal enuresis (about 14% of children will improve without treatment each year).

**V. ASSOCIATED PROBLEMS**

**A. Bacteriuria/Urinary Tract Infection** (see Chapter 6)

There is a strong association between bladder dysfunction and bacteriuria. However, it is not known whether the bacteria cause the bladder dysfunction first or vice versa. Probably, both are true, and this often leads to a vicious cycle.

**B. Bowel Dysfunction** (see Chapter 10)

**1.** Constipation

**2.** Encopresis (stool incontinence)

**C. Nocturnal Enuresis**

**D. Psychological Stressors**

Many studies have noted psychiatric disturbances associated with incontinence. However, whether the psychological factor or social pressure are the primary reason for the voiding problem, or if the incontinence leads to the psychosocial problems, is difficult to differentiate. Psychosocial or psychiatric help should only be the primary focus in severe cases (e.g., death of family member, sexual abuse).

**E. Vesicoureteral Reflux** (see Chapter 7)

Bladder dysfunction may lead to the development, persistence, and, when treated, resolution of vesicoureteral reflux. A child with dysfunctional voiding may have a functional obstruction and therefore high intravesical pressures during voiding. It is important to recognize the voiding dysfunction in children presenting with reflux, as surgical correction of the reflux will often not change their voiding habits and only part of the problem will be solved.

**VI. DIAGNOSIS**

**A. History:** Although difficult to illicit in this population, a good voiding history can often lead to diagnosis without further testing. The following are the most common history findings in children with the various causes of incontinence.

**1.** Voiding dysfunction

**a.** The potty dance (Fig. 8–2A–C): Dancing, squatting, holding, or posturing to avoid leakage. This is thought to be caused by a failure of the cerebral cortex to inhibit a reflex bladder contraction and, in response, either an involuntary void or a guarding sphincteric contraction (helped by squatting) that can temporarily prevent incontinence.

**b.** Urinary tract infections

**c.** Constipation

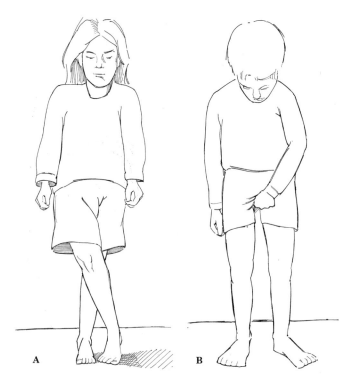

**Fig. 8–2. Schematic of various posturing in children with dysfunctional voiding. A: Vincent's curtsy. B: Holding.**

    **2.** Uninhibited bladder
        **a.** Frequency
        **b.** Urgency
        **c.** Potty dance
    **3.** Frequency disorders
        **a.** Lazy bladder
            **(1)** Infrequent voiding (one to three times per day)
            **(2)** Abdominal straining with voiding
            **(3)** Intermittent urinary stream and/or abrupt cessation of urinary stream
            **(4)** No sense of needing to void upon waking in the morning
        **b.** Benign urinary frequency
            **(1)** Sudden onset of urinating as often as every 5 to 15 minutes
            **(2)** Does not awaken the child at night
            **(3)** Child is continent of urine
    **4.** Vesicovaginal voiding
        Wet immediately after voiding, often described as *leaking*

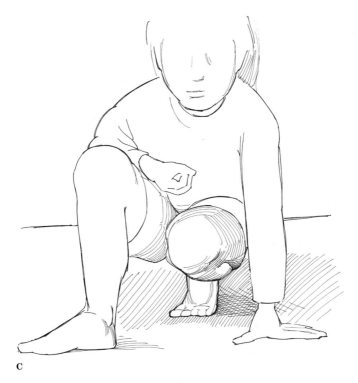

C

**Fig. 8–2.** (*Continued*) **C: Squatting with heel in perineum.**

   **5.** Giggle incontinence
        Only experiences incontinence with giggling,
        not with other types of Valsalva such as
        maneuvers, coughing, sneezing, or increased
        activity.
 **B. Physical Examination**
   **1.** General
      **a.** Self-esteem assessment
      **b.** Inspection of the underwear for dampness or
            fecal soiling
      **c.** Careful observation of the child's gait
   **2.** Abdomen
      **a.** Pay particular attention to kidneys (severe hy-
            dronephrosis) and bladder
      **b.** Assess for retained stool.
   **3.** Lumbosacral region: the following should be ex-
        cluded because they are signs of possible neuro-
        logic lesions.
      **a.** Hemangioma
      **b.** Hair patch
      **c.** Dimple

       **d.** Sacral agenesis

       **e.** Subcutaneous lipoma

    **4.** External genitalia

       **a.** Anatomy

       **b.** Rash

       **c.** Leakage of urine (at baseline and with straining)

       **d.** Perianal sensation and anal tone

       **e.** A rectal examination is very useful but generally not well tolerated.

       **f.** Attention to anomalies (e.g., epispadias, ureteral or urethral ectopy) is important.

**C. Urinalysis**

    The urinalysis should include measuring specific gravity (to rule out a concentrating defect and therefore high urinary volumes), dipstick for glucose (diabetes and high urinary output), protein, microscopic evaluation, and screening for an infection with a culture.

**D. Voiding Diary**

    **1.** When the voiding pattern cannot be differentiated well by history, some objective measures are needed to document the situation. The most noninvasive (and useful) of these is the voiding diary (Fig. 8–3). A diary is not only useful for the examining practitioner, it also will demonstrate the voiding pattern to the child and the family. Almost all urinary incontinence problems can be accurately diagnosed and subsequently treated with a comprehensive history, physical examination, and voiding diary.

    **2.** The child should record and document during at least two 24-hour periods the timing and amount of each void as well as the quantity of any incontinence. Correlation and evaluation of the diary can differentiate and recognize many voiding dysfunction problems. It is important to treat any constipation prior to administering the voiding diary.

**E. Urinary Flow Rate**

    **1.** A flow rate is a noninvasive diagnostic tool that can give additional objective information on how a child empties his or her bladder. This can be done with a machine that gives an objective printout, but can almost as effectively be done by merely observing the child voiding.

       **a.** Staccato voiding: another term for an *intermittent stream*. Usually there will be a delayed start. In contrast to normal voiding, in which there is relaxation of the sphincter, the staccato pattern is caused by bursts of pelvic floor activity during voiding, resulting in bladder pressure peaks and drops in flow rate. Often the bladder fails to completely empty.

       **b.** Fractionated and incomplete voiding: this micturation pattern is characterized by the use of

# Voiding Diary

### Day 1

| Time | Amount of Urine | Amount of Wetting Scale : 1 to 5* | Medication/ Comments | Soiling |
|------|------|------|------|------|
|      |      |      |      |      |
|      |      |      |      |      |
|      |      |      |      |      |
|      |      |      |      |      |
|      |      |      |      |      |
|      |      |      |      |      |
|      |      |      |      |      |
|      |      |      |      |      |
|      |      |      |      |      |

### Day 2

| Time | Amount of Urine | Amount of Wetting Scale : 1 to 5* | Medication/ Comments | Soiling |
|------|------|------|------|------|
|      |      |      |      |      |
|      |      |      |      |      |
|      |      |      |      |      |
|      |      |      |      |      |
|      |      |      |      |      |
|      |      |      |      |      |
|      |      |      |      |      |
|      |      |      |      |      |
|      |      |      |      |      |

*1 = spotting,  5 = soaked

**Fig. 8–3.  Voiding diary.**

abdominal straining to help void. The detrusor is hypoactive and therefore abdominal pressure is used to attempt to empty the bladder. Because of the assisted abdominal pressure, the reflex activity of the pelvic floor muscles make the urinary flow very irregular and interrupted, with increases in flow timed with breath holding (the Valsalva maneuver cannot be performed while breathing). The flow time is prolonged. It is sometimes difficult to differentiate this pattern in urinary flow from the typical staccato voiding.

### F. Sonogram

If the child has a history of infection, some upper tract imaging is important. It is important to obtain bladder images postvoiding, to assess residual urine volume noninvasively. Also a thick-walled bladder can be recognized (more than 5 mm). Most children with urinary incontinence will have a normal renal bladder ultrasound; however, obtaining the ultrasound can be very reassuring to the family as well as the practitioner that nothing more serious is being missed.

**G. X-Ray**

A x-ray may be obtained to assess for stool retention when history and physical examination are not sufficient.

**H. Voiding Cystourethrogram**

1. This study is reserved for children with a history of febrile urinary tract infections. A voiding cystourethrogram gives information on whether vesicoureteral reflux is present and if residual urine remains after voiding. It also demonstrates thickened or abnormal bladder musculature. However, when performed as an isolated study, bladder function can be evaluated by inference only.

2. If the morphologic and functional correlation with voiding dysfunction and recurrent urinary tract infection is appropriate, a video urodynamic study is much more useful.

**I. Video Urodynamic Study**

1. This is an invasive study and is used only in selected cases (e.g., children with complex symptoms, failure of the usual therapy, or a history of urinary tract infections). The urodynamic study observes the functional phenomenon of bladder filling, sensation, and the voiding process.

2. The cystometry part of the examination requires the placement of a bladder catheter, usually transurethrally. For measurement of external sphincter activity, perineal electromyography is the norm and is performed with surface electrodes placed around the anal sphincter. The bladder is filled at a moderate rate (1 to 2 mL/kg/min) with a room temperature or warm x-ray contrast fluid ($37°C$) and the anatomy is characterized simultaneously using fluoroscopy.

3. Studies in children with voiding dysfunction and recurrent urinary tract infections have been able to demonstrate a good correlation between the presence of unstable detrusor contractions and clinical symptoms (urge/squatting). Also, if vesicoureteral reflux was present there was a high correlation with very high-pressure, unstable detrusor contractions (higher than 70 cm $H_2O$).

4. It must be remembered that most children with voiding dysfunction will be able to be evaluated by less invasive methods.

**J. Cystoscopy**

Cystoscopy, although common in the past, usually with urethral dilation or meatotomy, is now clearly seen as unhelpful, potentially dangerous, and expensive.

**K. Spinal Radiography**

If one suspects significant neurogenic bladder dysfunction, sacral agenesis, or a spinal defect, a magnetic resonance imaging study of the spine (in addition to a full neurologic evaluation) is indicated.

## VII.   TREATMENT

A.   **Treat Constipation** (see Chapter 10)

It is imperative to diagnose and treat any constipation prior to moving forward with any treatment of urinary incontinence.

B.   After constipation has been treated, treatment depends on the diagnosis, which is usually obtained after reviewing the voiding diary.

C.   **Timed Voiding**

The most simple and effective treatment is timed voiding. Because many of these children either do not recognize or ignore the urge to void, a simple program of voiding by the clock at 2-hour intervals can be highly effective. This intervention is beneficial in both uninhibited and lazy bladders (but is easier said than done in the child).

D.   **Behavior Modification**

We typically reserve behavior modification until after a successful treatment plan has been developed. We do not reward children for being dry, only for following the recommended treatment plan. In the early stages, children do not understand how to be dry (but they do understand being rewarded for voiding at timed intervals and taking medication). We also do not want to set the child up for failure (reward the child for a treatment plan that does not work).

E.   **Medication**

1.   The use of drugs in the treatment of incontinence is only an adjunct to other bladder treatment regimens. It should be remembered that all medications have side effects and that the physician and parents must reach a collaborative decision that the benefits outweigh the risks. When medications are chosen, it should be emphasized that there is no magic pill, rather they should be combined with other treatments, for example, timed voiding.

2.   Anticholinergic medication

a.   This category of medications is used for the uninhibited bladder and generally has a significant effect.

b.   The most effective and bladder-selective anticholinergic drug is oxybutynin. It is both an anticholinergic and antispasmodic agent and has a good safety profile. It now comes in a timed-release tablet that needs only to be taken once per day.

c.   Side effects are common and include dry mouth, constipation, and occasionally drowsiness (often this will resolve after the first week of use). The medication also reduces perspiration and caution should be used in hot climates, where facial flushing is often seen as the first symptom of overheating. Fortunately, most of the side effects are short term, and few significant long-term side effects are recognized. Other anticholinergics are available for patients in whom oxybutynin is not feasible. The child and family will decide if the benefit (being dry) is worth the side effects.

**3.** $\alpha$-Blocker

$\alpha$-Blockers have been used for children with difficulty relaxing the external sphincter. Studies are limited and this use of $\alpha$-blockers is considered investigational at this time. Typically timed voiding will be enough for this patient population.

**4.** Methylphenidate

Methylphenidate has been used to treat giggle incontinence; however, it is investigational and most often the risks of the side effects do not outweigh the benefit.

**5.** Tricyclic antidepressants

Imipramine is used in selected cases, primarily for nocturnal incontinence. It has mild anticholinergic and mild $\alpha$-adrenergic effects. However, there is no evidence from properly controlled studies that this family of medications is effective in children with dysfunctional voiding. In addition, the high dosage of the medication necessary to obtain anticholinergic effects results in a significant risk of possible toxic side effects. It should be used only rarely for voiding dysfunction.

**6.** Low-dose prophylactic antibiotic medication

If febrile or nonfebrile recurrent urinary tract infection or bacteriuria are involved in the problem of dysfunctional voiding, it is advisable to add low-dose prophylactic antibiotic medications. This removes infection as a cause of voiding dysfunction and allows evaluation of baseline voiding function. Usually, trimethoprim and sulfamethoxazole or nitrofurantoin is recommended. One should emphasize to the child and parents that the most important way of eliminating bacteria is frequent voiding.

**F.** **Biofeedback**

Using biofeedback has become quite popular for the treatment of urinary incontinence; however, it is only shown to be effective for the voiding dysfunction cause of incontinence and in most cases voiding dysfunction can be treated with timed voiding alone just as effectively.

**G.** **Surgery**

Surgery is useful only in cases of congenital anomalies (e.g., ectopic ureters or epispadias).

H.  **Most Common Treatment Plans for Various Causes of Incontinence**
1.  Voiding dysfunction
    a.  Treat constipation first
    b.  Timed voiding
    c.  Voiding with relaxation
    d.  Possible prophylactic antibiotics
    e.  Clean intermittent catheterization: used rarely and only in the most severe (and rare) form, namely NNNB (Hinman syndrome)
2.  Uninhibited bladder
    a.  Timed voiding
    b.  Anticholinergic with frequent reassessment (symptoms worsen during times of stress but improve at other times; therefore, the child may not always need to be on medication)
3.  Transient wetting
    In the case of transient wetting, it is best to focus attention on the primary problem (infection, psychosocial stressor).
4.  Vesicovaginal voiding
    For younger children, voiding backward or, for older children, voiding with their legs in abduction is curative. This limits backflow of urine into the vagina.
5.  Voiding frequency disorders
    a.  Lazy bladder
        (1)  Timed voiding
    b.  Benign urinary frequency
        (1)  Reassurance with close follow-up
        (2)  Usually self-limited after 3 to 6 months

## RECOMMENDED READING

Skoog S, Scherz H. Office pediatric urology. In: *Adult and pediatric urology,* volume 3, 4th ed. Philadelphia: Lippincott Williams and Wilkins; 2002:2671–2718.

# Nocturnal Enuresis

Pamela A. Bogan

Enuresis is a common condition that affects all cultures and has been recognized for centuries. The etiology of and treatment for this condition are, to this day, not fully understood. This condition has many psychological ramifications for the patient, family, and treating practitioner.

I. **DEFINITION**
Enuresis is defined as the persistence of inappropriate voiding of urine beyond the age of anticipated control. This age varies in different cultures.
   A. **Diurnal or Nocturnal**
   Enuresis can occur both day and night, at night only, or, sometimes, only during the day. Although age dependent, approximately 15% of nocturnal enuretics are also wet during the day. Because the causes and treatments vary considerably based on the type of enuresis, this chapter focuses on nocturnal enuresis only.
   B. **Primary or Secondary**
   Primary enuretics have never had a dry period, whereas children with secondary enuresis have had a dry period of at least 6 months prior to beginning wetting again. Approximately 20% of nocturnal enuretics can be classified as secondary. Concern about secondary enuresis suggests a more extensive workup, but in most cases this is unnecessary.

II. **INCIDENCE**
   A. Although there are societal differences, approximately 15% to 25% of 5-year-old children have nocturnal enuresis.
   B. There is a spontaneous cure rate of 15% each year, independent of society or culture.
   C. Approximately 2% to 3% of older adolescents and 1% to 2% of adults have nocturnal enuresis. These data are confirmed by the number of army recruits rejected because of nocturnal enuresis.
   D. Nocturnal enuresis is more common in boys than girls ($\sim$3/2).

III. **ETIOLOGY**
Nocturnal enuresis is considered a symptom as opposed to a disease. Numerous causes may, therefore, explain this symptom. Most evidence suggests that the cause of nocturnal enuresis is multifactorial. Possibilities include the following.
   A. **Genetic**
   There is an increased incidence of nocturnal enuresis in children whose parents also had this condition.

1. Both parents, 77%; one parent, 44%; neither parent 15%.
2. In monozygotic twins the concordance rate is 68%; the rate for dizygotic twins is 36%.
3. The exact gene and what that gene encodes remain unclear.

B. **Maturational Delay**

Delayed functional maturation of the central nervous system may reduce the child's ability to inhibit bladder emptying at night.

1. The child's bladder fills, but the sensory output resulting from bladder stretching is not perceived or the message fails to reach the brain, failing, thereby, to inhibit bladder contraction.
2. Functional bladder capacity is small in some children with nocturnal enuresis.

C. **Sleep Disorders**

Most parents of enuretic children report that their children are deep sleepers. The findings of scientific studies of the sleep patterns of children with and without nocturnal enuresis however, show, wide variations.

D. **Upper Airway Obstruction**

Surgical relief of airway obstruction by tonsillectomy, adenoidectomy, or both is reported to have diminished nocturnal enuresis in 76% of cases, although these data are not well substantiated and are likely overly optimistic.

E. **Psychological Factors**

1. Nocturnal enuresis was once thought to be a psychological problem. In most cases, psychological problems now appear to be a result of nocturnal enuresis rather than the cause.
2. Low self-esteem has been associated with nocturnal enuresis.
3. In some cases of sexual abuse, psychological effects may be the primary cause of nocturnal enuresis.

F. **Urinary Tract Infections**

Wetting is the only symptom of urinary tract infection in approximately 1% of children with nocturnal enuresis. In the past, many of these children were classified incorrectly as having asymptomatic bacteriuria.

G. **Nocturnal Polyuria**

1. Nonenuretic children concentrate their urine overnight. This has been noted by first void morning specific gravity of below 1.015. There is a higher rate of poor first-void urine concentration in children with nocturnal enuresis.
2. Normal children show a circadian rhythm in the release of antidiuretic hormone (ADH) that increases nocturnally and is associated with lower urine outputs at night.
3. Children with nocturnal enuresis have been shown to have lower ADH levels at night, lower urinary osmolality, and higher urine volumes. It remains

unclear whether this is primary or secondary to increased daytime salt or fluid intake.
4. Even if pituitary dysfunction is abnormal, this fails to explain why enuretic children do not awaken and void in the toilet.

**H. Summary**

The exact etiology of nocturnal enuresis is often unclear. Therapy is, therefore, most often prescribed without regard to specific etiology.

## IV. EVALUATION

**A. History**

1. Documentation
   a. How many nights each week?
   b. How many times each night?
   c. Approximate volume each episode?
   d. What times during the night?
   e. Primary or secondary?
2. Voiding history
   a. Daytime frequency?
   b. Daytime urgency?
   c. Weak or intermittent stream?
3. Psychosocial history, especially in secondary cases
   a. Precipitating factors?
   b. History of sexual abuse?
   c. Family attitudes and response to enuresis?
4. General
   a. Family history of enuresis?
   b. General medical history?
   c. General family history?
   d. Developmental milestones?

**B. Physical Examination** (with attention to general demeanor and self-esteem)

1. General, including abdominal (feel for stool, percuss for bladder distension)
2. External genitalia
   a. Appearance (look for signs of abuse)?
   b. Is the perineum wet (sign of ectopic ureter, daytime incontinence)?
   c. Rash or excoriation?
3. Neurologic
   a. Spinal lesion (hemangioma, hairy patch, deep dimple, lipoma)?
   b. Rectal tone and sensation (generally, rectal examination is too traumatic and not useful)/anal wink?
   c. Gait and movement?
4. Urinary stream
   a. Observation when possible.
   b. Flow rate may be useful for pattern of voiding if observation is not feasible.

**C. Urinalysis**

1. Specific gravity (ability to concentrate urine)
2. Dipstick for glucose and protein
3. Dipstick and microscopic for infection (culture and sensitivity)

**D. Voiding Diary** (in select cases)
  1. Time of each void
  2. Amount of each void
  3. Documentation of incontinence
  4. Documentation of bowel movements
**E. Renal/Bladder Sonogram** (only in rare cases; may obtain bladder ultrasound for post-void residual urine)
**F. Voiding Cystourethrogram/Urodynamic Study** (only in very rare cases)
**G. Cystoscopy** (including urethral dilation and meatotomy; almost never!)

## V. TREATMENT

Treatment in each individual case must be tailored to the child, family, and social structure.

**A. Reassurance**

This may be all that is necessary for younger children and families who are particularly concerned about organic disease. Spontaneous cure occurs in 15% each year.

**B. Motivational Therapy**
  1. Should be encouraged in almost every case. It is useful in conjunction with other treatments.
  2. Positive reinforcement (stickers/stars on a calendar). Reward the child each time a goal is reached. At first the goal is to have a few dry nights.
  3. Limiting the amount of fluid the child drinks before bedtime helps. Especially true for fluids containing caffeine such as cola drinks.
  4. Waking the child to go to the bathroom periodically during the night prevents the child's bladder from becoming full.
  5. Cure rate is about 25%.
  6. Significant improvement in 70%.

**C. Pharmacologic Therapy**
  1. Anticholinergic medications are not effective unless there is also daytime frequency/urgency or small functional bladder.
  2. Antidepressants, principally imipramine hydrochloride
     a. Mechanism of action unclear (altered sleep cycles, mild anticholinergic effect).
     b. Give 0.5 to 1.5 mg/kg/d 1 to 2 hours before bed (may need to increase two to three times).
     c. Success rate is 50%, with a very high relapse rate when medication is discontinued.
     d. Side effects: daytime sedation, anxiety, insomnia, dry mouth, nausea, and adverse personality changes.
     e. Overdose can result in fatal cardiac arrhythmias, hypotension, respiratory distress, and convulsions.
     f. Currently used only rarely.
  3. Desmopressin acetate
     a. Synthetic ADH (more potent and longer lasting than ADH).

    **b.** Intranasal spray: 10 to 40 μg before bed (may fail to be absorbed when there is rhinitis) or tablets 0.2 to 0.6 mg before bed.

    **c.** Reduces urine output.

    **d.** May stimulate arousal during sleep.

    **e.** Reduces wet nights by 40% to 70% (but only 30% totally dry).

    **f.** Relapse rates can approach 80% to 100%.

    **g.** Danger of hyponatremia (very rare), but must limit fluids after dinner.

**D. Conditioning**

    **1.** Alarm attached to underwear or pajamas that goes off when urine connects the circuit.

    **2.** Works in the older child with a motivated family. Often the alarm is very disturbing to the family when the child who set off the alarm is a deep sleeper and needs to be awakened.

    **3.** This treatment can take 1 to 2 months.

    **4.** Mechanism of action is unclear (negative reinforcement versus heightened sensation and waking with bladder distention).

    **5.** Initial cure rate is 70%. Even with relapses, 50% achieve a long-term cure. Retreatment is often successful in relapsing patients.

    **6.** Disadvantages

        **a.** Most health insurance plans will not pay for the alarm.

        **b.** Difficult for families to follow through with.

**E. Miscellaneous**

    **1.** Avoid foods that cause allergic responses. Although this is unproven, occasional dramatic responses are seen (foods to avoid include colas, chocolate, and citrus products).

    **2.** Hypnosis and suggestion: Self-hypnosis works in some cases. There are, however, limited data available.

    **3.** Psychotherapy may be effective in selected, severe cases with associated psychosocial problems. Not appropriate for the average child.

    **4.** Positive reinforcement is a useful adjunct to all treatments!

**VI. COSTS**

It must be recognized that prices of all items may vary geographically and over time. The following estimates are approximate and for comparison only.

**A. Diapers:** $10.99/month

**B. Alarm:** $66 to $86

**C. Retraining program (with alarm):** $1,000 to $1,500

**D. Psychological treatment:** $1,400 to $1,700 per year

**E. Imipramine:** $17.79 per month

**F. Desmopressin acetate (DDAVP):** $377 for 90 tablets per month

**G. Tolterodine (Detrol LA) (4 mg):** $109.99 per month

**H. Oxybutynin (Ditropan XL) (10 mg):** $116.99 per month

## RECOMMENDED READING

Caldamone AA, Schulman S, Rabinowitz R. Outpatient pediatric urology. In: Gillenwater JY, Grayhack JT, Howards SS, et al, eds. *Adult and pediatric urology*, 3rd ed. St. Louis: Mosby; 1996.

Homsy YL, Austin PF. In: Belman AB, King LR, Kramer SA, eds. *Clinical pediatric urology,* 4th ed. London: Dunitz; 2002.

# Constipation and Urologic Conditions

Karla M. Giramonti and
Angelique C. Hinds

I. **INTRODUCTION**
Although constipation is not a urologic problem, interestingly, there is a strong correlation between constipation and urologic conditions. It is very important to always consider constipation when caring for children with the following urologic problems.

A. **Urinary Tract Infections**
1. Approximately one-third of children with recurrent urinary tract infections have associated bowel problems. Infections will recur in most of those not treated and only in a few of those treated.
2. Approximately 10% of constipated children have recurrent urinary tract infections.

B. **Uninhibited Bladder** (see Chapter 8)
Children with recurrent urinary tract infections and constipation often have uninhibited bladder contractions. After treatment for constipation, many children will have resolution of the uninhibited bladder and its associated symptoms (incontinence and recurrent infections).

C. **Vesicoureteral Reflux**
1. Vesicoureteral reflux is more likely to resolve if concurrent constipation is treated.
2. Constipated children with vesicoureteral reflux are more likely to have breakthrough urinary tract infections and more likely to have postoperative complications.

D. **Ultrasound Findings**
Constipated children have a significant increase in postvoid residual and upper renal tract dilation than children who are not constipated.

E. **Incontinence**
1. One-third of constipated children experience daytime urinary incontinence. If constipation is treated, most will have resolved daytime wetting.
2. One-third of constipated children will have nighttime urinary incontinence. If constipation is treated, two-thirds will have resolved nighttime wetting.

II. **DEFINITION**
*Constipation* consists of hard, small stools, infrequent bowel evacuations, abnormally large stools, difficult or painful defecation, or encopresis (smearing).

**III. ETIOLOGY**
  **A.** The most common cause of constipation in the other-wise healthy child is "withholding" of stool due to toilet teaching, dirty or public bathrooms, lack of privacy, too busy playing, past painful defecation, changes in routine or diet, or intercurrent illness.
  **B.** The action of withholding stool causes the rectum to expand to accommodate the increasing amount of stool. The stool increases in size and, as the body reabsorbs more water, the stool becomes increasingly hard. As the rectum expands, the normal urge to defecate diminishes. As the cycle is repeated, greater amounts of stool are built up in the bowel and motility, rectal elasticity, and sensation further decrease. Subsequently, some children begin to have encopresis due to looser stool leaking around a rectal impaction or because the muscles used to withhold become fatigued.
  **C.** No organic etiology is found in 90% to 95% of children with constipation.

**IV. PRESENTATION**
  A child will not typically present to the urology clinic with a complaint of constipation. These children more often present with urologic symptoms such as incontinence or recurrent urinary tract infections.

**V. INCIDENCE AND EPIDEMILOGY**
  **A.** Constipation accounts for 3% of pediatric outpatient visits and 25% of gastroenterology visits.
  **B.** Encopresis is present in 1.5% of children at school entry.
  **C.** Boys suffer from encopresis three to six times more often than girls. This is thought to be because of the standing versus sitting voiding position used by boys during urination. During urination, the pelvic floor muscles relax, when the pelvic floor muscles relax, stool in the rectum may be expelled. Because boys stand to urinate, when the pelvic muscles relax with voiding, they may soil their underwear.

**VI. DIAGNOSIS**
  **A. History**
    **1.** If an accurate clinical history can be obtained, then the diagnosis of constipation can usually be made by history alone. Unfortunately, an accurate bowel history in the school-aged child is close to impossible to obtain in most cases.
    **2.** Parental history of constipation can be incorrect in up to half of children. Children are also not good historians as to their own bowel and bladder habits.
  **B. Physical Examination**
    **1.** Abdominal examination may reveal hard stool in the abdomen.
    **2.** External examination of the anus and rectum may reveal large amount of stool in the rectum.

    **3.** A brief neurologic examination should assess perianal sensation, anal tone, and the presence of anal wink.

    **4.** Although controversial because it can be traumatic for some children, some clinicians include a formal rectal examination. This can determine the size of the rectum and the amount and consistency of stool.

**C. Radiologic Examination**

    **1.** Abdominal x-ray can further support the suspicion of constipation on history or physical examination. Fecal load can be estimated and objective scoring systems have been developed. An x-ray is especially useful in children for whom a digital examination can be difficult and/or traumatic.

    **2.** The problem with the x-ray is, of course, the radiation exposure. If there is a high suspicion of constipation, it might be better to treat without obtaining an x-ray.

    **3.** Ultrasound is promising, but guidelines have not been developed at this time.

**VII. TREATMENT**

**A. Treatment** for constipation can be very challenging. It is labor intensive and can take 6 months to 1 year. Our approach is a practical approach and includes two important phases: the clean-out phase and the maintenance phase.

**B. Clean-Out Phase:** The goal of the clean-out phase is to literally clean out the entire bowel of stool using medications. This will take anywhere from 3 to 7 days depending on the amount of retained stool. The success of the entire treatment depends on a successful initial clean out. This phase always requires medication. The medications we prefer for the clean out include the osmotic laxatives or a lubricant with or without a stimulant.

    **1.** Osmotic laxatives

        **a.** Polyethylene glycol 3350 (Miralax), an osmotic laxative, is our first choice for the clean-out phase because of its tolerability (does not taste bad), effectiveness, and limited side effects. The negatives are that it requires a prescription and is expensive.

        **b.** Magnesium supplements (magnesium citrate, Milk of Magnesia) are also osmotic laxatives. Although they are easy to obtain (over the counter), inexpensive, and effective, they do seem to cause more side effects.

    **2.** Lubricants

        Mineral oil is inexpensive and does not require a prescription. Side effects are minimal. One problem with mineral oil is some children refuse to take it; however, it can be made palatable by mixing with ice and fruit or ice cream in a blender. Another problem with mineral oil, but only as a clean-out medication, is it tends to ooze from the rectum long after the clean-out phase is complete.

**3.** Stimulants

      Stimulants [senna (Ex Lax, Ducolax)] can also be used in the clean-out phase. Chocolate Ex Lax tastes good, is inexpensive, and quite effective when used along with polyethylene glycol for the severely constipated child. The stimulants are best used only for the short term (clean-out phase). Some believe that chronic use of stimulants will take away the body's normal reflex to have a bowel movement.

**4.** Stool softeners

      We do not recommend using stool softeners [docusate (Colace)] for childhood constipation. Stool softeners are best used to treat constipation in patients who need to avoid straining (e.g., after surgery).

**5.** Enemas

      Enemas are rarely necessary in the otherwise healthy constipated child (see Special Circumstances).

**C. Side Effects**

      Side effects of all stool medications include soiling, gas, nausea, vomiting, abdominal pain, and diarrhea.

**D. Maintenance Phase:** The goal of the maintenance phase is to maintain the empty bowel by having one or two, continent, soft stools per day. This phase initially involves medication, but the medication is eventually weaned. This phase can take 6 months to 1 year. There are three steps in the maintenance phase: medications, diet and fiber, and the daily sit (behavior modification).

**1.** Medications: For the maintenance phase we recommend osmotic laxatives (enulose or polyethylene glycol 3350) or a lubricant (mineral oil).

    **a.** Polyethylene glycol 3350 can also be used as a maintenance medication (in smaller doses). The dose should be titrated to ensure one or two soft stools per day. As the bowel regains its elasticity and form over time the dose should be decreased.

    **b.** Mineral oil can also be used effectively as a maintenance medication, and with the smaller doses used in the maintenance phase, does not seem to cause soiling or oozing of stool that occurs when using mineral oil as a clean-out agent. It is important to have the child take the oil between meals because it decreases reabsorption of fat-soluble vitamins if taken with meals.

      **c.** Lactulose (Enulose) is another good maintenance medication. The dose needs to be slowly titrated up, however, until the desired effect is reached (one to two soft stools per day). Starting on too high of a dose increases cramping and gas. This medication is available by prescription only.

**2.** Diet and fiber

    **a.** Water

        Increased daily intake of water is important and will help to soften the stools.

    **b.** Fiber

      **(1)** Increased fiber intake is often recommended in the treatment of constipation; however, there is no direct evidence that increased dietary fiber intake is effective in childhood constipation.

      **(2)** Recommended fiber intake is the age of the child plus 5 grams of fiber. Our experience reveals that very few children can consume this much fiber. Therefore, we often recommend a fiber supplement.

      **(3)** There are many different types of supplemental fiber. For younger children, the powder form might be the best choice because it can easily be mixed in liquid. For the older child, who can swallow pills, the tablet or capsule form is probably the easiest. For the child somewhere in between, perhaps wafers are the best choice.

    **c.** The fluid/fiber ratio is important: not enough fluid with the fiber can make constipation worse.

**3.** Daily sit

    **a.** If the child suffers from encopresis then the daily sit is a crucial element of the bowel maintenance program. The goal is to have the child have a bowel movement at a socially acceptable time, in a socially acceptable place. This is done by sitting on the toilet for 15 to 20 minutes after a meal (due to the normal gastrocolic reflex that stimulates the bowel to move after eating).

    **b.** Many recommend that children sit on the toilet after every meal; however, this is very difficult for a school-aged child. Thus, in our practice, depending on the child's individual situation we have the child sit after breakfast, dinner, or both.

    **c.** Children whose feet do not touch the floor must use a stool for support.

    **d.** Positive reinforcement and reward systems improve success. Reward for following the program rather than success, because success takes too much time.

**E. Biofeedback**

Biofeedback has become quite popular in the treatment of stool and urinary incontinence; however, at this point in time there is only limited evidence showing a short-term benefit. It appears that there is no long-term benefit from adding biofeedback training to conventional treatment of constipation in children.

**VIII. SPECIAL CIRCUMSTANCES**

**A. Medications:** Commonly used medications, such as oxybutynin (Ditropan), imipramine (Tofranil), tolterodine (Detrol), and hyoscyamine (Levsin), cause constipation.

**B. Neurogenic Bowel:** Constipation in the neurologically challenged child is different from constipation in the otherwise healthy child.

  1. A neurogenic bowel has a lack of nerve innervation caused by spina bifida, spinal cord lesions, tethered spinal cords, or trauma.
  2. The major problems of the neurogenic bowel are constipation and stool incontinence due to the following reasons:
    a. Lack of awareness that the rectum is filled with stool
    b. Slow motility
    c. Inability to effectively empty bowel completely
  3. Treatment goals vary depending on the age of the child and chronicity of constipation.
    a. Infants and Toddlers (pre–potty teaching age): The goal in this age group is to prevent constipation. Children who have never experienced long periods of constipation achieve continence later in life with fewer problems than children who have been constipated.
    b. Older Child (post–potty teaching age): The goal of the bowel program in the older child is to wear underwear. Length of treatment depends greatly on how long the child has been constipated. If the family or child is not ready for the commitment to a bowel program, then every effort should be made to at least keep the child free from constipation until the child and family are ready for a continence program.
  4. Treatment in the neurogenically challenged patient includes the same clean out and maintenance phase as the otherwise healthy child with the following additions.
    a. Clean out: Oral medications alone may not be sufficient to clean out the older neurogenic child with severe constipation. Often it

is necessary (and more successful) to admit the child to the hospital for a clean out using high-dose osmotic laxative via nasogastric tube.

**b.** Maintenance: The medications and fiber and diet stages of the maintenance phase will be the same as the otherwise healthy child. However, the daily sit will often not be successful with mere sitting on the toilet after a meal. Often it is necessary to add an enema or suppository at the time of the daily sit to ensure a positive stool.

## RECOMMENDED READING

Dohil R, Roberts E, Jones FK, et al. Constipation and reversible urinary tract abnormalities. *Arch Dis Childhood* 1994;70:56–57.

Koff SA, Wagner TT, Jayanthi VR. The relationship among dysfunctional elimination syndromes, primary vesicoureteral reflux and urinary tract infections in children. *J Urol* 1998;160:1019–1022.

Loening-Bauke V. Urinary incontinence and urinary tract infection and their resolution with treatment of chronic constipation of childhood. *Pediatrics* 1997;100:228–232.

Loening-Bauke V. Encopresis. *Curr Opin Pediatr* 2002;14:570–575.

Youseff NN, Di Lorenzo V. Childhood constipation—evaluation and treatment. *J Gastroenterol* 2001;33:199–205.

# Spina Bifida, Myelomeningocele, and the Neurogenic Bladder

Ronald S. Sutherland

*Spina bifida* comprises a group of congenital and acquired abnormalities of the spinal cord generally referred to as *spinal dysraphism* (Table 11–1). It is the most common primary cause of neurogenic bladder dysfunction in children, affecting approximately 1 in 1,000 in the United States. About 95% of children with spina bifida have abnormal innervation of the bladder. As a consequence, they are at risk not only for urinary incontinence but also for damaging their kidneys because of increased bladder pressure, vesicoureteral reflux, obstruction, and infection. Early recognition of neurovesical abnormalities enables prompt intervention and usually prevents damage to the kidneys.

*Spinal dysraphism* arises from a defect in the formation of the neural tube. The etiology is uncertain, but various teratogens such as alcohol and zinc as well as some medications (e.g., valproic acid) have been implicated. Most recently, evidence has suggested that deficient maternal intake of folic acid is associated with development of spina bifida, and that supplementation may reduce the chances of acquiring such birth defects by sevenfold.

Urologic goals to consider in the care of children with spina bifida are to (a) preserve renal function; (b) achieve urinary and fecal continence (defined as out of diapers at a developmentally appropriate age); and (c) promote the development of healthy sexual function when age appropriate. In attaining these goals we hope to enable these patients to develop a sense of autonomy and better self-esteem.

## I. Diagnosis
### A. Prenatal Assessment
1. Serum $\alpha$-fetoprotein (AFP): Open spina bifida or anencephaly should be suspected if maternal serum AFP is elevated more than 3 standard deviations from the norm before 24 weeks' gestation (Table 11–1).
2. Fetal sonography: Fetal sonography and elevated serum AFP combined are highly sensitive (80%) and specific (99%) in diagnosing spina bifida.
3. Method of birth: Although vaginal delivery is safe, some recent studies have suggested that cesarean section may limit neurologic injury.

### B. Newborn Assessment
After delivery, it is important to have a well-trained support staff consisting of, but not limited to, a pediatrician, neurosurgeon, orthopedic surgeon, pediatric

**Table 11–1. Spinal dysraphism: classification and characteristics**

**Cystic:** Posterior protrusion of spinal elements through spinal defect

| | |
|---|---|
| Myelomeningocele | Cyst contains meninges, spinal cord and/or nerve roots, and CSF |
| Meningocele | Cyst contains meninges and CSF |
| Lipomeningocele | Cyst contains meninges, CSF, and fat |
| Myeloschisis | Extensive open neural plate or cleft spinal cord |
| Rachischisis | Complete cleft of vertebral bodies and cord |

**Noncystic:** No protrusion of spinal elements; presence of hair tuft, sinus or dimple, discoloration, or lipoma the only sign

| | |
|---|---|
| Intradural lipoma | Fatty infiltration of the spinal cord |
| Diastematomyelia | Bony spicule or fibrous band splitting the cord |
| Dermoid and epidermoid cyst/sinus | Invagination of surface epidermis |
| Cauda equina tumor | Cord compression |
| Anterior sacral meningocele | Anterior herniation of spinal elements into pelvis |
| Tethered cord | |
| Primary | Broad, thickened cord preventing upward migration |
| Secondary | Fixation or compression of cord from postoperative adhesions, fibrous bands, lipoma, and cysts |
| Syringomyelia | Cystic degeneration of cord |

urologist, neonatologist, experienced nurses, physical therapists, and social services personnel.

1. Neurosurgical intervention: For open defects, neurosurgical intervention is performed as soon as possible. Ideally, abdominal ultrasound and a functional evaluation of the bladder (urodynamic study) should be performed before closure of the back defect, but often this is not feasible. Because many of these infants experience spinal shock and urinary retention after closure, urologic intervention is often necessary before urodynamic study.

2. Evaluate for occult spinal dysraphisms. Although open spinal dysraphism is the most common variant observed, closed spinal defects (Table 11–1) also occur frequently. Suggestive signs include a sacral pit or dimple, a hairy patch, hemangiomas, aberrant gluteal cleft, lipoma, and laxity of anal sphincter tone. Spinal defects are also associated with other conditions including anorectal anomalies and cloacal exstrophy.

## II. CARE OF THE NEWBORN
### A. Evaluation

1.  Urodynamics: The goal of urodynamic assessment is to characterize the compliance and contractility of the bladder and the function of the outlet (the bladder neck and external sphincter). These tests evaluate bladder pressure (cystomyography), sphincter activity (electromyography), emptying ability, and radiographic appearance of the lower urinary tract. In addition, vesicoureteral reflux may be detected on fluoroscopy during urodynamic assessment. Urodynamic testing is done as soon as the infant can be placed in the supine position, prior to discharge from the hospital. Some centers may prefer watchful waiting and follow the infant with sonography alone, deferring urodynamic evaluation until hydronephrosis is detected, or continence is desired.

2.  Sonography: This is performed to detect hydronephrosis, that may be the result of vesicoureteral reflux or a hostile, noncompliant bladder, and to monitor renal growth.

3.  Urinalysis and culture: Urinalysis and urine culture may be performed only if the child is symptomatic for a urinary tract infection.

### B. Treatment of the Newborn

1.  Treatment is based on the urodynamic findings.
    a.  Weak sphincter, normal bladder: observation
    b.  Flaccid bladder: clean intermittent catheterization (CIC)
    c.  Hyperreflexic and/or noncompliant bladder: CIC plus anticholinergic medication

2.  Some centers start all babies who have abnormal urodynamics (more than 95%) on CIC immediately at birth. These centers, ours included, do this because it is easier to start a CIC program in infancy and eventually most children require CIC. It is our experience that older children who were started on CIC as infants appear to tolerate and be more compliant with the CIC than children who begin CIC at a later age. For example, if a baby has a weak sphincter in infancy, there is no medical reason to catheterize the baby. However, later, this same baby will be incontinent and the urologist may choose to operate to tighten the sphincter, after which the child will need to be catheterized. This surgery is usually done close to the age of normal toilet teaching or prior to entry to kindergarten. Unfortunately, the timing of the surgery is at one of the worst ages, developmentally, to start a CIC program, the best approach is to give the parents all the information, such as urodynamic results, chance of needing catheterization in the future and information on the ease in starting an infant on CIC

as compared to a 5 year old. Then the parents can make an informed choice for their family.

3. Early institution of CIC every 3 hours is preferred over the *Credé maneuver* (suprapubic compression to express urine), which is not physiologic, causes markedly increased bladder pressures, and is not appropriate for long-term management. The addition of anticholinergic medication (see below) in the neonatal period is safe and well tolerated. In the infant who has progressive urinary tract deterioration despite maximal medical therapy, a temporary vesicostomy (surgical diversion of the bladder to the lower abdominal wall) will prove effective.

4. Avoid the use of latex-containing products.

## III. LONG-TERM MANAGEMENT
### A. Bladder Function.

1. CIC: When taught to family and patients early, CIC is very well tolerated and accepted, and easily becomes a lifelong habit. More importantly, a consistent policy of early CIC helps to prevent renal deterioration and may preserve some bladder function (decreasing the need for major bladder surgery in the future).

2. CIC plus anticholinergic medication: Increased bladder pressure and inadequate capacity may become manifest as incontinence, hydronephrosis, urinary tract infection, and occasionally suprapubic discomfort. Medical therapy with anticholinergic medication (such as oxybutynin 0.1 mg/kg tid), coupled with intermittent catheterization, is usually sufficient to provide both a low bladder pressure and continence. In some children, higher doses may provide additional detrusor relaxation with enhanced continence. If side effects arise, intravesical instillation can be utilized. In addition, newer forms of administration (prolonged-release tablets or patches) have equal efficacy and fewer side effects.

3. Surgical bladder augmentation: When medical therapy fails to achieve adequate low-pressure capacity, surgical enlargement of the bladder may be achieved by various methods (Fig. 11–1). Because of the potential complications of this procedure, it should be undertaken only when the other options have failed.

   a. Use of ileum and colon: These are the most commonly used segments that successfully provide surgical expansion of the bladder capacity. Unfortunately, complications are common, including electrolyte and acid/base derangements (chronic acidosis), chronic mucus production, and problems resulting from open bowel surgery (peritonitis and bowel obstruction).

   b. Use of stomach (gastrocystoplasty): Because of its ability to secrete acid, using a segment

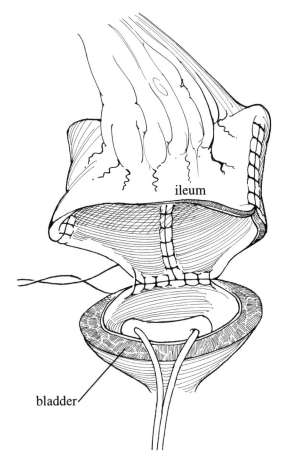

ileum

bladder

**Fig. 11–1.  Augmentation of the bladder is performed using a segment of ileum as a patch to increase the capacity and decrease the pressure of the bladder.**

of stomach may benefit children with chronic acidosis (particularly those with renal impairment). Mucus is much less of a problem with this segment. Occasionally children may develop hematuria and dysuria due to marked acidity. This is usually treated with antacids and H2 blockers; however, the procedure should not be used in children with anuria.

**c.** Use of ureter: Occasionally, the dilated ureter of a nonfunctional renal unit can be used as a patch after removal of the kidney. When such a segment is present, it allows for placement of a urothelium-lined structure onto the bladder and avoids interruption of the bowel, reabsorption of urine, and mucus production.

**d.** Follow-up of patients after augmentation

**(1)** Metabolic evaluation: These patients are at risk for metabolic disturbances because of absorption or secretion of electrolytes and through the bowel segments. With ileum and colon, hyperchloremic metabolic acidosis is most common; with stomach, hypochloremic, hyperkalemic metabolic alkalosis can occur. Chronic acidosis alters calcium metabolism and thus bone development. Therefore, serum electrolytes (including bicarbonate) and calcium, phosphorous, and magnesium levels should be checked annually or as needed.

**(2)** Renal function: Assess serum creatinine and electrolytes at least annually.

**(3)** Urine microscopy: In children who perform self-catheterization the urine will most likely be colonized with bacteria and may have a few leukocytes and red blood cells. Moreover, after an augmentation with an intestinal section, the urine will almost always be filled with mucous and bacteria. Unless the child is symptomatic or has vesicoureteral reflux, this should not be treated with antibiotics.

**(4)** Continent catheterizable stomas: After augmentation of the urinary bladder, catheterization is nearly always required to facilitate complete drainage. In patients who are wheelchair-bound or those who have severe scoliosis/lordosis, catheterization may be physically challenging. Others may not be able to see or reach the urethra. In these individuals, a catheterizable, continent stoma may be created to provide an easily accessible route of bladder emptying (Fig. 11–2). This may be created from appendix, ileum, or colon. Boys with intact urethral sensation, in whom self-catheterization may not be well tolerated, may also benefit from an abdominal catheterizable stoma.

**B. Continence** (sphincter function)

**1.** Medication: Urinary incontinence related to inadequate outlet resistance rather than inadequate storage may occasionally be amenable to control by $\alpha$-adrenergic medication (phenylpropanolamine or pseudoephedrine). Although these agents may provide minor improvement due to contraction of

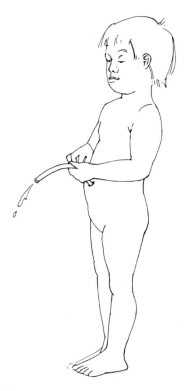

**Fig. 11–2.** Child inserting a catheter into a continent catheterizable channel from the umbilicus to the bladder.

smooth muscle, most often sphincter function will be improved only by surgical correction.

2. Periurethral injection therapy: Injection of substances such as collagen, Teflon, or Deflux around the bladder neck may result in short-term improvement in continence; long-term results are lacking at this time. The advantage of this technique over open surgical reconstruction to improve outlet resistance is the minimally invasive nature of this endoscopic procedure. Unfortunately it is only rarely successful long term.

3. Bladder neck suspension and sling procedures: Suspension of the bladder neck and proximal urethra to the pubis using sutures or compression by a sling of rectus fascia, can be coupled with bladder neck reconstruction. Success rates in achieving continence are reported as high as 70%. Patients who experience only partial improvement can be

supplemented by collagen injections. Most patients with a sling will need to catheterize using a continent abdominal stoma.

4. Artificial urinary sphincter: Placement of an inflatable cuff around the bladder neck offers up to 90% improvement in continence in both girls and boys (Fig. 11–3). Although highly successful, complications include device failure (in about 12% because of erosion of the cuff) and the conversion of a low-pressure bladder to a noncompliant, hostile reservoir (seen in as many as 30%). For best results, only patients with normal bladder capacity

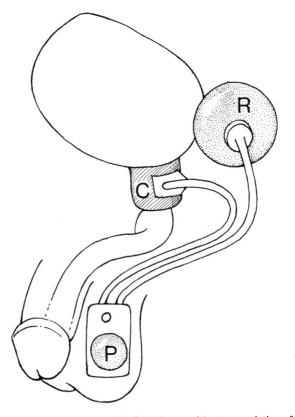

Fig. 11–3. Diagram of an artificial urinary sphincter consisting of three parts. The cuff (*C*) is placed around the bladder neck or prostatic urethra (in boys) and is connected to a pump (*P*) in either the scrotum or labium, and a fluid reservoir (*R*) implanted beneath the rectus muscle. Fluid is pumped from the cuff into the reservoir which then passively refills the cuff over 60 to 90 seconds. In children who perform CIC, the cuff is pumped open and catheterization is easily done.

and compliance should be selected for sphincteric implantation; alternatively, augmentation should be performed simultaneously. It is unclear if this complication is exclusive to artificial sphincters or whether any continence procedure may predispose the bladder to this form of deterioration.

C. **Vesicoureteral Reflux:** Between 40% and 65% of patients with spina bifida will have vesicoureteral reflux. This is usually due to increased intravesical pressures resulting from detrusor sphincter dyssynergia or a poorly compliant bladder. Treatment is directed toward improvement of storage and elimination of urine, usually by instituting anticholinergic agents and intermittent catheterization. Persistent reflux must then be managed on an individual basis. Low-dose antibiotic prophylaxis should be given to all children with reflux. Surveillance should be offered to children with low-grade reflux who do not have symptomatic urinary infections or renal scarring, and are compliant with bladder management. Should surgical intervention become necessary because of breakthrough infections or worsening hydronephrosis, an endoscopic antireflux procedure (subureteric injection of collagen or Deflux) may be a reasonable first choice. However, the gold standard remains ureteral reimplantation. If surgical intervention is undertaken to improve capacity or continence, it is prudent to consider reimplantation at that time.

D. **Bacteriuria:** Bacteriuria is found in many children with spinal dysraphism, especially those who perform CIC, and is termed *asymptomatic bacteriuria.* These patients do not require antibiotic therapy or prophylactic suppression unless there is documented vesicoureteral reflux or symptoms such as fever, dysuria, or new-onset incontinence. In the absence of vesicoureteral reflux, there is little risk of renal scarring.

E. **Renal Function:** Elevated detrusor pressures and recurrent urinary tract infections are the primary risk factors for renal deterioration and may be prevented by appropriate care of the lower tract. Because serum creatinine and renal sonography may not provide a consistent measure of early renal injury, a more accurate measure may be obtained with a technetium-dimercaptosuccinic acid (DMSA) renal scan. It is advisable then to obtain a DMSA renal scan as a baseline in children who have not been evaluated in the neonatal period and repeat them as often as indicated by noninvasive studies or clinical parameters. We recommend renal sonography and urinalysis every 3 months for the first year of life and every 12 months thereafter in all cases, as well as at the time of any change in status (incontinence, infection, problems with catheterization).

F. **Bowel Management:** The management of fecal elimination can be a significant challenge to patients and

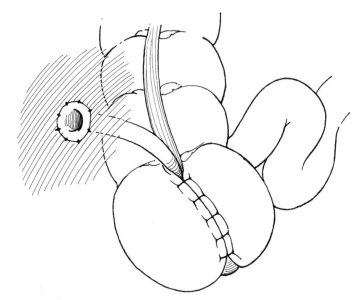

**Fig. 11–4.** The Malone ACE procedure (antegrade continence enema) utilizes the appendix as a continent catheterizable channel to deliver a bolus of fluid (such as tap water) to help flush out the colonic contents in patients with severely refractory neuropathic constipation.

caregivers. All patients require a bowel program that includes dietary modification, cathartics and/or enemas, and possible digital stimulation and manipulation. For patients in whom conservative management fails, creation of a continent abdominal conduit to the colon may enable antegrade delivery of a large-volume enema to clear the colonic contents (Malone antegrade continence enema; ACE procedure) (Fig. 11–4). We have found that children in whom we have aggressively treated constipation early on (birth to 3 years) have greater success with training for stool continence. Therefore, all constipation should be treated aggressively in this population despite age or desire for continence.

G.  **Sexual Function and Fertility:** The majority of adults with spina bifida report being sexually active. Adolescents, however, have more than the usual problems of developing a sexually desirable identity when concerns about bowel or bladder continence persist into the teenage years. For this reason, we encourage measures to improve continence before the onset of puberty, which commonly comes about early in female spina bifida patients. Caregivers should to pay careful attention to this often overlooked area. These patients frequently have no role model and need open dialogue to support their growth and independence.

Fertility in men with spina bifida is less likely than in the general population due to inadequate erectile function, semen quality, and factors of socialization. However, each male patient must be approached individually with a goal of maximizing his available function and counseled regarding the possibility of paternity. Modern treatment of erectile dysfunction and infertility may improve the possibilities for these patients greatly. All these patients should be given appropriate counseling regarding sexually transmitted diseases and pregnancy. Both boys and girls need to be given information on how to obtain nonlatex condoms.

   **H.  Latex Precautions:** Life-threatening anaphylactic reactions attributable to an allergy to latex are more likely to occur in children with spina bifida who undergo general anesthesia. The anaphylaxis experienced by this group has been linked to IgE-mediated hypersensitivity to latex. Latex allergies occur in up to 40% of patients with spina bifida presumably due to chronic exposure to latex-containing products. Suggestive signs of latex allergy include skin rash and itching, rhinorrhea, and conjunctival irritation after exposure to latex. Products containing latex include gloves, urethral catheters, tourniquets, IV injection ports, anesthesia ventilation bags, blood pressure cuffs, and adhesive tape. Because this population is at risk, it is now recommended that exposure to latex products be avoided at all times (use only plastic or silicone catheters for intermittent catheterization).

**IV.  OCCULT SPINAL DYSRAPHISM** (Table 11–1)

   **A.  Signs:** Sometimes defects of the spinal cord may not be apparent on physical examination and become manifest only after the onset of urologic, neurologic, or orthopedic problems. Occasionally the only clue is a prominent sacral dimple or sinus tract, a tuft of hair or prominent pigmentation, or presence of a lipoma. Any of these signs should prompt further evaluation. The presenting signs and symptoms are often insidious. New onset of urinary incontinence, changes in voiding pattern, or urinary tract infection in an individual who has been voiding normally or who has a known diagnosis of spina bifida suggests the possibility of occurrence. The underlying problem is usually a tethered spinal cord characterized by a short, thickened filum terminale, which prevents the ascent of the conus medullaris during development.

   **B.  Workup**
   1.  Spinal ultrasound: In the neonate or infant, spinal ultrasound examination can reliably reveal low position and a nontapered, bulbous appearance of the conus, dorsal location of the cord within the bony canal, solid or cystic masses in the distal canal or

soft tissue of the back extending toward the canal, patulous distal thecal sac, and a thick filum terminale. This study is only possible in infants.

2. Magnetic resonance imaging (MRI): MRI characterizes spinal cord involvement more accurately. It is the diagnostic procedure of choice in older children in whom bone maturation precludes accurate sonography.

C. **Intervention:** Whether or not early neurosurgical intervention ameliorates voiding dysfunction by relieving spinal cord compression or tethering remains controversial. If detected in infancy, it is reasonable to think that urologic deterioration can be prevented in most and improved in many of those who present with dysfunction (expect a 70% improvement in voiding symptoms and more than 50% resolution of detrusor hyperreflexia). Older patients who present with neurologic changes are unlikely to improve. Overall, patients with neuropathic bladders from occult lesions should be managed in the same fashion as those with overt spinal dysraphism.

V. **PRENATAL INVENTION FOR MYELOMENINGO-CELE**

As noted, urologic morbidity in patients with myelomeningocele (MMC) is significant secondary to a poorly compliant bladder, sphincteric dysfunction, secondary vesicoureteral reflux, a predisposition to urinary tract infections, possible renal scarring, and renal failure. Urologic morbidity is the sequela of neurologic injury. The neurologic deficit seen in MMC is believed to be due to several factors. The first and most obvious is defective nerve development. There is also evidence of damage when the spinal cord is exposed to amniotic fluid. Indeed, lower limb movements observed on ultrasound studies at 16 to 17 weeks, have been seen to diminish subsequently. These observations have led to an attempt to repair the defect in utero with fetal surgery to close the open neural tube defect. In utero repair of MMC has been attempted both endoscopically and through open surgery via a hysterotomy. Presently, open fetal surgery is the technique of choice. A standard neurosurgical closure is performed through a small hysterotomy. A randomized prospective trial is now in progress to determine the efficacy of this approach.

Finally, some have argued that vaginal delivery itself may cause trauma to the spinal cord. In centers that believe in this possibility, elective cesarean section is recommended in most cases. Overall, this is still controversial.

VI. **CONCLUSION**

Urologic care of patients with spinal dysraphism focuses on preserving renal function, establishing urinary and bowel continence, promoting the development of normal sexuality, and a commitment to minimizing surgical intervention. Early intervention (both diagnostically and therapeutically) and patient education help to guarantee the most successful outcome. Intermittent catheterization with close clinical follow-up should be instituted early to prevent, rather than treat, the complications of neurogenic bladder dysfunction.

## RECOMMENDED READING

Mingin GC, Nguyen HT, Mathias R, et al. Growth and metabolic consequences of bladder augmentation in children with myelomeningocele and bladder exstrophy. *Pediatrics* 2002;110:1193–1198.

Sutherland RS, Mevoarch RA, Baskin LS, et al. Spinal dysraphism in children: an overview and an approach to prevent complications. *Urology* 1995;46:294–304.

# Prenatal Urologic Diagnosis and Maternal Counseling

Barry A. Kogan

With the advent of the widespread use of prenatal ultrasound in clinical practice, urologic conditions are being diagnosed in many infants before birth. Because ultrasound is performed so commonly, the impact of these diagnoses has been enormous. It remains unclear, however, whether this early diagnosis results in benefit to the neonate or merely increased anxiety over testing. In the majority of cases, parents can be reassured that postnatal evaluation is all that is needed and that their infant will have a good prognosis.

I. **INCIDENCE**
Urologic anomalies are found in about 0.4% of pregnancies. Of these, hydronephrosis is found in about half (see Chapter 13).

II. **FINDINGS**
Urologic findings may range from mild hydronephrosis that is essentially a normal finding to significant hydronephrosis resulting from any type of obstructive uropathy (Figs. 13-1, 13-2, and 13-3). In rare cases, renal tumors can be found or congenital anomalies like exstrophy and epispadias.

III. **GENERAL TREATMENT**
After initial diagnosis, a more extensive ultrasound survey is performed to confirm the diagnosis, look for associated findings, and, in the case of renal anomalies, to monitor the amount of amniotic fluid. In a few cases, some intervention is warranted in utero; for example, aspiration of an enormous cystic mass or, in very rare cases, placement of a vesicoamniotic shunt. It is almost never indicated to deliver the baby early. In most cases no intervention is needed before birth. In the majority, a postnatal evaluation is recommended, as well as prevention of urinary tract infection prior to postnatal evaluation. However, the overall benefits of prenatal diagnosis are unproven.

IV. **SPECIFIC DIAGNOSES**
   A. **Hydronephrosis:** Easy diagnosis in utero. The following parameters are important.
      1. The amount of amniotic fluid (correlates loosely with renal function)
      2. Unilateral or bilateral (unilateral less concerning because of the normal contralateral kidney)
      3. Evaluate the amount of hydronephrosis [generally by measuring the anteroposterior (AP) diameter of the renal pelvis]. An AP diameter greater than

10 mm of the renal pelvis in the third trimester warrants a postnatal evaluation (see below).

4. Amount of renal parenchyma
5. Corticomedullary differentiation (when present, suggests good renal function)
6. Echogenicity (when present this suggests renal dysplasia)
7. Cortical cysts (when present this suggests renal dysplasia)
8. Ureteral dilation (suggests a problem at the bladder or urethral level) and requires a postnatal evaluation
9. Bladder distention (suggests a problem at urethral level)
10. These diagnoses rarely, if ever, require in utero treatment. Another example of the very rare scenario where intervention would be considered is a massively obstructed solitary kidney from an ureteropelvic junction obstruction with progressive decrease in amniotic fluid.
11. Postnatally, patients with significant prenatal hydronephrosis as defined by an AP diameter greater than 10 mm in the third trimester or ureteral dilation should have a sonogram and a voiding cystourethrogram (VCUG; 33% incidence of reflux) at several weeks of age.
12. Prophylactic antibiotics [amoxicillin or cephalexin (Keflex)] should be given until proven that there is no reflux.
13. As a corollary, a prenatal diagnosis of hydronephrosis with an AP diameter less than 10 mm in the third trimester rarely if ever results in a clinically significant postnatal outcome such as loss of renal function, pain, or progressive hydronephrosis. These patients have a slightly dilated yet normal functioning kidney. They do not need postnatal evaluation unless clinical suspicion such as a urinary tract infection, hematuria, or pain results.
14. Circumcision is not contraindicated for boys with significant prenatal hydronephrosis. It may be beneficial because it may reduce the rate of urinary tract infections.
15. Generally, patients with prenatal hydronephrosis have an excellent prognosis.

B. **Urethral Valves**
1. Diagnosed by hydronephrosis, bladder distention, and the key-hole sign on ultrasound. The same findings as above are important, but especially amniotic fluid and renal parenchymal changes.
2. If these are okay, then the most appropriate treatment is to defer treatment until after birth.
3. At that time the neonate should have catheter drainage, VCUG, and resection of valves if he is

large enough; alternatively, a temporary vesicostomy can be used to bypass the blockage.

4. In rare cases, consider fetal intervention (see below).

5. Prognosis depends on the degree of renal dysplasia and is generally determined after birth if amniotic fluid is normal.

### C. Multicystic Kidney

1. Easily diagnosed in utero. The main findings are chaotic configuration of the kidney, multiple cysts that do not communicate, and no normal renal parenchyma.

2. Generally associated with a normal contralateral kidney and normal amniotic fluid.

3. Postnatally, we recommend prophylactic antibiotics until ultrasound and VCUG (25% of children have contralateral reflux into the solitary kidney). This condition will generally not affect life expectancy or health. In most institutions, nephrectomy has become rare as most of these kidneys involute on their own.

### D. Duplications, Ectopic Ureters, or Ureteroceles

1. Often diagnosed in utero by hydronephrosis of one pole of a kidney (typically the upper pole), ureteral dilation, and/or a classic ureterocele configuration in the bladder.

2. Provided amniotic fluid is normal, no further in utero treatment is needed. Prophylactic antibiotics and postnatal ultrasound and VCUG are appropriate (see Chapter 14 for treatment).

## V. PRENATAL TREATMENT AND MATERNAL COUNSELING

### A. Urinary Tract Obstruction

1. Prenatal intervention is appropriate in only the exceptional urologic case.

2. The most common circumstance is in cases of severe bilateral hydronephrosis with reduced amniotic fluid. In those instances, a careful fetal survey (to rule out other anomalies) and amniocentesis (for chromosome analysis) are essential before consideration of intervention.

3. Analysis of the degree of renal injury is the next step and this is done first by ultrasound. In general, acceptable renal function is associated with normal amniotic fluid; however, when the fluid is reduced other assessments are needed.

4. The amount of renal parenchyma can be assessed easily. More specifically, though, the lack of corticomedullary differentiation and the presence of increased echogenicity and cortical cysts are all associated with renal dysplasia.

5. If the kidneys are acceptable by ultrasound, fetal urine samples are obtained (some feel it is best to drain the bladder 3 days in a row to obtain fresh urine).

6. Although many tests have been proposed, low sodium and low osmolarity (indicative of enough tubular function to reabsorb urine) are associated with salvageable renal function.

7. In these highly selected patients, after counseling of maternal as well as fetal risks, consideration may be given to in utero intervention.

8. Although there are reports of fetal cystoscopic treatment, the accepted intervention is a fetal vesicoamniotic cavity shunt (usually via percutaneous catheter placement). This is done under local anesthesia with maternal sedation and with careful monitoring and medications to reduce the risk of premature delivery. Despite this, many of these infants do deliver early.

9. Long-term results are mixed. There is a clear benefit in preventing pulmonary hypoplasia (and thereby increasing neonatal survival), but it is still unclear whether renal functional improvement is achieved. This brings up the ethical concern that these children may be surviving due to therapy, but doomed to neonatal renal failure with all its attendant problems.

B. **Myelodysplasia**

1. Prenatal diagnosis of this condition is increasing owing to increased use of maternal screening for $\alpha$-fetoprotein.

2. Based on this, prenatal open surgical hysterotomy and fetal myelomeningocele repair is being done in several centers as part of a multiinstitutional study sponsored by the National Institutes of Health.

3. Early results suggest that the rate of ventriculoperitoneal shunting is reduced in these patients, but neurogenic bladder dysfunction is still a problem. However, these results are still too early and too limited to draw firm conclusions.

VI. **SUMMARY**

A. Fetal diagnosis of urologic anomalies is common.

B. Although the benefits are not proven fully, the prevalence of prenatal ultrasound means that many children will be diagnosed.

C. In most instances, parental education should emphasize the excellent prognosis and the need for nonemergent postnatal evaluation.

D. In extremely rare cases, fetal intervention may be warranted.

## RECOMMENDED READING

Coplen DE. Prenatal intervention for hydronephrosis. *J Urol* 1997;157:2270–2277.

Holmes NM, Nguyen HT, Harrson MR, et al. Fetal intervention for myelomeningocele: effect on postnatal bladder function. *J Urol* 2001;166:2383–2386.

Holmes N, Harrison MR, Baskin LS. Fetal surgery for posterior urethral valves: long-term postnatal outcomes. *Pediatrics* 2001;108:E7.

Liang CC, Cheng PJ, Lin CJ, et al. Outcome of prenatally diagnosed fetal hydronephrosis. *J Reprod Med* 2002;47:27–32.

Woodward M, Frank D. Postnatal management of antenatal hydronephrosis. *BJU Int* 2002;89:149–156.

# 13

# Neonatal Hydronephrosis (UPJ Obstruction) and Multicystic Dysplastic Kidneys

Ahmet R. Aslan

**NEONATAL HYDRONEPHROSIS (UPJ OBSTRUCTION)**

**I. DIAGNOSIS**

The diagnosis of neonatal hydronephrosis is most often made based on an incidental finding detected on prenatal ultrasound done for another reason. Occasionally, an infant may be brought to the physician with a flank mass, urinary tract infection, or rarely with hematuria. Older children most often present with intermittent pain and vomiting.

**A. Incidence**

1. The incidence of hydronephrosis varies depending on the cut-off level for renal anteropelvic diameter that is used during prenatal sonographic evaluation.

2. Because of high false-positive rates, pelvic diameters below 10 mm are generally not considered significant.

3. Although the incidence of some renal enlargement on prenatal ultrasound is 1.0% to 1.4%, most of these cases resolve after birth and the incidence of significant urinary tract disease is 0.2% to 0.4%.

**B. Differential Diagnosis of Prenatal Urinary Tract Dilation** (Fig. 13–1)

1. Ureteropelvic junction (UPJ) tract hydronephrosis (UPJ Obstruction) (about two-thirds of cases)

2. Vesicoureteral reflux (about one-fourth of cases)

3. Ureterovesical junction (UVJ) obstruction (will have a dilated ureter)

4. Multicystic dysplastic kidneys (multiple renal cysts that do not connect to each other)

5. Posterior urethral valves (will have a markedly abnormal bladder also)

6. Other diseases like prune-belly syndrome or polycystic kidney disease (rare)

**C. Etiology of UPJ Obstruction** (Fig. 13–2)

1. The exact cause is debatable, but a scarred or adynamic segment of the proximal ureter often leads to a kink at the UPJ that may be responsible for the obstruction.

2. Less common causes are congenital mucosal folds or polyps of the upper ureter or in older children a crossing artery to the lower pole of the kidney. Figure 13–2A compares UPJ type hydronephrosis to ureterovesical junction (UVJ) type hydronephrosis 13–2B.

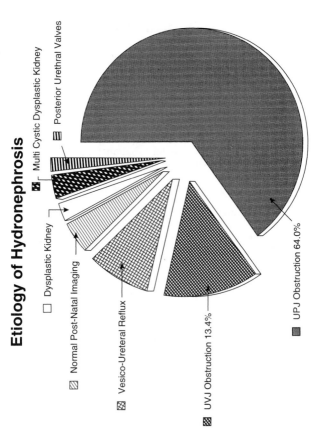

**Fig. 13–1.** Common etiologies of hydronephrosis in children.

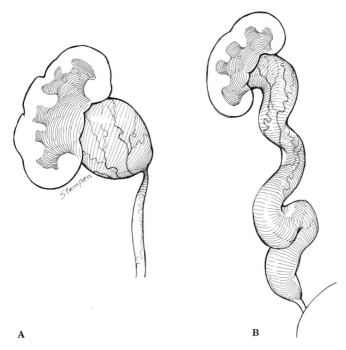

**Fig. 13–2.** Schematic of ureteropelvic junction obstruction (A) as compared to congenital megaureter (B).

## II.  EVALUATION OF NEONATAL HYDRONEPHROSIS
### A.  Ultrasound
1.  Unless there is severe bilateral hydronephrosis, dilated ureter, or dilated posterior urethra on prenatal sonograms, postnatal ultrasound should be postponed until the physiologic dehydration of newborn has resolved (usually after 72 hours). Earlier testing may underestimate the degree of hydration.
2.  The grading system of the Society of Fetal Urology may be used as a guideline to determine the degree of hydronephrosis (Fig. 13–3 and Table 13–1). Another way to define hydronephrosis is to simply measure the greatest dimension of the renal pelvis. As mentioned, renal pelvic diameters greater than 10 mm (grade 2 on the Society of Fetal Urology grading system) should be considered clinically relevant and require further evaluation. Clearly, quantification of the hydronephrosis is dependent on the ultrasound operator and the hydration status of the patient. The status of the urinary bladder can also affect the degree of hydronephrosis (when

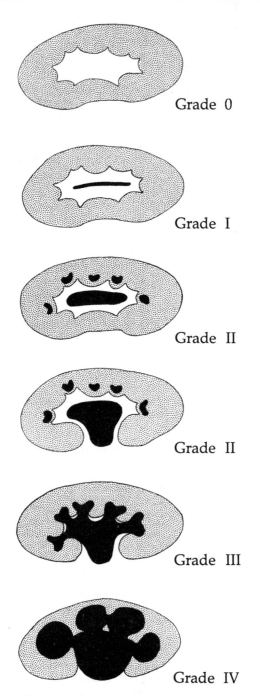

Grade 0

Grade I

Grade II

Grade II

Grade III

Grade IV

Fig. 13–3. Ultrasound grading system of hydronephrosis (see text).

**Table 13–1.   Ultrasound grading system for hydronephrosis**

| Grade of Hydronephrosis | Central Renal Complex | Renal Parenchymal Thickness |
|---|---|---|
| 0 | Intact | Normal |
| 1 | Slight splitting | Normal |
| 2 | Evident splitting Complex confined Within renal border | Normal |
| 3 | Wide-splitting pelvis Dilated outside renal Border and calices Uniformly dilated | Normal |
| 4 | Further dilation of renal pelvis and calices | Thin |

possible, hydronephrosis should be assessed when the bladder is both full and empty.)

**B.   Voiding Cystourethrography** (VCUG)

1. Most clinicians recommend a VCUG in every infant with neonatal hydronephrosis because sonography is not a good predictor of vesicoureteral reflux and 25% to 33% of these children will have reflux.

2. Some will counterargue that this reflux is not clinically significant.

3. We perform a VCUG at 3 to 4 weeks of age and recommend prophylactic antibiotics until the diagnosis of vesicoureteral reflux is ruled out.

**C.   Radionuclide Scanning**

Not all urinary tract dilation is a sign of significant obstruction. Although the size of the renal pelvis is of some value, it is not definitive in most cases. To help distinguish "obstructed" kidneys from those that are merely dilated, the most commonly used test is the diuretic renogram. This test estimates the relative renal function of the two kidneys and gives an estimate of the "washout" of radioisotope from the kidney. This washout correlates with the degree of obstruction (although the size of the renal pelvis and the amount of diuresis are also critical in determining the rapidity of the washout). The test requires hydration and the injection of a radioisotope that is excreted in the urine. The two principle choices are:

1. 99m-technetium-diethylenetriaminepentaacetic acid (DTPA): DTPA is cleared by glomerular filtration and is not reabsorbed or excreted by tubules. Thus, it provides a good measurement of glomerular filtration rate.

2. 99m-Technetium-mercaptoacetyltriglycine (MAG-3): MAG-3 is the first choice in children with poorly

functioning kidneys because it is mostly cleared by tubular excretion. It is also a good indicator of effective renal plasma flow.

It is important to recognize the technique and related pitfalls. After the administration of radiopharmaceutical agent (DTPA or MAG-3) and taking serial images with a gamma camera, the regions of interest (ROI) over both kidneys and the background are defined. The amount of radioisotope excreted in the urine (the number of counts in each ROI) over time is calculated; then the background activity is subtracted from the kidney counts. Furosemide is administrated 20 minutes after renogram (F+20) to develop time–activity washout curves. The rapidity of washout is correlated with the degree of obstruction. Some authors have tried to use the half-time clearance of radioisotope from the collecting system ($t_{1/2}$) as an indicator of obstruction ($t_{1/2}$ of more than 20 minutes, obstructed; $t_{1/2}$ of 10 to 20 minutes, indeterminate; $t_{1/2}$ of less than 10 minutes, nonobstructed), but there are many problems with the calculation as well as its dependence on the anatomy. $t_{1/2}$ should be interpretted with caution. Overall, the technique is affected by the following items:

**a.** The degree of obstruction (severe obstruction may cause in delays in peak renal activity with reduction in renal filtration pressure)

**b.** The compliance of renal pelvis (a highly dilated or compliant pelvis may not respond well to diuretic)

**c.** The dosage and timing of furosemide (F+20 and F-15 have different effects)

**d.** The degree of hydration (dehydration may delay excretion)

**e.** Drainage of the bladder (a full bladder may delay renal washout)

In sum, the data collected in radionuclide scanning must be interpreted depending not only on computer analysis, but also on clinical status of the patient. The test is particularly unreliable before 4–6 weeks of age.

Although not useful in determining the degree of obstruction, DMSA is the most reliable technique to show the relative renal function (it remains bound to proximal tubular cells especially before 1 month of age.)

**III. MANAGEMENT OF UPJ HYDRONEPHROSIS AND OBSTRUCTION IN INFANTS**

**A. Natural History of UPJ Hydronephrosis** (conservative management)

The ultimate goal of therapy is to preserve renal function in these children and, at the same time, to prevent unnecessary surgery. Unfortunately, there are no clearcut methods to predict whether a hydronephrotic kidney will deteriorate or remain unaffected. In fact, the majority of these infants do very well over a long period of time when observed. However, there are some data to provide guidelines.

1. In children with significant hydronephrosis who are observed, there is a need for future surgery in ~25%.
2. Kidneys with renal pelvic diameter of greater than 50 mm have a high likelihood of renal deterioration; hence, early repair seems to be the best choice for this group.
3. Kidneys with renal pelvic diameter of less than 20 mm rarely need intervention and may be followed using serial ultrasounds and, sometimes, diuretic renography.
4. When the hydronephrotic kidney has a relative renal function less than 40% or has a loss of function greater than 10% in serial scans, surgery is generally recommended.
5. In routine follow-up, there should be a high index of suspicion for urinary tract infections, as there are no specific symptoms in this age group. Infections in the face of obstruction may cause rapid renal deterioration. The use of a prophylactic antibiotic is controversial in cases with isolated hydronephrosis without ureteral dilatation or reflux. We generally do not use antibiotics in these cases.
6. Both infections and stone formation are also indications for surgery.

B. **Surgery**
1. Anderson-Hynes dismembered pyeloplasty is the gold standard of techniques used for the repair of UPJ with an overall success rate of more than 95%.
2. Endopyelotomy (either balloon cautery or cold knife) is feasible in older children, but the success rate is only about 80% and it is not routinely used in pediatric population. Also it may be particularly dangerous when an extrinsic obstruction (usually an aberrant vessel) is present.
3. Laparoscopic pyeloplasty is becoming a reasonable alternative to the open surgery in pediatric population. In children, however, the advantages of a shorter hospital stay and faster recovery time are small.

## MULTICYSTIC DYSPLASTIC KIDNEYS (MCDK)

Multicystic dysplastic kidneys are a severe form of renal dysplasia in which the kidney has virtually no function. On ultrasound, there is very thin and abnormal renal parenchyma, surrounded by multiple cysts of various sizes that do not connect, nor do they connect to the renal pelvis.

## I. DIAGNOSIS
Most cases of MCDK are diagnosed incidentally during prenatal sonography. In more unusual cases, it may be

diagnosed after discovery of a palpable or visible abdominal mass in the infants. MCDK must be distinguished from the hydronephrosis caused by UPJ obstruction because the latter may be repairable. The diagnosis may be made by ultrasound with good reliability. The existence of infundibular connections between calyces and the renal pelvis is good evidence of hydronephrosis, instead of MCDK.

II. **EVALUATION**

A. **Renal Scan**

There is an increased incidence of UPJ hydronephrosis and obstruction (3% to 12%) in the contralateral (solitary functional) kidney. A radionuclide scan is also recommended if there is any question of UPJ obstruction in the affected kidney. In hydronephrosis, a rim of functioning parenchyma is seen. In MCDK, there is little or no uptake of radionuclide.

B. **VCUG**

Because there is a high rate of reflux in the contralateral (solitary functioning) kidney (18% to 43%), most clinicians recommend a VCUG.

III. **NATURAL HISTORY**

A. When multicystic kidneys occur bilaterally, this condition is not compatible with life and these children die immediately after birth from pulmonary hypoplasia.

B. Most cases are unilateral and virtually all become smaller over time. When the involution occurs, the cyst fluid disappears and the dysplastic cells may remain in place; however, in most cases the involution is severe enough that there is generally not any identifiable tissue on ultrasound. It is highly likely that involution occurs in most cases, as the condition is extremely rare in adults.

C. Hypertension occurs in rare cases, so the infant's blood pressure should be checked periodically. When hypertension has been reported, nephrectomy has been curative.

D. The presence of dysplastic cells has lead to the theory that these children have an increased risk of malignancy. In fact the development of Wilms tumor in these patients has been reported only once. Removal of a multicystic dysplastic kidney is rarely indicated with the occasional indication of respiratory compromise from a huge multicystic kidney.

IV. **MANAGEMENT**

A. When detected prenatally, unilateral multicystic kidney should be followed relatively unaggressively. Unless it is massive in size, there is no need for any change in the routine treatment prenatally or in the mode of delivery.

B. Postnatally, an ultrasound should be obtained to confirm the diagnosis (and a VCUG to be certain there is no contralateral reflux). Once the diagnosis is confirmed, observation is usually recommended. Most clinicians recommend annual sonography; however, there are no objective data to indicate that this is needed. Indeed, the length of time that a patient with multicystic kidney should be monitored remains unknown. In an era of evidence-based medicine, routine annual ultrasound may be found to be costly and of minimal benefit.

C.  Families should be counseled because the child has a solitary functional kidney. It is generally recommended that they avoid contact sports out of concern for injuring the solitary kidney. On the other hand, injuries sufficient to result in nephrectomy are vanishingly rare in contact sports (see Chapter 28).

## RECOMMENDED READING

Coplen DE. Prenatal intervention for hydronephrosis. *J Urol* 1997;157:2270–2277.

Ouzounian JG, Castro MA, Fresquez M, et al. Prognostic significance of antenatally detected fetal pyelectasis. *Ultrasound Obstet Gynecol* 1996;7:424–428.

Roth JA, Diamond DA. Prenatal hydronephrosis. *Curr Opin Pediatr* 2001;13:138–141.

# Hydroureteronephrosis: Ureteroceles, Duplications, and Ureteral Ectopy

Michael DiSandro

I. **DEFINITIONS**
   A. **Hydronephrosis:** an *anatomic* entity describing an enlargement, or dilation, of any portion of the collecting system of the kidney.
   B. **Pelviectasis:** dilation of the renal pelvis
   C. **Caliectasis:** dilation of the renal calyces
   D. **Pelvocaliectasis:** dilation of both the pelvis and calyces
   E. **Pyelocaliectasis:** equivalent to caliectasis
   F. **Hydroureteronephrosis:** includes dilation of any portion of the collecting system of the kidney, plus dilation of the ureter.
   G. **Ureterectasis:** dilation of the ureter
   H. **Obstruction:** a restriction of urinary outflow. A complete obstruction will lead to renal damage. An incomplete obstruction may be *physiologic* (i.e., normal and not affecting renal function) or *pathologic* (i.e., abnormal and leading to renal injury). Obstruction and hydronephrosis are not synonymous. A patient may have an enlarged renal collecting system but not have a pathologic obstruction.

II. **INCIDENCE**
   Hydronephrosis is present in up to 1.4% of fetuses, and persists postnatally in half (0.7%).

III. **SIGNIFICANCE**
   One must distinguish whether the hydronephrosis is secondary to an ongoing obstruction (in which case there may be progressive renal deterioration) or secondary to a prior obstructive event that both occurred and resolved antenatally (in which case there will be no further renal damage). In the former, if the obstruction is severe, surgical treatment to correct the obstruction may be necessary to preserve renal function; in the latter, surgical treatment is unnecessary.

IV. **ETIOLOGY**
   A. Before one can debate whether the child with hydronephrosis needs surgical treatment, one must first determine the etiology of the hydronephrosis. Sometimes the etiology is straightforward (e.g., posterior urethral valves, ureteroceles) and thus the treatment options are clear (relieve the obstruction). In most cases, however, the hydronephrosis is secondary to a ureteropelvic (64%) or ureterovesical (13%) junction

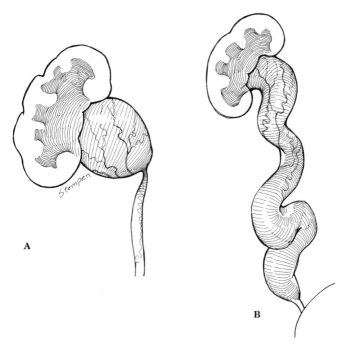

**Fig. 14–1.  UPJ obstruction (A) as compared to congenital megaureter (B).**

obstruction. In such cases, the treatment options are less clear. Many of these patients are not truly pathologically obstructed, and surgical intervention is not warranted or necessary.

**B.** Vesicoureteral reflux and posterior urethral valves are discussed in Chapters 7 and 15, and therefore will not be included here.

**A.  Ureteropelvic Junction (UPJ) Obstruction**

    **1.**  Incidence: The UPJ is the most common site of obstruction in the upper urinary tract (Fig. 14–1). Approximately 64% of the 0.7% of children born with hydronephrosis will have a UPJ obstruction.

    **2.**  Pathophysiology

        **a.**  Successful conduction of urine from the renal pelvis to the ureter requires an anatomically patent UPJ as well as an undisturbed transmission of peristaltic contractions in the proximal ureter. Thus, UPJ obstruction can result from an anatomic abnormality, or from poor conduction of peristalsis (Fig. 14–1A). The abnormality can be either *extrinsic* or *intrinsic*.

     **b.** Intrinsic obstruction secondary to a narrow segment with muscular discontinuity is the most common cause.

     **c.** Extrinsic causes include aberrant vessels, kinks, or a high insertion of the ureter into the pelvis.

     **d.** There may also be a combination of intrinsic and extrinsic obstruction—for example, an intrinsic ureteral obstruction leading to a dilated pelvis, which then results in a kink in the ureter (extrinsic).

**3. Clinical Presentation**

     **a.** Infants: Most cases of UPJ obstruction are diagnosed in utero. If not noted in utero, infants present with abdominal mass, hematuria, urinary tract infection, or gastrointestinal discomfort. Of all abdominal masses in infants younger than 1 year of age, 50% are renal in origin and 40% of these are secondary to a UPJ obstruction.

     **b.** Older children: Older children present with abdominal or flank pain, chronic nausea, hematuria following mild trauma, or urinary tract infection. Younger children tend to have more generalized lower abdominal pain, and older children will have more conventional flank pain. The flank pain may worsen with diuresis (e.g., after ingesting caffeinated beverages). Any child with gross hematuria after minor trauma should be evaluated for a UPJ, as should any boy with a frank urinary tract infection.

**4.** Associated anomalies: Patients with imperforate anus, contralateral multicystic kidney disease, congenital heart disease, VATER syndrome, or esophageal atresia should be screened with a renal ultrasound to rule out hydronephrosis. Also, 10% of patients with UPJ obstruction have ipsilateral ureterovesical reflux.

**5.** Workup

     **a.** Hydronephrosis discovered antenatally

          **(1)** Postnatal ultrasound: If hydronephrosis (defined as a renal pelvic diameter of greater than 7 to 10 mm, caliectasis, or ureter dilation) is discovered in utero, a follow-up renal and bladder ultrasound should be performed at 3 to 7 days of age (after normal physiologic diuresis has begun), unless the in utero hydronephrosis is massive or bilateral, in which case the ultrasound should be performed as soon as possible after birth. If the postnatal ultrasound shows dilation of the collecting system, then a voiding cystourethrogram (VCUG) and renal scan should be obtained (see below). If there is no hydronephrosis on postnatal ultrasound, there is no need for further ultrasound studies. However, a VCUG should still be performed to rule out reflux (33% of cases).

**(2)** VCUG: A urinary catheter must be inserted for this procedure, and the patient must void. The main role of the VCUG is to rule out vesicoureteral reflux, and in boys to evaluate the posterior urethra. It should be performed in every child with a suspected UPJ obstruction.

**(3)** Diuretic renography: Diuretic renography is a functional study that has the ability to diagnose UPJ obstruction, and to assess differential renal function (see also Chapter 13). The radiopharmaceutical used is MAG 3, so the test is commonly referred to as a *MAG 3 Lasix Renogram.* The MAG 3 Lasix Renogram can distinguish total and individual renal function as well as determine the drainage time of the radioisotope from the renal pelvis. In the newborn, if the hydronephrosis is unilateral and not severe, then the test should be performed at 1 month of age for the most meaningful results. If the hydronephrosis is bilateral or unilateral and severe, then the test should be performed after the infant is 3 days old. A bladder catheter should be inserted for the test.

**(a)** Interpretation of results: The washout curve gives an indication of the extent of obstruction, if present (Fig. 14–2). In the dilated system, if the washout time is rapid ($t_{1/2}$ less than 15 minutes) after diuretic is given, the patients are said to have a *dilated non-obstructed system.* If the washout time is delayed ($t_{1/2}$ is longer than 20 minutes), then the patients have an *obstructed pattern.* If the washout time ($t_{1/2}$) is between 15 and 20 minutes, then the study is *indeterminate.*

**(b)** Differential renal function is also important. If one kidney shows an obstructed pattern, and the relative renal function of that kidney is less than 40% of overall renal function, then the patient is thought to have a pathologic UPJ obstruction and is therefore at high risk for further renal deterioration.

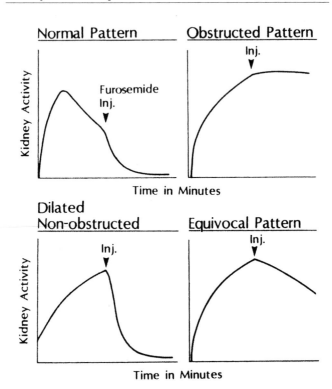

Fig. 14–2. **Obstructed versus nonobstructed washout curves on diuretic renography.**

  **(4)** Intravenous urogram (IVU): In the infant, the usefulness of IVU is less clear. The combination of renal ultrasound and diuretic renography is performed on almost all children with suspected UPJ, and the IVU rarely reveals any additional useful information. If performed, the child must be at least 2 to 4 weeks of age. Dilation of the renal pelvis, caliectasis, delayed excretion of contrast, and nonvisualization of the ipsilateral ureter are hallmarks of obstruction.

 **b.** In older children

  **(1)** Ultrasound: Although an ultrasound should be performed as a screening test for an older child with a suspected UPJ obstruction, it may not always show hydronephrosis. If it does not show hydronephrosis, it should be repeated when the patient is experiencing pain. If the ultrasound is done during an episode of pain, it will almost always show hydronephrosis if a UPJ obstruction is present.

**(2)** Diuretic renography: A MAG 3 Lasix Renogram is performed if the ultrasound shows hydronephrosis. Like the ultrasound, the renogram should be performed during an episode of pain. Refer to the section above regarding interpretation of results.

**(3)** VCUG: As in infants, a VCUG must be performed to rule out reflux in all children with a suspected UPJ obstruction.

**(4)** IVU: An IVU is also a good initial study for the older child with intermittent flank pain. Ideally, the study should be performed during an acute attack of pain. If the study shows the hallmarks of a UPJ obstruction, then obstruction is almost certainly present, especially if there is increased hydronephrosis when compared to an IVU or ultrasound when there is no pain.

**(5)** CT scan: With the ubiquitous use of CT scans in the emergency room setting UPJ obstruction may be diagnosed in the workup for acute abdominal pain. A follow-up sonogram or diuretic renogram may be near normal once the pain/obstruction has resolved.

**6.** Treatment

  **a.** Natural History and Patient Selection

   **(1)** Symptomatic: An older child with a UPJ obstruction may have *intermittent abdominal or flank pain,* at times associated with nausea and vomiting. Younger children tend to have more generalized lower abdominal pain, and older children will have more conventional flank pain. The pain may worsen during a brisk diuresis (after caffeine or alcohol intake). MAG 3 Lasix Renogram is the cornerstone of diagnosis in this group of patients. If the pain is intermittent, the renogram should be performed during an attack of pain. If the renogram reveals the hallmarks of a UPJ obstruction, then surgery is indicated to relieve the obstruction and consequently the pain.

   Patients with a UPJ obstruction may also present with *pyelonephritis.* These patients are initially treated with antibiotics, and surgical repair of the obstruction is performed once the infection has resolved. If the pyelonephritis is acute and unresponsive to antibiotic treatment, percutaneous pyelostomy tube placement should be performed to temporarily relieve the obstruction until the infection has resolved and pyeloplasty can be performed.

In some cases, *kidney stones* may develop in the obstructed pelvis. In this situation, whether symptomatic or not, pyelolithotomy should be performed at the same time as pyeloplasty.

In all cases, a follow-up renal ultrasound is obtained approximately 4 to 6 weeks postoperatively. If the ultrasound shows improved hydronephrosis, then a renogram is performed 3 to 6 months after surgery. Most patients (up to 95%) will have a definite improvement in the renogram and resolution of their symptoms after surgery.

(2) Asymptomatic: The asymptomatic child with an incidental UPJ obstruction poses somewhat of a management dilemma. On the one hand, some patients with an apparent UPJ obstruction experience complete recovery without surgical intervention (a physiologic obstruction), whereas others deteriorate to the point of significantly reduced renal function (a pathologic obstruction). Obviously, surgery to relieve the obstruction is necessary only in the latter group. Unfortunately, no diagnostic test alone can reliably predict which kidneys will improve and which will not. However, using the current tests available, observation and treatment protocols have been developed which minimize both the amount of unnecessary operations performed and the number of patients who will suffer renal deterioration. These are general guidelines, and each patient's renal scan, ultrasound, and overall condition should be carefully assessed prior to making any decisions.

(a) Observe if there is significant hydronephrosis on ultrasound, yet renal scan reveals greater than 40% of function from the obstructed kidney, even if the washout is delayed.

(b) Operate if there is significant hydronephrosis on ultrasound, and the renal scan reveals less than 40% of function from the obstructed kidney, especially if the washout is delayed.

**b.** Observation protocol: Yearly renal ultrasound and diuretic renogram until certain the obstructed kidney's function is stabilized. Prophylactic antibiotics are appropriate for infants until they reach 1 year of age. The ultrasound and renogram may be performed more frequently if the patient's renal function is borderline or significant hydronephrosis is present.

**c.** Surgery: The success rates for open dismembered pyeloplasty are 90% to 95%, even in neonates. Follow-up ultrasound is obtained approximately 4 to 6 weeks postoperatively. If the ultrasound shows improvement in the hydronephrosis, then the patient can be followed safely with ultrasound at increasing intervals (initially each year, then every 2 to 3 years). If the postoperative sonogram has not improved then a follow-up Lasix renogram is indicated to rule out continued obstruction. A second ultrasound and renogram are obtained approximately 3 months later. Minimally invasive procedures such as percutaneous and retrograde endopyelotomy and laparoscopic pyeloplasty can also be performed in children. Although these procedures are now well established in the adult, they remain experimental in most children. Select teenagers may be good candidates for laparoscopic pyeloplasty in centers of excellence, and thus laparoscopic surgery should be discussed with the parents of teenagers.

**B. Other Causes of Hydronephrosis**

**1.** Congenital megaureter

**a.** Definition: The presence of an enlarged ureter (more than 7 mm in diameter) with or without concomitant dilation of the upper collecting system (Fig. 14–1B).

**b.** Types

**(1)** Nonrefluxing, obstructed

**(2)** Refluxing, nonobstructed

**(3)** Refluxing, obstructed

**(4)** Nonrefluxing, nonobstructed

**c.** Pathology: The nonrefluxing, obstructed megaureter is thought to be caused by an abnormality in the distal ureteral muscle, which causes an aperistaltic segment. This leads to a partial obstruction that may or may not be significant. In some cases, the ureterovesical tunnel will be abnormal as well, and urine will reflux up the ureter but be unable to come back down (refluxing, obstructed). In other cases, the urine will reflux and drain freely (refluxing, nonobstructed; see Chapter 7). Interestingly, some patients will have neither reflux nor obstruction identified, yet have persistent ureteral dilation (nonrefluxing, nonobstructed).

**d.** Presentation: Megaureter accounts for approximately 20% of cases of hydronephrosis in the newborn, second only to UPJ obstruction as the most common cause of hydronephrosis in the newborn. Most cases are secondary to the refluxing, nonobstructed type (see Chapter 7). The condition is mainly found incidentally on prenatal sonography, and typically the physical examination is normal, as is the urinalysis and serum creatinine. If the condition is not discovered early with prenatal sonography, patients mainly present later in life with a urinary tract infection, hematuria, abdominal pain or mass, or uremia. It is important to determine the etiology of the megaureter once discovered because many will require treatment.

**e.** Evaluation: The main goal is to determine which patients are obstructed, which have reflux, and which have both. Even the patients with neither obstruction nor reflux need to be identified because they must be followed carefully. Obviously the treatment options will be much different depending on the final diagnosis. The patient must have an ultrasound confirming a dilated ureter (greater than 7 mm in diameter). A VCUG must then be performed to rule out reflux and to be certain there is no evidence of urethral obstruction. If there is reflux, and it is severe in grade and drains poorly, *refluxing obstructed* megaureter must be considered. If there is no reflux, then the patient either has *nonrefluxing obstructed* or *nonrefluxing nonobstructed* megaureter. A diuretic renogram is then obtained to help distinguish between the two.

**f.** Management: The management of primary refluxing megaureter is discussed in Chapter 7. Management of obstructed and nonobstructed megaureters is discussed below; the two are distinguished mainly on the basis on symptomatology.

   **(1)** If symptomatic: The presenting signs and symptoms are usually the most important determinants as to whether surgical correction is necessary. If the child presents with recurrent urinary tract infections, pyelonephritis, persistent flank pain, or hematuria, and a megaureter is discovered, then surgical correction is warranted.

(2) If asymptomatic: If the megaureter is discovered incidentally, and the patient has no symptoms, then nonoperative treatment is warranted. This consists of regimented surveillance with annual ultrasound and diuretic renography. If the megaureter remains stable, and there is no decrease in renal function, then surveillance may end after 2 to 4 years. These patients are considered to have a *nonobstructed* system, and there is a rather high spontaneous resolution rate in this group of patients. If there is increasing hydronephrosis on ultrasound, or decreasing renal function on the affected side, or if any of the above symptoms develop, then surgery is warranted. These patients have an *obstructed* system. Because of the high risk of infection, all children should be placed on prophylactic antibiotics while on surveillance.

**g.** Surgery: If necessary, the *primary obstructed megaureter* can be treated surgically by excision of the distal obstructed segment, tapering of the dilated ureter and reimplantation into the bladder by a reflux prevention technique. The success rate approaches 97%, even in small infants. However, the success rate decreases substantially if this procedure is performed on the other types of megaureter, thus, proper evaluation is essential. Postoperatively, renal ultrasound and diuretic renogram should be performed every 6 months to 1 year. The drainage may remain delayed for up to 1 year postoperatively, therefore, renal function is paramount. If renal function decreases and the drainage remains delayed postoperatively, there should be suspicion of obstruction. A VCUG should be performed 6 months following surgery to rule out reflux.

**2.** Ureteroceles

**a.** Definition: A cystic dilatation of the terminal intravesical segment of the ureter (Fig. 14–3).

**b.** Incidence: On autopsy, 1 in 500 cases. They occur 4 to 7 times more frequently in women and are more common in white patients. Ureteroceles are bilateral in 10% of cases. Eighty percent are associated with the upper pole of a duplex system, and 60% have an orifice located ectopically in the urethra.

**c.** Classification: Ureteroceles are classified as being either *intravesical* (Fig. 14–3A) (within the bladder) or *ectopic* (Fig. 14–3B) (some

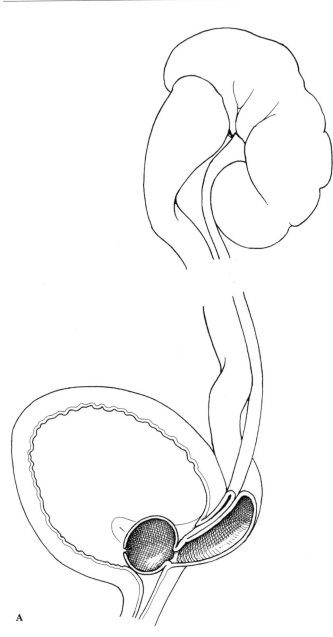

A

**Fig. 14–3.** Intravesical (A) versus ectopic (B) ureterocele.

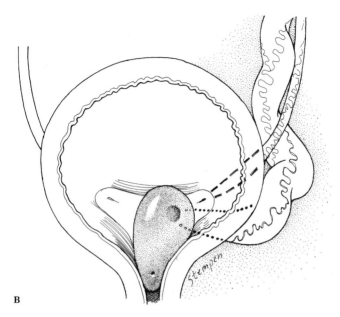

**B**

**Fig. 14–3.** (*Continued*)

portion extends beyond the bladder neck). Other terms commonly encountered include *stenotic* (intravesical with a small orifice), *sphincteric* (ectopic with the orifice within the urethral sphincter), *sphincterostenotic* (same as sphincteric with a stenotic orifice), and *cecoureterocele* (some part extends beyond the bladder neck, but the orifice is in the bladder).

  **d.** Presentation: The most common presentation is urinary tract infection in the first few months of life. Some are detected incidentally on antenatal ultrasonography. Some patients may have a palpable abdominal mass secondary to an obstructed kidney. Although urethral obstruction is rare, the most common cause of urethral obstruction in girls is urethral prolapse of a ureterocele.

  **e.** Workup

    **(1)** Abdominal ultrasound should be performed first. This will usually reveal a well-defined cystic intravesical mass in the posterior portion of the bladder. A dilated proximal ureter may also be seen. There will most often be a duplex kidney on the ipsilateral side, and the upper pole may be dysplastic.

(2) Renal scan is used to determine the relative function of all the renal segments, and the washout time as well.

(3) IVU is not mandatory, but if performed will reveal a negative shadow of the ureterocele within the bladder, a drooping lily sign in the kidney (downward displaced lower pole), a lower pole collecting system with missing upper pole infundibulum and a laterally displaced lower pole ureter that loops around the dilated upper ureter in the pelvis.

(4) VCUG must be performed in all patients. Up to 50% of the ipsilateral lower pole and 25% of the contralateral renal units will have vesicoureteral reflux. Also, the ureterocele can usually be seen as a round filling defect within the bladder on the initial filling films.

(5) Cystoscopic findings are variable. The ureterocele is usually seen best when the bladder is empty and the flank is being compressed. When the bladder is full, the ureterocele may become completely decompressed, or it may appear as a bladder diverticulum if there is poor bladder wall backing. In a duplicated system, the upper pole ureter will be associated with the ureterocele, and the lower pole ureter will be seen above and lateral to the ureterocele, if it can be seen at all.

**f.** Treatment: The type of treatment depends on the type of ureterocele and the mode of presentation. Most patients require surgery, which ranges from endoscopic puncture to complete open reconstruction. If the patient presents with sepsis secondary to obstruction, then immediate drainage of the kidney is necessary. Often, endoscopic puncture of the ureterocele is the first step. This is a definitive procedure in 90% of the cases of intravesical ureterocele, and 50% of ectopic ureteroceles. If endoscopic puncture fails, then open reconstruction needs to be performed. If there is no function in the upper pole moiety, then upper pole nephrectomy is performed, usually laparoscopically.

**3.** Ectopic ureters

**a.** Definition: When the ureteral orifice lies in a position caudal to the normal insertion of the ureter on the trigone, the ureter is said to be *ectopic* (Fig. 14–4).

**b.** Location of the orifice: The ectopic orifice is always along the pathway of normal development of the mesonephric system. Thus,

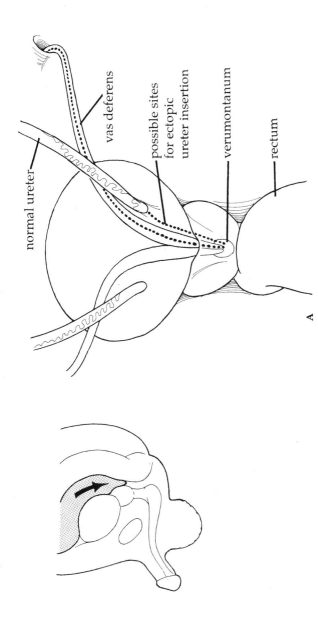

**Fig. 14-4.   Potential sites of an ectopic ureteral orifice. A: Male.**

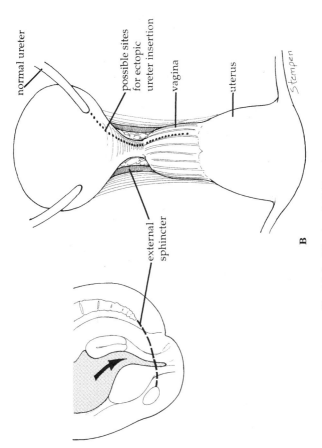

**Fig. 14-4.** (Continued) **B: Female.**

in boys, the orifice may lie in the bladder neck, prostate (to the level of the ejaculatory duct orifice), or even along the course of the male genital system, including the epididymis (Fig. 14–4A). In girls, the orifice may lie in the bladder neck, urethra, vagina, or rarely in the cervix and uterus (Fig. 14–4B).

c. Incidence: Ectopic ureters are much more common among girls than boys (ratio of 6 to 1). Approximately 70% of ectopic ureters are associated with complete ureteral duplication. Boys are more likely than girls to have single-system ectopia. There is a high incidence of associated renal parenchymal dysplasia in the segment drained by the ectopic ureter. Also, the incidence of contralateral duplication is as high as 80%.

d. Presentation

(1) In boys: Usually discovered during an evaluation for urinary tract infections. Epididymoorchitis is possible if the ureter enters the genital ducts. Boys never present with incontinence because the ectopic ureter is always cephalad to the external urethral sphincter (Fig. 14–4A). Boys may also present with prenatal hydronephrosis on ultrasound if the ureteral orifice is obstructed (e.g., lies within the epididymis).

(2) In girls: In infancy, girls usually present with urinary tract infection. However, older girls tend to present with incontinence. This is usually described by the parent as the child always being wet even though she has normal voiding habits, or the patient becoming more wet when sitting on the parent's lap (urine pooling in the dilated ureter or vagina). Some patients may present with pyonephrosis if the ureter is extraurethral and the kidney dysplastic. Girls may also present with prenatal hydronephrosis on ultrasound if the ureteral orifice is obstructed (e.g., lies within the sphincter).

e. Workup

(1) Abdominal ultrasound should be the initial screening test. The ureter is most often dilated down to its abnormally low position. It may be followed proximally to a dysplastic or normal upper segment moiety of a duplex system. In single-system ectopia, the kidney may be dysplastic and difficult to visualize.

(2) Computed tomography (CT) or magnetic resonance imaging (MRI) of the abdomen

and pelvis with contrast is helpful if the ureter is not dilated (e.g., in older girls where the ureter drains into the vagina). The CT or MRI scan can usually pinpoint the location of the ectopic ureter.

(3) IVU is not usually necessary because the CT scan usually provides the best information, but it can be helpful if the involved segment of renal tissue functions sufficiently to excrete contrast material. Findings usually include a dilated upper segment with a functioning lower segment displaced inferiorly and laterally. If the upper segment is nonfunctioning, the diagnosis is more difficult. There may be a large, nonvisualized ureter to the upper segment that causes the lower pole ureter to be displaced and tortuous. This can usually be seen better on ultrasound.

(4) VCUG should be part of the evaluation for a suspected ectopic ureter. Reflux may occur into the abnormally positioned upper segment of a duplicated system.

(5) Dye tests can be used if the above imaging studies fail to establish the diagnosis. The bladder is filled with dye, and a cotton ball is inserted into the vagina. The patient then ambulates and the cotton ball is checked for dye.

(6) Diuretic renography is important to assess renal function, the moiety associated with the ectopic ureter.

(7) Cystoscopy usually does not make the diagnosis alone but can be helpful in identifying the ureteral orifice within the urethra. If the orifice is within the vagina, it is very difficult to localize on cystoscopy.

f. Management

(1) Ectopic ureter in a duplex system: Because most cases are associated with a dysplastic upper pole renal segment, excision of this segment along with the proximal ureter is usually curative. In select case this surgery can be performed laparoscopically.

(2) Ectopic ureter in a single system: In girls, the kidney associated with the ectopic ureter is usually small and poorly functional. A hemitrigone is present in the bladder. If the kidney is functional, the treatment is resection of the distal ectopic ureter and reimplantation. Otherwise nephroureterectomy is performed, either open or laparoscopically.

## RECOMMENDED READING

Coplen DE. Management of the neonatal ureterocele. *Curr Urol Rep* 2001;2:102.

DiSandro MJ, Kogan BA. Neonatal management. Role for early intervention. *Urol Clin North Am* 1998;25:187.

King LR. Management of neonatal ureteropelvic junction obstruction. *Curr Urol Rep* 2001;2:106.

Noe HN. The wide ureter. In: Gillenwater JY, ed. *Adult and pediatric urology,* 4th ed. Philadelphia: Lippincott Williams and Wilkins; 48:2002.

Schlussel RN, Retik AB. Ectopic ureter, ureterocele, and other anomalies of the ureter. In: Campbell MF, ed. *Campbell's urology,* 8th ed. Philadelphia: WB Saunders; 2003:58.

# Posterior Urethral Valves

## Michele B. Ebbers

Posterior urethral valves are the most common congenital cause of bladder outlet obstruction, resulting in a spectrum of damage to the entire urinary tract. Valves are obstructing membranes within the lumen of the urethra, extending from the verumontanum distally. They occur only in boys (Fig. 15–1). They are, in fact, the number one congenital cause of renal failure and renal transplantation in the pediatric population.

I. **Epidemiology**
   A. The incidence of posterior urethral valves has been estimated to be approximately 1 per 5,000 to 8,000 male infants, although some recent studies report it as commonly as 1 in 1,250 fetal ultrasounds.
   B. There does not appear to be any known ethnic or familial predisposition toward the development of valves.

II. **CLINICAL PRESENTATION**
   The presentations of patients with valves display a wide clinical spectrum depending on the degree of in utero obstruction. Patients may present prenatally or postnatally.
   A. **Prenatal Presentation**
      Modern application of prenatal ultrasound examination is responsible for the detection of the majority of posterior urethral valves cases.
      1. Prenatal ultrasound features
         a. Distended, thick-walled fetal bladder
         b. Hydronephrosis: This can be due to bladder outlet obstruction and/or the presence of vesicoureteral reflux.
         c. Oligohydramnios: An assessment of the amniotic fluid volume is an important prognostic indicator. Because most of the amniotic fluid volume depends on fetal urine production after 16 weeks, oligohydramnios is an indication of either poor fetal renal function or bilaterally obstructed kidneys. Severe oligohydramnios predisposes the infant to Potter syndrome and pulmonary hypoplasia. The timing and degree of oligohydramnios plays an important role in the severity of postnatal outcomes.
      2. Prenatal intervention
         a. Prenatal diagnosis of posterior urethral valves has allowed pediatricians and pediatric urologists an opportunity to plan for and initiate treatment immediately after birth.
         b. Although some authors had expressed initial enthusiasm with in utero treatment of valves by the placement of a vesicoamniotic shunt or

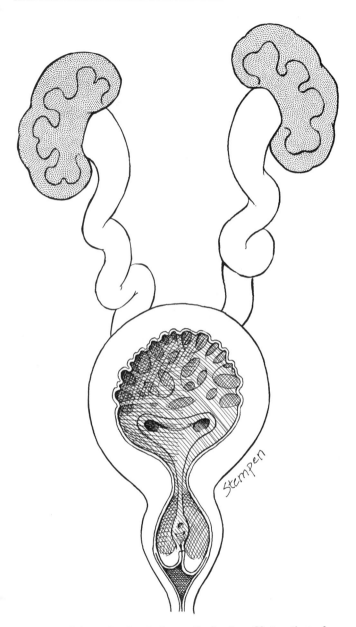

**Fig. 15–1.** Schematic of posterior urethral valves. Obstructing valve is seen in the dilated posterior urethra at the bottom of the diagram. Note thickened bladder and bilateral hydroureteronephrosis.

fetal open surgery, there is now little evidence to suggest a favorable risk to benefit ratio in terms of the preservation of renal or bladder function.

c. Similarly, early delivery has failed to show significant benefit.

**B. Postnatal Diagnosis**

Postnatal diagnosis may occur either immediately postnatally or may be delayed several years, owing to the wide spectrum of the disease and its manifestations.

1. Respiratory distress: Infants with severe oligohydramnios usually present immediately postnatally because of the consequences of life-threatening pulmonary hypoplasia.

2. Sepsis and azotemia: The most severely affected infants may also present in the neonatal period with fulminate sepsis and azotemia, due to longstanding obstruction and renal dysplasia.

3. Abdominal distention: In the neonatal period, the presence of valves is suggested by the finding of a palpable distended bladder. The presence of urinary ascites or markedly distended upper tracts can also result in a tensely distended abdomen.

4. Voiding dysfunction: Some neonates may have difficulty in generating a normal urinary stream or fail to void during the first 48 hours of life. In rare cases, less severely affected patients may present during early childhood with incontinence or recurrent infections. Abnormalities in voiding dynamics and bladder compliance are responsible for the persistence of what is commonly called the *valve bladder syndrome*, a condition manifested by a spectrum of bladder and renal dysfunction.

**III. INITIAL MANAGEMENT OF POSTERIOR URETHRAL VALVES**

Once the diagnosis of posterior urethral valves is suspected, the first step in the management often consists of the stabilization of acute illness (Fig. 15–2). The patient should be medically stabilized as much as possible before proceeding with urologic evaluation and treatment.

A. Acute illnesses associated with posterior urethral valves

1. Respiratory distress
2. Sepsis
3. Dehydration
4. Electrolyte abnormalities

B. Immediate urologic relief can usually be accomplished with temporary drainage of the urinary tract accomplished by placement of a pediatric feeding tube per urethra into the bladder. Foley catheters should not be used in these infants because the balloon can cause significant bladder spasms and obstruction of the ureteral orifices. If the urethra is difficult to catheterize secondary to a dilated posterior urethra, the clinician

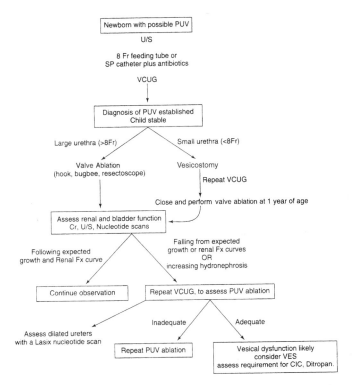

**Fig. 15–2.** **Treatment algorithm for patients with posterior urethral valves.**

should attempt to pass a Coude catheter, which may more easily negotiate the high bladder neck.

C. Radiologic evaluation of valves

Until an assessment of vesicoureteral reflux can be performed, the neonate should be kept on prophylactic antibiotics.

1. Voiding cystourethrogram (VCUG): The diagnosis of posterior urethral valves cannot be made reliably by cystoscopy. The VCUG is considered the gold standard examination used in the diagnosis of posterior urethral valves. Characteristic findings on VCUG include the following:

a. A dilated, thick-walled, trabeculated bladder, *and*

b. An elongated, dilated prostatic urethra with a relatively narrow bladder neck, *and*

c. It may be possible to visualize the billowing folds of the valves as filling defects emanating from the verumontanum within the prostatic urethra.

2. Associated anomalies: The VCUG also allows identification of the numerous anomalies commonly associated with valves.

   a. Vesicoureteral reflux: reflux has been noted in approximately one-third to one-half of patients with valves.

   b. Valves unilateral reflux and renal dysplasia (VURD) syndrome: denotes massive unilateral reflux into a nonfunctioning dysplastic renal unit.

   c. Manifestations of elevated intravesical pressure

      (1) Bladder diverticula

      (2) Poor bladder compliance (high pressure/trabeculated bladder)

      (3) Renal forniceal rupture, resulting in urinary ascites

   d. Pseudoresidual: Often posterior urethral valve patients have capacious upper tracts (either due to vesicoureteral reflux or high urine flow) that hold significant amounts of urine. This urine will fill the bladder after the patient voids, thereby giving the appearance of having a postvoid residual despite complete emptying.

D. Surgical relief of obstruction: Once the diagnosis of posterior urethral valves has been established with a VCUG and all acute medical issues have been stabilized, definitive relief of the obstructing valves should be performed.

   1. Primary valve ablation: In this technique, a pediatric cystoscope is carefully passed into the infant's urethra and the obstructing valves are visually identified and ablated using either a single wire or small electrode, thus relieving the obstruction. This approach is advocated by most pediatric urologists as the preferred treatment of valves in full-term, normal-sized infants.

   2. Cutaneous vesicostomy and delayed valve ablation: Occasionally, a premature infant presents with posterior urethral valves, and because of the small caliber of the urethra, endoscopic manipulation should be avoided. A vesicostomy is performed in these infants by creating an incontinent stoma from the dome of the bladder to the abdominal wall. This allows the urine to drain freely into the infant's diaper when the bladder pressure increases. When the infant has grown enough to allow a pediatric cystoscope to pass into his urethra, endoscopic valve ablation can be performed without excessive urethral trauma. Alternatively, valve ablation can be performed from an antegrade approach through the vesicostomy. To prevent urethral stricture and to maximize bladder potential with cycling, the

vesicostomy should be closed at the time of valve ablation.

3. Temporizing upper tract diversion: Following adequate valve ablation or vesicostomy, the dilated bladder and ureters may continue to demonstrate poor peristalsis and emptying, thus predisposing the infant to urinary stasis, infection, and worsening renal function. Worsening sepsis or azotemia may be indications of poor drainage of the upper urinary tract. In these instances, some authors advocate temporary drainage of the upper urinary tract by performing high-loop cutaneous ureterostomy. It has been argued that upper tract diversion prevents normal cycling of the bladder, which may contribute to future voiding dysfunction. Furthermore, these infants generally have significant renal disease, requiring peritoneal dialysis and early transplantation. Most have severe reflux and closing the ureterostomies and reconstructing these patients prior to transplantation is a major challenge, therefore upper tract diversion should be undertaken only with careful consideration. Alternatively, temporary drainage can also be accomplished with bilateral nephrostomy tubes, which can be easily removed if there is not immediate improvement. Currently, there is no clear-cut evidence that upper tract diversions improve long-term outcomes.

## IV. LONG-TERM MANAGEMENT OF POSTERIOR URETHRAL VALVES

Many valve patients will continue to have residual effects from bladder outlet obstruction even following definitive valve ablation. The various manifestations of bladder dysfunction together make up what is commonly referred to as the *valve bladder syndrome*. It has been estimated that up to one-third of all valve patients will have significant lower urinary tract dysfunction most commonly manifested by urinary incontinence. In a small but significant number of patients, bladder dysfunction may be so severe as to lead to further deterioration of renal function. Valve patients may also have progressively poor renal concentrating ability, leading to obligatory polyuria, that, in turn, worsens the incontinence.

### A. Desired Goals in Bladder Management

1. Preservation of renal function: Serum creatinine and renal bladder ultrasound should be followed regularly.

2. Compliant low-pressure storage of urine: Urodynamic studies should be performed in patients who are failing clinically (either elevated renal function, infection, increased hydronephrosis on ultrasound, or incontinence). If needed, anticholinergic medications and/or clean intermittent catheterization may be used to improve bladder function.

3. Avoidance of infection: Vigilant investigation of fever, flank pain, or change in voiding habits is required. Some patients may require prophylactic antibiotics, especially in cases of vesicoureteral reflux.
4. Socially acceptable urinary continence: This can usually be accomplished by timed voiding habits, and may need to be supplemented with clean intermittent catheterization and less often with surgery.

**B. Radiologic Follow-up**
1. Patients should be followed with serial ultrasounds to document appropriate renal growth and hydronephrosis.
2. All patients are recommended to have a follow-up VCUG 2 months after definitive valve ablation to ensure that there is no residual urethral obstruction.
3. In addition, all patients with vesicoureteral reflux must be maintained on prophylactic antibiotics and followed with as needed with VCUG exams until they demonstrate resolution of reflux.
4. Approximately one-third of patients who initially present with reflux will have spontaneous resolution of their reflux after relief of obstruction.
5. Another one-third can be safely maintained on chemoprophylaxis to allow for the ureters to decrease in caliber over time.
6. The last one-third of patients will have repeated complications of reflux (infection, decreased renal growth, renal function deterioration), and require more aggressive intervention, including in some cases reimplantation.

**C. Urodynamic Evaluation**
1. It is of critical importance to precisely define the nature of lower tract dysfunction by performing urodynamic evaluation in all valve patients who are not doing well clinically.
2. Long-term management of valve patients depends on the type of bladder dysfunction exhibited on urodynamic evaluation.

**D. Medical Management**
1. Timed voiding: Poorly emptying bladders can be treated with a regimen of frequent timed voiding to reduce urinary residual and stasis.
2. Anticholinergic medications may be instituted to treat those patients who manifest low-capacity, hyperreflexic bladders on urodynamic evaluation. Close monitoring of urine output and postvoid residual are necessary for those on anticholinergics to avoid urinary retention as these patients may be exquisitely sensitive to anticholinergic medications. If retention is suspected, the patient should be treated with clean intermittent catheterization as necessary to maintain low-pressure storage of urine.

3. Clean intermittent catheterization may be necessary to ensure complete emptying.

4. Nighttime drainage: Because of high urine output, some patients will need to use an indwelling catheter at night to allow for maximum, continuous low-pressure drainage during sleep.

5. Antibiotic prophylaxis: The persistence of vesicoureteral reflux should be treated with antibiotic prophylaxis. The decision to correct vesicoureteral reflux surgically should be considered carefully secondary to the high complication rate in these patients. If high-pressure bladders are not treated concurrently, recurrence of reflux after surgery is likely.

6. Treatment of renal insufficiency: Some children with posterior urethral valves continue to have deterioration of renal function resulting in chronic renal insufficiency. This can lead to a variety of metabolic abnormalities and growth retardation.

   a. Polyuria: Progressive decreased concentrating ability in the collecting ducts contributes to polyuria, which can predispose the child to dehydration and electrolyte imbalance, especially in the face of gastrointestinal losses or fever. High urinary flow rate also causes persistent ureteral dilation and can amplify the average resting bladder pressure. The treatment of polyuria consists of timed voiding in conjunction with low renal solute load diets. Antidiuretic hormone (given as dDAVP) is not effective in treating this type of polyuria because the collecting ducts are damaged and no longer respond to the dDAVP.

   b. Salt-losing nephropathy: Long-term effects of obstruction of the renal tubules may result in a tubular concentrating defect and salt loss. Dietary sodium supplementation appears to be of benefit in these patients.

   c. Metabolic acidosis: Metabolic acidosis enhances calcium loss from the bones and contributes to growth retardation. Dietary supplementation with bicarbonate salts should be used to correct metabolic acidosis.

   d. Renal osteodystrophy: Children with chronic renal failure may require dietary restriction of phosphates or the addition of phosphate binders such as calcium carbonate to prevent bone demineralization. Calcium carbonate can also provide supplemental dietary calcium.

   e. Growth retardation: Treatment involves correction of poor dietary intake and the previously mentioned metabolic abnormalities. Recombinant human growth hormone is now available to treat severely affected children.

### E. Surgical Management

1. Vesicoureteral reflux: This should be observed for a significant period of time, and many cases will resolve on their own. However, in some cases, such as children with recurrent pyelonephritis, surgical correction of the reflux should be considered. Until resolution of the reflux is accomplished, the child should remain on prophylactic antibiotics. Prior to correction of vesicoureteral reflux, care must be taken to ensure that the patient voids regularly and to completion because the correction of the reflux will be compromised by a high-pressure bladder. In the presence of high bladder pressures, the ureter may be recruited to act as a pop-off valve, which would compromise the antireflux mechanism further.

2. Bladder augmentation: For children with severely contracted small capacity bladders that fail to respond to maximal medical therapy, it may be necessary to surgically augment the bladder to achieve appropriate bladder capacity and urinary continence, and to preserve renal function. Surgical bladder augmentation is usually performed using a detubularized segment of ileum as a patch on the dome of the bladder. Bladder augmentation using gastrointestinal segments can result in its own set of metabolic complications. There may also be a significant risk of malignancy with long-term follow-up in these patients. As an option, some have recommended gastric bladder augmentation in these cases because the stomach segment will secrete acid and thereby improve the metabolic acidosis. This type of augmentation is, however, prone to other problems and the decision to proceed to augmentation in these patients should not be taken lightly.

## V. SUMMARY

Posterior urethral valves is one of the most common urologic perinatal emergencies. The immediate survival of the infant depends on early recognition and stabilization of the acute metabolic abnormalities. Following definitive relief of the obstructing lesion, patients with posterior urethral valves often continue to manifest a variety of urologic dysfunctions, and should be closely followed throughout childhood. Accurate characterization by urodynamic studies and careful management of bladder dysfunction are the keys to the long-term prognosis of these patients.

## RECOMMENDED READING

Gonzales Jr ET. Posterior urethral valves and other urethral anomalies. In: Walsh PC, Retik AB, Vaughan ED, et al, eds. *Campbell's urology,* 8th ed. Philadelphia: WB Saunders; 2002:2207–2230.

Smith GHH, Duckett JW. Urethral lesions in infants and children. In: Gillenwater JY, Grayhack JT, Howards SS, et al, eds. *Adult and pediatric urology,* 3rd ed. St. Louis: Mosby-Year Book; 1996:2411–2444.

# Congenital Anomalies (Urachal Anomalies, Exstrophy–Epispadias Complex, Imperforate Anus, and Prune-Belly Syndrome)

Ronald S. Sutherland

I. **URACHAL ANOMALIES (Fig. 16–1)**
   A. **Background.** The *urachus* is a fibrous band that extends from the anterior bladder wall to the umbilicus as the remnant of the allantoic duct. Ordinarily, this tract obliterates by the end of the first trimester; it rarely remains partially or completely open.
   B. **Presentation.** Complete failure of urachal obliteration results in a persistent communication from the bladder with constant leakage of urine. Although this may occur as a result of bladder outlet obstruction such as posterior urethral valves, more often there is no associated anomaly. The usual presentation is a neonate who has a constant wet umbilicus that worsens during crying or straining. If the urachal lumen is only partially obliterated, it may present later in childhood because of enlargement (due to accumulation of desquamated products) or infection. Symptoms and signs include pain, fever, mass, umbilical drainage, and signs of urinary tract infection (voiding frequency, urgency, and dysuria). Included in the differential diagnosis of such a presentation are infected urachal cyst, sinus, or diverticulum; vitelline cyst; umbilical hernia; and ovarian cyst. Usually there is an associated urinary tract infection if there is a communication with the bladder.
   C. **Workup.** If one suspects a urachal anomaly, an ultrasound of the abdomen is usually diagnostic. Other forms of urachal anomalies may require placement of a probe into the urachal tract or instillation of contrast for fistulography. Occasionally, a voiding cystourethrogram will delineate the communication, but is more useful for ruling out other etiologies or associated lower urinary tract anomalies.
   D. **Treatment.** Complete extraperitoneal excision of the urachal malformation is indicated in most cases. Occasionally, infected cysts may benefit from simple drainage and antibiotics; however, most require removal eventually because of the high likelihood of recurrence. Although rare, adenocarcinoma of the urachus has been reported to arise in patients with a history of infected cysts.

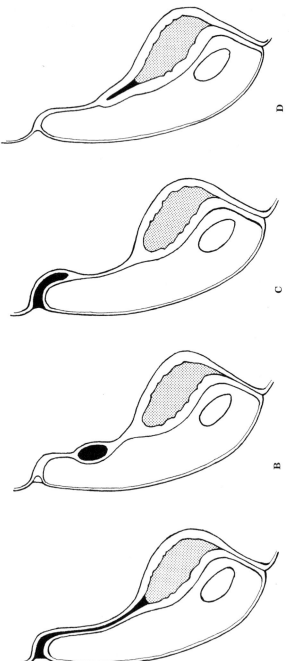

Fig. 16–1.   Urachal anomalies. A: Patent urachus. B: Urachal cyst. C: Umbilical sinus. D: Vesical diverticulum.

## II. EXSTROPHY–EPISPADIAS COMPLEX (Fig. 16–2)

A. **Background.** This anomaly of the bladder and urethra includes a range of abnormalities from minor epispadias to cloacal exstrophy. Occurring in between 1 and 30,000 to 40,000, it affects boys three to four times more often. Within this spectrum of anomalies, classic bladder exstrophy occurs in 60%, epispadias (all forms) in 30%, and complex cloacal exstrophy and other variants in 10%.

B. **Embryogenesis.** Persistence of the cloacal membrane after the 4th week of gestation prevents the lateral mesoderm from migrating medially. Once the membrane disappears by the 9th week, the posterior wall of the bladder is exposed to the outside with the umbilicus adjacent to the bladder wall. There is also failure of urethral folding dorsally that causes the epispadiac appearance. The most severe form, cloacal exstrophy, occurs when an abnormally large cloacal membrane perforates prior to division of the cloaca itself by the urorectal septum. When this occurs, an exstrophied bladder separated by an exstrophied ileocecal bowel area results.

C. **Anatomy.** At birth, the exposed bladder and urethra are obvious malformations (Fig. 16–2A). The bladder plate may vary in size from a small vestigial structure to 6 to 7 cm in diameter. Pubic separation is present in all cases. The upper urinary tracts are generally normal except in cloacal exstrophy patients in whom up to 66% may have abnormalities. Exposure of the bladder results in bacterial colonization, thickening of the bladder with squamous metaplasia, and resultant fibrosis. Once the bladder has been closed, vesicoureteral reflux occurs in the vast majority of patients due to the abnormal placement of the ureters and lack of muscular backing by the bladder. Inguinal hernias are common (both direct and indirect), especially in boys. The testes are descended normally in most cases. Some children may have rectal prolapse (10% to 20%) due to weakness in the perineal floor and the anterior aspect of the levator muscle complex. Adequate bladder closure and approximation of the symphysis may help prevent this.

   In girls, the clitoris is divided on both sides of the urethra; the vagina is tilted anteriorly and may be stenotic. There is a higher incidence of müllerian abnormalities such as duplication. Despite this, girls are potentially fertile. In boys, the penis usually is significantly curved upward and shortened. The corporal bodies of the penis are separate (unlike the normal penis in which the corpora communicate) and diverge to attach to the inferior pubic rami that are rotated laterally and anteriorly. Thus, osteotomy performed to restore normal symphyseal distance results in further shortening of the already stubby penis.

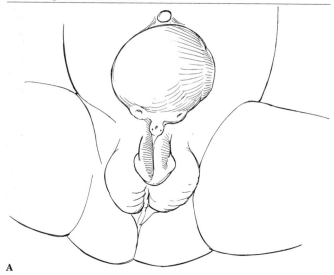

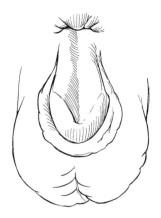

Fig. 16–2.   A: Bladder exstrophy. B: Epispadias.

D. **Initial Evaluation of the Newborn**
1. Although upper urinary tract anomalies in classic exstrophy are rare, abdominal ultrasound is important as a baseline. This is especially true for cloacal exstrophy patients.
2. To prevent injury to the bladder, it should be covered with silastic or smooth plastic (e.g., Saran wrap) to avoid contact with diapers and clothing. Ideally, a silk suture should be used to ligate the umbilical stump rather than a plastic or metal clamp to prevent scraping of the bladder.

E. **Treatment**
1. **Classic bladder exstrophy.** In the distant past, urinary diversion was usually performed by detaching the ureters from the bladder and attaching them to the sigmoid colon (ureterosigmoidostomy). This technique was popular because the presence of an intact rectal sphincter mechanism rendered the children continent. Unfortunately, it became apparent that there was an increased risk for tumor formation at the site of the ureterosigmoid anastomosis and there is a high rate of pyelonephritis with renal loss over time.

Presently, patients are closed either in a staged approach or most recently, with primary complete bladder and epispadias repair. Primary complete closure or a staged approach provide adequate drainage of kidneys and may enhance the potential for continence after reconstruction.

a. **Primary bladder and epispadias closure.** In the newborn period, the bladder and epispadias are closed in a single operation. After the immediate newborn period, the pelvic bones may be inflexible and osteotomies are required to bring together the pubic bones. The goal of complete primary closure is to add urethral resistance to the newly closed bladder that should result in bladder cycling and thereby increase bladder capacity and improve long-term continence results. Long-term outcomes determine whether this approach is justified compared to the staged repair.

b. **Staged approach to bladder exstrophy and epispadias**
(1) **Primary bladder closure.** Performed during the newborn period, this effectively converts the exstrophied bladder to an epispadias. Some feel that closure in the newborn does not necessitate iliac osteotomies to bring the divergent pubic rami together because of the pliability of the innominant bones and the sacroiliac joint. Others recommend osteotomy strongly, claiming that it contributes to continence in the future by making

bladder and abdominal wall closure tension free (thus less prone to dehiscence), placing the urethra within the pelvic ring, and reapproximating the urogenital diaphragm to enhance voluntary urinary control.

(2) **Epispadias closure** (Fig. 16–2B) is performed between 6 months and 1 year of age. Repair involves correction of intrinsic dorsal curvature (chordee) of the corporal bodies followed by urethral reconstruction that incorporates the same principles utilized in hypospadias repair. Modern repairs bring the urethra from its dorsal position to a more normal ventral position on the penis.

(3) **Bladder neck reconstruction and ureteral reimplantation.** The next stage involves bladder neck tightening along with bilateral ureteral reimplantation to correct reflux. Generally this is performed at 3 to 5 years of age. Bladder capacity at this stage is a significant prognostic feature for future continence. Reconstructing the bladder neck should result in a raised pressure at which urine leaks (called the *opening* or *leak point* pressure, which should be about 30 cm $H_2O$). Sometimes a suspension procedure of the bladder neck is done to increase the opening pressure.

(4) **Primary epispadias** (Fig. 16–2B). The most common form is that of a proximal urethral opening (penopubic), but other variations may exist including a very mild form of dorsal glanular epispadias. Generally, the more proximal the meatus, the more likely the chance for maldevelopment of the external sphincter and bladder neck continence mechanism. Repair is performed as mentioned for epispadias after bladder exstrophy closure and can be done in the first year of life. Addressing the surgical correction of incontinence should wait until the child is 3 to 5 years old.

(5) **Cloacal exstrophy.** In the past, patients with this most severe and rare form (incidence of 1 per 200,000 live births) of the exstrophy–epispadias complex were usually left to die. Significant problems associated with this include omphalocele, numerous gastrointestinal anomalies (including malrotation, duplication,

duodenal atresia, and Meckel diverticulum), and significant genitourinary (GU) anomalies (including separate bladder halves and bifid genitalia). Newborn boys were occasionally gender converted to female as a result of inadequate genital development and the poor prognosis for developing a normal male phenotype. With modern surgical techniques and a multidisciplinary approach to their care, children with this complex disorder can achieve acceptable lifestyles. The advisability of gender conversion has also been called into question.

**F. Prognosis**

1. **Continence.** With the current staged approach, continence rates of up to 50% and 60% have been reported, although this varies among treatment centers and surgeons. Many factors influence the outcome, including experience of surgeon, capacity and compliance of the bladder, and the expectations of the family. Continence may improve in boys in adolescence when growth of the prostate occurs. In the majority of patients who remain incontinent after the staged procedures, limited bladder capacity is the cause. Surgical bladder augmentation or creation of a bladder reservoir using bowel can be performed to solve this problem. In a minority of patients the bladder outlet is weak, and placement of an artificial urinary sphincter or urethral augmentation with collagen or Teflon injection may be beneficial.

2. **Renal Function.** Renal deterioration is prevented if bladder pressures remain relatively low and if the child remains on antibacterial prophylaxis because of reflux. In children with more severe forms of exstrophy who may require urinary diversion, upper tract damage can occur and varies according to the type of diversion: 82% for ileal conduits, 22% for nonrefluxing colonic conduits, and 33% for ureterosigmoidostomies.

3. **Obstetric complications**. A common complication in girls with exstrophy is uterine prolapse during pregnancy and delivery. This is thought to be due to a weakened pelvic floor, an abnormally shortened vagina, and failure of development of the cardinal ligaments. Patients who have had prior bladder neck reconstruction or ureterosigmoidostomy should be delivered by cesarean section; those who have had urinary diversion to a stoma should be delivered vaginally if possible to avoid inadvertent injury to the urinary reservoir or conduit. Vaginal delivery is associated with a higher risk of incontinence.

### III. IMPERFORATE ANUS (Fig. 16–3)

**A. Background.** Imperforate anus comprises a spectrum of anorectal anomalies ranging from simple anal fistula to complex cloacal malformations involving multiple organ systems.

1. **Associated anomalies** are seen in up to 50% of cases and urologic involvement in 26% to 50%. Generally, the more severe the defect (i.e., the higher the rectourethral or rectovaginal communication), the higher the incidence of associated anomalies.

   a. **Spinal malformations** include hemivertebra, sacral agenesis or deformation, and spinal dysraphism (spina bifida).

   b. **VACTERL syndrome.** Previously known as VATER (*v*ertebral, *a*norectal, *t*racheoesophageal fistula, *r*adial abnormalities), the terminology has been updated to include *c*ardiac, *r*enal, and *l*imb anomalies.

   c. **GU anomalies.** Major malformations include renal agenesis (20%), vesicoureteral reflux (23%), hydroureter (12%), neurogenic bladder (6%), cystic or dysplastic kidney (5%), renal ectopia (5%), ureteral ectopia (4%), and ureteropelvic junction obstruction (3%). Minor malformations include cryptorchidism (4%), ureteral duplication (3%), hypospadias (3%), and renal malrotation (2%).

2. **Embryology.** By the 8th week of gestation, the primitive hindgut becomes separated into the rectum and the urogenital sinus by the descending urorectal septum. Incomplete migration of the septum with persistence of the cloacal membrane may result in communication (fistula) between the rectum and the urinary tract as well as malformations of the pelvic musculature (sphincter).

3. **Classification.** Anorectal anomalies can be divided into high, intermediate, or low defects based on the level of the fistula between the rectum and the urinary tract or the level of the rectal agenesis (Fig. 16–2).

4. **Morbidity.** Factors contributing to morbidity in these patients relate mainly to GU anomalies, spinal (especially sacral) anomalies, other malformations, and the quality of bowel and urinary sphincters. GU factors include sepsis, absorptive hyperchloremic metabolic acidosis (from absorbed urinary electrolytes via the bowel mucosa), progressive pyelonephritic scarring exacerbated by vesicoureteral reflux, neurovesical bladder dysfunction, and urethral obstruction.

**B. Prenatal diagnosis.** Although a subtle finding on ultrasound, a dilated distal bowel segment can be a sign. Occasionally, intraluminal calcification is present, which occurs as a result of mixed stagnant urine and meconium.

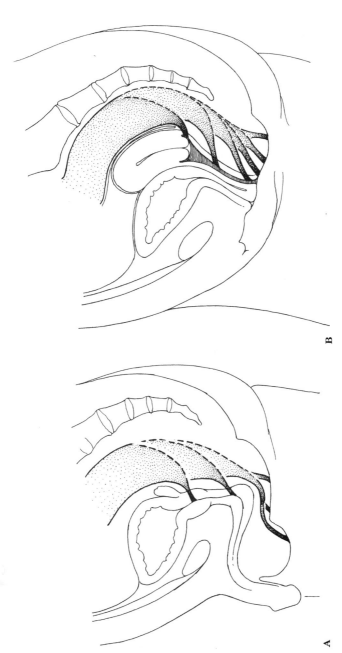

Fig. 16-3.   Imperforate anus. Possible location of rectal genital fistula: (A) boys; (B) girls.

C. **Diagnosis and Management**
  1. **Perineal inspection.** The initial evaluation of the perineum yields much information about the severity of the defect and the type of intervention necessary for the infant. In boys, addition of a urinalysis to assess for meconium determines whether a colostomy is needed. If there is any question regarding the diagnosis, a cross-table lateral plain x-ray with the patient in the head down position and with skin marker at the level of the anus (or where it should be), should be done (*invertogram*).
  2. **Surgical management.** Most patients with high lesions require a colostomy to divert the fecal stream temporarily until a more distal repair can be accomplished. Distal repair is most often done using the posterior sagittal approach for the anorectoplasty and repair of the rectourinary fistula. The posterior approach is advantageous in preserving the sphincteric musculature (puborectalis sling portion of the levator muscles). In lower or more minor lesions, a posterior anorectoplasty may accomplish the job without having to resort to a colostomy.
  3. **Urodynamic evaluation** (see Chapter 11). This is an important part of management because of the possibility of spinal dysraphism or sacral agenesis, and operative injury to bladder innervation.
  4. **Urologic interventions**
     a. **Antibiotic prophylaxis.** Until lower urinary tract anomalies are ruled out or reconstructed, all patients should be placed on prophylactic antibiotics to avoid urosepsis.
     b. **Catheterization difficulties.** Often, fistula repair results in urethral narrowing, scarring, or possibly the presence of a diverticulum, all of which make catheterization a challenge. Use of a curved-tip (coudé) catheter may be helpful. If a patient is unable to negotiate the urethra with any catheter and requires intermittent catheterization, placement of a continent catheterizable channel to the bladder (Mitrofanoff appendicovesicostomy) may be a suitable alternative.
     c. **Augmentation cystoplasty.** If bowel segments are necessary to enlarge the capacity of the bladder, avoid using the sigmoid colon so as not to devascularize the distal bowel. Also, the ileocecal valve should be preserved to avoid exacerbating stool incontinence as a result of marginal sphincteric function.

IV. **PRUNE-BELLY SYNDROME (Fig. 16–4)**
  A. **Background.** Referred to as Eagle-Barrett, triad, or mesenchymal dysplasia syndrome, all share three major pathologic anomalies: a deficiency, or absence of, abdominal wall musculature; a variety of ureteral,

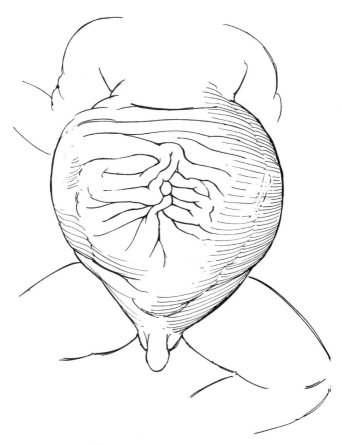

**Fig. 16–4.  Prune-belly syndrome.**

bladder, and urethral anomalies, manifested in most cases by marked dilation; and bilateral undescended testes. Other coexisting orthopedic, pulmonary, and cardiac anomalies have been noted as well. The incidence ranges from 1 in 35,000 to 1 in 50,000 live births with most cases occurring in boys (3% to 5% of cases are in girls).

**B.  Pathogenesis.** The definitive origin of this syndrome remains controversial, but two theories predominate.

    **1.  Obstructive theory.** This suggests that severe bladder outlet obstruction existed early in gestation and was subsequently relieved after irreversible damage had occurred. This obstruction resulted in bladder distention, ureteral dilation, hydronephrosis, and atrophy of the abdominal wall muscles by the increased pressure, mechanical distension, and interference with the blood supply of the organs involved. Most patients with prune-belly syndrome lack anatomic obstruction at the time of birth, however.

2. **Mesodermal defect theory.** Because obstruction is rarely present at birth and there is a lack of bladder hypertrophy and hyperplasia, a second theory suggests that a primary defect in mesenchymal development occurs early in gestation.

C. **Clinical Manifestations**

1. **Kidney.** Renal abnormalities are the major determinants of survival, with a 20% chance of stillbirth or death in the neonatal period from renal dysplasia and the associated pulmonary hypoplasia. An additional 30% of patients develop urosepsis, renal failure, or both in the first 2 years of life.

2. **Ureter.** Severely dilated, and tortuous, the ureters are most severely affected at the lower end and appear histologically to have patchy areas of fibrosis. Vesicoureteral reflux is present in 75% of these patients. Although their radiographic appearance is alarming, drainage is generally adequate.

3. **Bladder.** The bladder is generally capacious, smooth walled, and irregularly thick, without trabeculation. Often a urachal remnant or diverticulum creates an hourglass configuration. Functionally, patients with these bladders exhibit a diminished sensation of fullness and have a large capacity with poor contractility, decreased voiding pressures, and thus a poor ability to empty.

4. **Prostate and posterior urethra.** The prostatic urethra is elongated and characteristically tapers to the membranous region, which gives rise to the typical radiographic appearance of a triangular posterior urethra.

5. **Anterior urethra.** Although the urethra is most often normal in prune-belly syndrome, both urethral atresia and megalourethra can be seen.

6. **Testicles.** Cryptorchidism is seen universally in boys with prune-belly syndrome, the gonads characteristically being found high in the abdomen. Because the gonads are intraabdominal and may be injured further in bringing them down and in addition, the prostate is underdeveloped and the bladder neck open, infertility is the rule. However, in recent years, pregnancies have been achieved using intracytoplasmic sperm injection after retrieval of the occasional sperm.

7. **Abdominal musculature.** The most characteristic manifestation of the syndrome is the wrinkled, prunelike skin of the abdomen in the newborn infant. Skeletal muscle hypoplasia is seen in all three layers of the abdominal wall muscles. Complications are surprisingly minimal. The inability to sit up directly from the supine position may delay the

onset of walking, but it rarely affects normal physical activity.

8. **Other associated anomalies.** Other anomalies are found in over 65% of patients, the most common being cardiopulmonary and gastrointestinal, and including orthopedic and developmental problems. Pulmonary abnormalities range in severity, with the most significant arising in cases with associated antenatal oligohydramnios. Children who survive the neonatal period usually have no associated pulmonary problems.

D. **Fetal diagnosis and treatment.** Antenatal ultrasound is capable of detecting abnormal urinary tract dilation as early as 14 weeks. However, it is difficult to differentiate prune-belly syndrome from other causes of urinary tract dilation. In the presence of oligohydramnios, prenatal intervention has been advocated to decompress the dilated bladders and restore the amniotic fluid volume. However, although prenatal intervention may improve pulmonary function, its effectiveness in improving renal function is uncertain. Furthermore, intervention in cases of prune-belly syndrome is difficult to justify because in utero obstruction may not exist.

E. **Management of the Neonate**
1. **Immediate evaluation**
   a. **History and physical.** Rule out life-threatening cardiac and pulmonary problems first. The abdominal examination is made much easier by the thin, relaxed belly, which permits easy palpation of the intraabdominal and retroperitoneal contents.
   b. **Serum creatinine** levels in the first days of life reflect maternal values, but a progressive increase (or failure to decline) suggests some degree of renal insufficiency.
   c. **Bladder stimulation test.** Simple bladder massage can be used to stimulate a detrusor response, and one can use this as a test of voiding.
   d. **Imaging**
      (1) Begin with an ultrasound that can provide information on renal potential and bladder emptying.
      (2) Voiding cystourethrography (VCUG) should be postponed to avoid introducing bacteria into a stagnant system. However, if renal function is abnormal, a VCUG should be done early. Aggressive antibiotic treatment is essential around the time of VCUG as the introduction of even a few bacteria can result in sepsis in the stagnant urinary tract.
      (3) A dimercaptosuccinic acid scan may be done to evaluate for renal malformation and scarring.

2. **Treatment.** Management is decided based on whether patients are severely affected (oligohydramnios, pulmonary hypoplasia, or pneumothorax); moderately affected with typical external features and uropathy of the full-blown syndrome, but without immediate problems with survival; or have a mild form unlikely to develop urosepsis or azotemia. The third category of patients show internal features that may be mild or incomplete. Uropathy is less severe and renal function is stable.

   a. **Severely affected** patients in the first category usually do not survive the neonatal period; however, for the few who do survive, urinary diversion by vesicostomy, cutaneous pyelostomy, or ureterostomy is often recommended to provide optimal urinary drainage.

   b. **Moderately affected.** The approach to the second category of patients with prune-belly syndrome is variable, but is usually nonoperative unless infection (despite antibiotic prophylaxis), failure of adequate renal growth, or decreasing renal function is encountered. In these cases the urinary tract is reconstructed with ureteral tailoring and correction of reflux to reduce stasis. Reconstruction of the abdominal wall as well as orchidopexy are often performed simultaneously.

   c. **Mildly affected** patients in category three who have good renal function do not usually require surgical intervention. However, lifelong antimicrobial prophylaxis should be instituted (in neonates, amoxicillin or first-generation cephalosporin; later, trimethoprim-sulfamethoxazole or nitrofurantoin). Orchidopexy may be delayed until such time as any other reconstructive procedures may become necessary or at about 6 months.

F. **Management into childhood and beyond.** Abnormalities of bladder drainage are the principal source of problems that may lead to renal deterioration.

   1. **Evaluation: urodynamics.** The child with a low urinary flow rate and a significant residual volume should be evaluated with urodynamics (see Chapter 12).

   2. **Treatment**

      a. In some cases, endoscopic evaluation of the urethra with internal urethrotomy of pseudovalves may be attempted to reduce the outlet resistance, although this remains controversial.

      b. **Ureteral surgery.** Although pyelonephritis or renal deterioration may prompt one to reimplant and perhaps tailor the ureters to improve drainage and prevent reflux, these procedures are complicated by the poor peristaltic nature of these ureters and the abnormal bladder into which they are reimplanted. Although the radiographic appearance of the urinary tract improves after surgery, it remains to be seen whether there is any long-term functional improvement. Because of persistent stasis postoperatively, nearly all these patients are maintained on lifelong antibacterial prophylaxis.

   **c. Clean intermittent catheterization.** Adequate drainage can be obtained with clean intermittent catheterization, but this can be difficult because these patients have normal urethral sensation and some have urethral anomalies. For this reason, a continent abdominal stoma may be useful. If the family cannot catheterize the patient, a urinary diversion, usually a cutaneous ureterostomy, can be life saving until the child is mature enough to perform the catheterization.

**3. Prognosis**

   **a. Renal function.** Patients who survive infancy with mildly impaired renal function may develop renal failure as a result of chronic pyelonephritis and reflux nephropathy. In these individuals, renal transplantation can be performed successfully. All these patients should perform clean intermittent self-catheterization to alleviate chronic retention.

   **b. Testicles.** Early intraabdominal orchidopexy is warranted in boys with prune-belly syndrome because repair in infancy allows placement of the testes into the scrotum without division of the spermatic vessels, which may not be possible later in life. Although likely to be infertile, these patients may benefit from advances in fertility techniques. In addition because these patients have the same risk for testicular malignancy as normal boys with undescended testes, having gonads in the scrotum will facilitate examination.

   **c. Abdominal wall.** Major reconstruction of the abdominal wall repair can be done at the same time as orchiopexy. This procedure includes excision of redundant prunelike folds of skin and fascia to create a satisfactory waistline. In milder cases, observation may be best because of the tendency for the abnormal abdominal wall to stretch out again.

## RECOMMENDED READING

Sheldon CA. Imperforate anus, urogenital sinus, and cloaca. In: Belman AB, King LR and Kramer SA, eds. *Clinical Pediatric Urology*. London: Dinitz, 2002:811–858.

Caldemone AA. Exstrophy-epispadias complex. Anomalies of the bladder and cloaca. In: Gillenwater JY, Grayhack JT, Howards SS, et al, eds. *Adult and pediatric urology*. St. Louis: Mosby Year Book, 1991:2023–2054.

Sutherland RS, Mevorach RA, Kogan BA. Prune belly syndrome: The prune belly syndrome: current insights. *Pediatr Nephrol* 1995;9:770–778.

# Adolescent Urology: Testicular Torsion, Varicoceles, and Gynecologic Problems

Michael DiSandro

## I. THE ACUTE SCROTUM

The acute onset of scrotal pain, swelling, or both in the adolescent boy is a urologic emergency. Up to 60% of adolescent patients will have testicular torsion, and the best chance for testicular salvage occurs if testicular blood flow is restored within the first 8 hours (97%). There is a higher incidence of testicular atrophy if the ischemia lasts longer than 8 hours. In addition to torsion, the differential diagnosis for acute scrotal pain in the adolescent includes epididymitis (20%), torsion of the appendix testis or epididymis, mumps orchitis, trauma, and, rarely, tumors. It is important, but sometimes difficult, to distinguish the above conditions from torsion. Table 17–1 highlights some of the distinguishing features. If there is any doubt in the diagnosis, an immediate urologic consultation is mandatory.

A. **Distinguishing Testicular Torsion from Epididymitis** (Table 17–1)

B. **Additional tests.** Although testicular *radionuclide scans* and *Doppler sonography* have the ability to delineate testicular blood flow, they are not accurate enough to distinguish torsion from epididymitis reliably. Surgical exploration should not be delayed to obtain these tests.

   A testicular scan may be helpful in a very late presentation of epididymitis (beyond 24 hours) because scrotal exploration and orchiectomy will need to be performed if testicular infarction is present.

C. **Treatment for torsion.** After the diagnosis of torsion is made, surgery should be scheduled immediately.

   1. In the meantime, *manual detorsion* may be attempted to temporarily relieve the ischemia. The testis are rotated laterally by 360 degrees. If there is no relief of pain, an additional 360-degree rotation is performed (Fig. 17–1). If this results in relief of pain, the patient should be admitted to the hospital and the operation may then be performed on an urgent rather than emergent basis.

   2. *Surgical exploration* is via a midline scrotal incision. The torsed testicle is detorsed, and observed for 30 minutes. In the meantime, a contralateral orchiopexy is performed. If after 30 minutes the ipsilateral testicle does not recover, then an orchiectomy is performed. If there is recovery, then ipsilateral orchiopexy is carried out.

**Table 17–1. Distinguishing testicular torsion from epididymitis**

|  | Torsion | Epididymitis |
|---|---|---|
| **Incidence** | Accounts for 50% to 60% of acute scrotum cases in adolescents, and 25% to 30% of all pediatric patient cases. | Accounts for 20% of the acute scrotum cases in adolescents, and <1% in prepubertal boys. |
| **History** | Acute onset of scrotal pain. The patient can usually state the exact time the pain began. Patients may or may not be sexually active. Urethral discharge not usually present. Usually not associated with any voiding complaints. | Gradual onset of symptoms. Patients are usually sexually active. The most common etiologic agent in adolescents is chlamydia. Urethral discharge may be present; thin and watery suggests chlamydia; thick and creamy suggests *Neisseria gonorrhea.* Irritable voiding symptoms may be present. Not all cases, however, are associated with an infectious agent, and therefore, above symptoms may not be present. |
| **Physical examination** | Patients appear uncomfortable and restless. Nausea and emesis may also be associated with the pain. High riding testicle. Absence of cremasteric reflex (although rare, there are cases of torsion with a cremasteric reflex). | *Early:* An enlarged and tender mass posterior to and very distinct from the testis. *Later:* Entire testicle enlarged and tender, without an apparent distinction between epididymis and testis. Most adolescents present at this stage. It may be extremely difficult to distinguish this stage of epididymitis from testicular torsion. |
| **Laboratory** | Urinalysis usually negative. | Urinalysis usually reveals numerous leukocytes. Urethral swab may reveal infectious agent. |

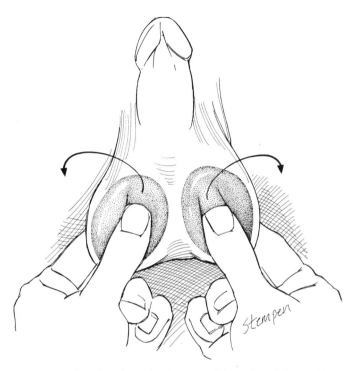

**Fig. 17–1.** **Direction of rotation for manual detorsion of the testicle.**

    **D.** **Treatment for epididymitis.** Upper urinary tract evaluation is not necessary in the adolescent because, in contrast to prepubertal boys, epididymitis is not associated with a higher incidence of structural anomalies.

        Any urethral discharge should be gram stained and then cultured for *Neisseria*. If gonorrhea has been excluded, then the patients can be treated empirically for chlamydia with doxycycline 100 mg PO BID for 10 days. If gonorrhea is present, treatment should include one IM dose of 250 mg of ceftriaxone followed by a 10-day course of doxycycline (up to 20% of patients infected with gonorrhea also have a chlamydial infection.)

        Patients should also be encouraged to avoid physical activity until the symptoms abate. A scrotal support may help to alleviate some of the discomfort.

    **E.** **Other Conditions That May Lead to an Acute Scrotum**

        **1.** **Torsion of the testicular or epididymal appendix.** The appendix testis, or less commonly the appendix epididymis (Fig. 17–2), may become torsed and lead to significant testicular pain. If

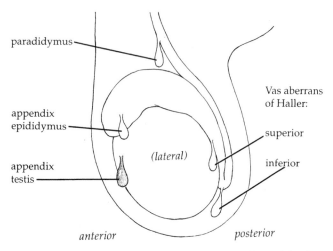

**Fig. 17–2.  Location of appendix testis and appendix epididymis.**

the presentation is early enough, the diagnosis can usually be made with a good history and physical examination. Early on, the patients will localize the pain to one spot on the testis. If the presentation is delayed, inflammation can spread and the entire testicle can become painful and tender. Any motion aggravates the pain, so the patients sit very still and walk with a characteristic wide gait. The patients usually point to the upper, outer pole of their testis if asked where they hurt.

On physical examination, the tenderness can usually be localized to this one point, especially early on. Some patients have a "blue dot" sign where the infarcted appendix can be seen though the skin. If there is any doubt in the diagnosis, the patient should undergo surgical exploration for torsion of the testicle. Otherwise, patients can be treated conservatively with analgesics.

2.  **Tumors.** Although unlikely, testicular tumors can present with acute scrotal pain. Follow-up within 1 month after treatment for epididymitis is therefore extremely important to reexamine the testicle for masses. If a testicular mass is present after treatment, a scrotal ultrasound should be obtained. If a solid intratesticular mass is present, a radical orchiectomy should be performed.

II.  **GENITAL ULCER SYNDROME (HERPES AND SYPHILIS)**
   A.  **Epidemiology.** Of the adolescent population, 25% to 35% are sexually active and unlikely to utilize condoms. The overall incidence of genital ulcer syndrome is

rising, especially in the inner cities where the number of reported syphilis cases has increased markedly over the past 5 years. Herpes and syphilis account for 95% of the cases of genital ulcer syndrome in the United States.

**B. Physical Findings**

1. *Herpes* is characterized by the presence of painful vesicles on an erythematous base.

2. The classic *syphilis* ulcer is a single, firm, painless lesion with rolled edges. There may be associated inguinal adenopathy.

**C. Laboratory Evaluation.** If syphilis is suspected clinically, order either the rapid plasma reagin (RPR) or the Venereal Disease Research Laboratory (VDRL) test. If the screening RPR or VDRL is positive, a microhemagglutination *Treponema pallidum* antibody assay should be ordered to confirm the diagnosis (there can be false positives with the RPR or VDRL). Treatment, however, should be started based on the results of the screening test.

**D. Treatment** consists of benzathine penicillin 2.4 million units IM for one dose. If penicillin allergic, erythromycin base 2 g PO BID for 10 days can be used. RPR or VDRL should be repeated in 1 month and should be negative. Because open ulcers leave male and female patients vulnerable to HIV infection, an adolescent with a genital ulcer should be tested for HIV infection.

**III. URETHRAL BLEEDING (URETHRORRHAGIA)**

In most patients, urethrorrhagia is a benign, self-limiting condition usually discovered as blood stains on the patient's underwear. There are usually no associated symptoms, although some have terminal hematuria or dysuria. The symptoms can last longer than 1 year and the mean duration of symptomatology is 17 months. A fractionated (three-glass) urinalysis as well as a urine culture should be performed. If the urine culture is positive or microscopic hematuria is present in all three fractions, an abdominal and pelvic ultrasound should be performed. If the symptoms are present for longer than 6 months, a voiding cystourethrogram may be performed. Cystoscopy is not usually necessary. Reassurance of both family and patient is necessary; most symptoms resolve with time.

**IV. VARICOCELE**

**A. Background.** A varicocele is a dilation of the pampiniform venous plexus and the internal spermatic vein (Fig. 17–3). Varicoceles are quite common; the incidence in adolescent boys ranges from 19% to 26%. They occur on the left side 90% of the time. They are a concern in adolescents because in some adults, varicoceles are associated with an abnormal semen analysis and infertility and are the most common correctable cause of male infertility. However, 85% of adults with an uncorrected varicocele are fertile, and in most patients, a varicocele is of no clinical significance. There are currently no parameters to reliably predict which

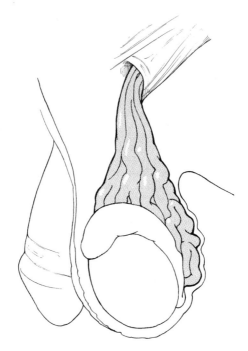

**Fig. 17–3. Varicocele.**

adolescents with a varicocele will develop infertility as adults, but there are several diagnostic tests to help in the decision-making process.

1. Major determinants
   a. *Testis size.* The testis can be measured with a goniometer. If there is ipsilateral testis atrophy with a volume of at least 3 mL less than the contralateral testis, surgical repair is indicated.
   b. *Pain.* Although pain is uncommonly associated with a varicocele, rarely it can be an indication for surgery.
2. Other determinants
   *Semen analysis.* In adults, semen analysis is an excellent determinant of testicular exocrine function and semen parameters are used to determine whether surgery is indicated. A semen analysis from an adolescent would also prove useful; however, it is difficult to obtain a semen sample from this sensitive age group and normal values are not clear.

B. **History and Physical Examination**
   1. History: The patient may notice a painless sac adjacent to his testicle on the left side that was not

present before puberty. An examining physician notes most varicoceles incidentally. Few patients present with pain secondary to the varicocele.

2. Physical findings: The classic finding is a nontender "sac of worms" adjacent to the left testicle that is more prominent when the patient is standing and usually decreases in size when supine. Grade I varicoceles are palpable only when the patient does a Valsalva maneuver; grade II varicoceles are palpable without any maneuvers; grade III varicoceles are visible to the examiner's eye.

   a. Management

     (1) Grades I, II, and III varicoceles without testicular atrophy mandate annual examinations to check for new-onset testicular atrophy.

     (2) Grade III varicoceles with testicular atrophy (as defined) usually require surgical correction.

   b. Surgical options: The three most common approaches to varicocelectomy include surgical ligation and division of the veins within the inguinal canal (Ivanissevitch procedure), high retroperitoneal approach (Palomo procedure; can be performed laparoscopically), and the subinguinal microsurgical approach. Angiographic embolization can also be utilized and is especially useful in recurrent cases.

## V. DELAYED PUBERTY

The average age for the onset of puberty for United States boys is 11.5 years with a range from 9 to 14 years. Delayed puberty is defined as any boy over age 14 who has failed to initiate the development of secondary sexual characteristics. However, 0.6% of the normal population enter puberty after their fourteenth birthday (*temporary delayed puberty*), and they ultimately enter and pass through puberty.

  A. Evaluation

   1. Physical examination: Testicular examination (evaluate for cryptorchidism); Tanner staging.

   2. Endocrine workup: Serum testosterone, luteinizing hormone (LH), and follicle-stimulating hormone (FSH) levels should be ordered. If there is low or absent serum testosterone and markedly elevated LH and FSH ($3\times$ normal), then the testis are absent or damaged. If these tests are normal, then human chorionic gonadotropin is administered and testosterone, LH, and FSH levels are repeated. If LH and FSH rise and the testosterone does not, then the testis are absent or damaged.

  B. **Differential diagnosis** includes isolated gonadotropin deficiency, Kallman syndrome, congenital hypopituitarism, craniopharyngiomas, and hypergonadotropic hypogonadism (testicular failure secondary to chemotherapy and radiation, vanishing testis syndrome, mumps orchitis).

## VI. PEDIATRIC GYNECOLOGY
### A. Genital Anomalies

Anomalies of the female genitalia are relatively rare. They are most often diagnosed by a careful physical examination.

1. Clitoral hypertrophy: Usually seen in premature infants. It resolves with differential growth. In term babies, clitoral enlargement (>6 mm) should be evaluated for intersex. Severe vulvovaginitis and neurofibromatosis are also causes for clitoral hypertrophy.

2. Labial anomalies
   a. Labial adhesions are mainly asymptomatic, but sometimes associated with postvoid dribbling. If severe enough, they may also predispose to urinary tract infections. They can usually be treated with short counsel of estrogen cream.
   b. Ectopic labium are unusual, and associated with renal agenesis.
   c. Intralabial masses
      (1) Paraurethral cysts: The urethral meatus is displaced from the midline by a whitish-appearing mass, which is often difficult to visualize on physical examination. Posterior compression of the urethra through the vagina may produce a pussy urethral discharge. They are usually asymptomatic, and rupture and drain spontaneously.
      (2) Urethral prolapse: Usually found in young black girls, they usually present with blood spotting on the underwear. The urethral mucosa protrudes beyond the meatus, and a portion of the anterior urethral mucosa may be necrotic and edematous (Fig. 17–4). If symptomatic, topical steroids will usually alleviate the symptoms. Surgical excision and reduction is sometimes necessary.
      (3) Prolapsed ectopic ureterocele: Patients usually present with incontinence, voiding dysfunction, urinary tract infections, or all three. On examination, there is a whitish lesion extending from the inferior aspect of the urethral meatus. Patients require radiologic evaluation of the kidneys and ureters to assess for duplication and function. Voiding studies to assess for reflux should also be obtained. Surgical correction is usually necessary.
      (4) Sarcoma botryoides or rhabdomyosarcoma of the bladder or vagina appear as a lobulated mass arising from the introitus. There may be blood spotting on the underwear. Direct biopsy of the mass confirms the diagnosis.

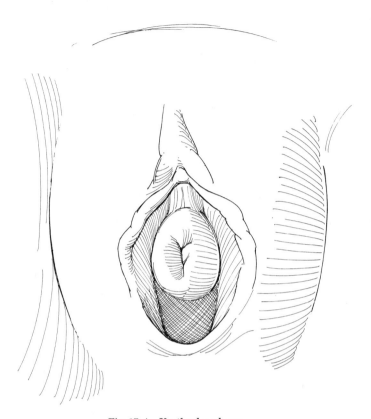

**Fig. 17–4.   Urethral prolapse.**

(5) Neonatal vaginouterine prolapse is rare. Most cases (over 80%) are associated with congenital spinal defects such as myelomeningocele or spina bifida.

3. Anomalies of the female genital tract

a. Vaginal obstruction, vaginal agenesis: The presentation occurs either in the newborn period as an abdominal mass, or in the pubertal period during evaluation for amenorrhea. The abdominal mass is secondary to an accumulation or secretions in the obstructed vagina (*hydrocolpos*) or in the vagina and uterus (*hydrometrocolpos*). If the patient presents at puberty, then there is cyclic abdominal pain and amenorrhea. The urinary tract must also be evaluated as unilateral renal agenesis is common.

b. Urogenital sinus anomalies result from an abnormal formation of the urorectal septum. On physical examination, there is an anteriorly displaced anus and a common opening for the urethra and genital tract. A genitogram (the retrograde injection of contrast into the urogenital sinus) is useful to define the anatomy. This is a common finding in the more severe forms of congenital adrenal hyperplasia. Surgical reconstruction is required. If there is a cloacal malformation, then there will be a combination of urogenital sinus anomalies and anorectal anomalies. They present at birth with abdominal distention and an abnormal perineum. Again, surgical reconstruction is necessary after evaluation of the urinary tract.

   **c.** Ovarian masses are rare in childhood. The most common presenting symptom is abdominal pain and the second most frequent symptom is a palpable abdominal mass. In almost one-half of patients, the acute onset of symptoms results from torsion, hemorrhage, or perforation. In childhood, 23% to 45% of ovarian masses are nonneoplastic. There are rare neoplastic ovarian lesions as well.

**B. General Vulvovaginal Complaints**

   **1.** Recurrent urinary tract infections and daytime accidents: Common complaints from the parent are "she pulls at herself," or "she says it hurts down there," and this is associated with the symptoms of dysfunctional voiding and bladder instability. Whether the patients have chronic skin irritation and vulvitis secondary to the dysfunctional voiding, or whether they have dysfunctional voiding to avoid urinating onto an inflamed vulva, is sometimes difficult to delineate.

   In early infancy, vulvovaginitis is relatively uncommon. However, as the child ages, the vaginal pH and mucosal lining change, and the tissue becomes more prone to irritation and abrasion, and more susceptible to vulvovaginitis.

   **a.** Nonspecific vulvovaginitis (no certain infections or etiology can be found)

   **(1)** Possible causes

   **(a)** Dysfunctional voiding due to bladder instability, leading to chronic urinary leakage.

   **(b)** Vaginal voiding from voiding with the knees together, especially in obese children, can lead to chronic skin exposure to urine. Urea-splitting bacteria in the vulvovaginal area can convert urea into ammonia, which can cause irritation when exposed to the skin.

   **(c)** A somewhat hypospadiac urethral meatus may predispose to vaginal voiding.

      **(d)** Overzealous rubbing between the labia during routine hygiene can lead to dysuria and then dysfunctional voiding.

  **(2)** Treatment

      **(a)** Avoid irritants (urine; rough toilet paper; harsh soaps; tight, irritating clothing)

      **(b)** An individualized bladder retraining program (see Chapter 8)

      **(c)** Symptomatic relief with warm bath soaks followed by good air drying of the vulva. Cool, loose cotton underpants also help. A 1% hydrocortisone cream, in brief applications, may also help.

      **(d)** "Tea baths" are useful in the treatment of nonspecific vaginitis in childhood. Three to five black tea bags are added to the bath water. Soak for 15 minutes; repeat daily for 3 to 5 days.

      **(e)** If symptoms persist despite treatment, a vaginal culture is necessary. If performing a vaginal culture it is important to rule out all sexually transmitted diseases; therefore, one must order a swab of the vagina to specifically rule out gonorrhea in addition to the routine culture and then a second swab using the correct chlamydia medium. In children, including adolescents, it is recommended to perform true cultures rather than screening tests because of legal issues with regard to child sexual abuse.

**b.** True vulvovaginitis

  **(1)** Requires the identification of specific pathogens that are not normal inhabitants of the vagina. Normal flora includes diphtheroids, *Staphylococcus epidermidis*, α-hemolytic streptococci, lactobacilli, *Escherichia coli*, β-hemolytic (non-group A or B) streptococci, group B streptococcus, and *Candida tropicalis*.

  **(2)** The most common pathogens in vulvovaginitis are *Streptococcus pyogenes, Streptococcus pneumonia,* and *Shigella*. Other pathogens include *Candida* (most commonly seen after the child is treated with antibiotics for an unrelated infection), *Neisseria gonorrhea, Chlamydia trachomatis,* and *Herpes simplex*. The latter three should all be reported and should arouse suspicion of sexual abuse (herpes, however, can be acquired by maternal–neonatal transmission). Pinworms (*Enterobius vermicularis*) can also cause vulvitis (the diagnosis is made by identifying the eggs in the perianal areas collected in the morning on sticky tape.

(3) Treatments

    (a) *S. pyogenes, S. pneumoniae:* Penicillin V 50 mg/kg/d QID for 10 days

    (b) *Shigella:* Trimethoprim/sulfamethoxazole 8/40 mg/kg/d for 7 days

    (c) *Candida:* Topical nystatin, miconazole, or clotrimazole cream

    (d) Pinworms: Mebendazole (Vermox) 100 mg orally at the time of diagnosis and at 1 to 2 weeks

    (e) For treatment of sexually transmitted diseases, see Table 17–2.

2. Other vaginal problems

    a. Chronic vaginal discharge: In the near pubescent girl, this is a normal physiologic leukorrhea. It starts before menarche in the form of a white mucoid watery or thick discharge. A wet mount shows only epithelial cells without inflammatory cells. It is self-limiting.

    b. Lichen sclerosis of the vulva: Characterized by small white patchy lesions involving the labia minora or majora, it may be symptomatic with pruritus, pain, dysuria, vaginal discharge, painful intercourse, and bleeding. Treatment is mainly symptomatic with topical corticosteroid cream and avoidance of trauma to the lesions. Referral to a dermatologist is recommended because the condition is usually chronic and adolescent and adult women need further counseling and treatment with regard to painful intercourse.

    c. Prepubertal vaginal bleeding: Most commonly a result of vulvovaginitis with group AB-strep and *Shigella* or scratching from pinworms. Precocious puberty, tumors, and sexual abuse are other less common etiologies that must be excluded. Foreign bodies inserted intravaginally may also cause bleeding without discharge.

    d. Amenorrhea

        (1) **Definitions**

            (a) *Primary amenorrhea* is the absence of any menstruation by the age of expected menarche (16 to 17 years in the United States) in the presence of breast development or by age 14 to 15 years in the absence of any breast development.

(b) *Secondary amenorrhea* is the post-menarchial cessation of menses for more than 6 consecutive months in those with previous regular menses or for more than 12 months in those with previous irregular menses. In the adolescent, the clinical approach to both primary and secondary amenorrhea are similar and are discussed together.

**(2)** Etiology

(a) Central causes: Hypothalamic causes are secondary to partial or complete inhibition of gonadotropin-releasing hormone (GnRH) release. This may be secondary to nutritional deficiencies, stress, endocrinopathies, specific drugs, or local lesions of the hypothalamus. Isolated GnRH deficiency is sometimes associated with absence of smell (anosmia; Kallman syndrome). Pituitary causes may be secondary to tumors, granulomas, or infarction. The most common cause of amenorrhea in reproductive-age women is the prolactin-secreting tumor, which is commonly associated with galactorrhea.

(b) Gonadal causes: Amenorrhea may be secondary to ovarian failure caused by gonadal dysgenesis, premature ovarian failure, infection, or hemorrhage, or following radiation therapy for childhood cancers. Over 10% of cases of primary amenorrhea are due to gonadal dysgenesis, including Turner (XO) syndrome. Anatomic defects may also be the cause of primary amenorrhea. These include imperforate hymen, vaginal atresia, or absence of the uterus, cervix, or both. Some rare but important causes of primary amenorrhea include gonadotropin-resistant ovary syndrome (abnormal ovarian receptors), defects in estrogen synthesis, and androgen insensitivity syndrome (abnormal androgen receptors). The latter two causes can result in an XY genotype, but a phenotypic female with primary amenorrhea.

(c) Evaluation: Physical examination includes assessment of Tanner

**Table 17–2. Treatment of sexually transmitted diseases (from http://www.cdc.gov/std/treatment/default.htm); California STD treatment guidelines for adults and adolescents 2002**

| Disease | Recommended Regimens | Dose/route | Alternative Regimens |
|---|---|---|---|
| **Chlamydia** | | | |
| Uncomplicated Infections Adults/Adolescents[1] | • Azithromycin **or**<br>• Doxycycline[2] | 1 g po<br>100 mg po bid × 7 d | • Erythromycin base 500 mg po qid × 7 d **or**<br>• Erythromycin ethylsuccinate 800 mg po qid × 7 d **or**<br>• Ofloxacin[2] 300 mg po bid × 7 d **or**<br>• Levofloxacin[2] 500 mg po qd × 7 d |
| Pregnant Women[3] | • Azithromycin **or**<br>• Amoxicillin **or**<br>• Erythromycin base | 1 g po<br>500 mg po tid × 7 d<br>500 mg po qid × 7 d | • Erythromycin base 250 mg po qid × 14 d **or**<br>• Erythromycin ethylsuccinate 800 mg po qid × 7 d **or**<br>• Erythromycin ethylsuccinate 400 mg po qid × 14 d |
| **Gonorrhea[4]** | | | |
| Uncomplicated Infections Adults/Adolescents | • Cefixime[5] **or**<br>• Ceftriaxone **plus**[4]<br>• A chlamydia regimen listed above | 400 mg po<br>125 mg IM | • Spectinomycin[4,5] 2 g IM **or**<br>• Ciprofloxacin[2,4,6] 500 mg po **or**<br>• Ofloxacin[2,4,6] 400 mg po **or**<br>• Levofloxacin[2,4,6] 250 mg po **or**<br>• Azithromycin[6] 2 g po |
| Pregnant Women | • Ceftriaxone **or**<br>• Cefixime[5] **plus**[4]<br>• A chlamydia regimen listed above | 125 mg IM<br>400 mg po | • Spectinomycin[4,5] 2 g IM |

| Disease | Recommended Regimens | Dose/route | Alternative Regimens |
|---|---|---|---|
| **Pelvic inflammatory disease[7]** | **Parenteral[8]** <br> • **Either** Cefotetan **or** Cefoxitin **plus** Doxycycline[2] **or** • Clindamycin **plus** Gentamicin | <br> 2 g IV q 12 hrs <br> 2 g IV q 6 hrs <br> 100 mg po or IV q 12 hrs <br> 900 mg IV q 8 hrs <br> 2 mg/kg IV or IM followed by 1.5 mg/kg IV or IM q 8 hrs | **Parenteral[8]** <br> • **Either** Ofloxacin[2,9] 400 mg IV q 12 hrs **or** Levofloxacin[2,9] 500 mg IV qd **plus** Metronidazole 500 mg IV q 8 hrs **or** • Ampicillin/Sulbactam 3 g IV q 6 hrs **plus** Doxycycline[2] 100 mg po or IV q 12 hrs |
| | **Oral/IM** <br> • **Either** Ceftriaxone **or** Cefoxitin **with** Probenecid **plus** Doxycycline[2] | <br> 250 mg IM <br> 2 g IM <br> 1 g po <br> 100 mg po bid × 14 d | **Oral** <br> • **Either** Ofloxacin[2,9] 400 mg po bid × 14 d **or** Levofloxacin[2,9] 500 mg po QD × 14 d **plus** Metronidazole 500 mg po bid × 14 d |
| **Mucopurulent cervicitis[7]** | • Azithromycin **or** • Doxycycline[2] | 1 g po <br> 100 mg po bid × 7 d | • Erythromycin base 500 mg po qid × 7 d **or** • Erythromycin ethylsuccinate 800 mg po qid × 7 d **or** • Ofloxacin[2,9] 300 mg po bid × 7 d **or** • Levofloxacin[2,9] 500 mg po qd × 7 days |
| **Nongonococcal urethritis[7]** | • Azithromycin **or** • Doxycycline | 1 g po <br> 100 mg po bid × 7 d | • Erythromycin base 500 mg po qid × 7 d **or** • Erythromycin ethylsuccinate 800 mg po qid × 7 d **or** • Ofloxacin 300 mg po bid × 7 d **or** • Levofloxacin 500 mg po qd × 7 days |

(*Continued*)

**Table 17–2.** (*Continued*)

| Disease | Recommended Regimens | Dose/route | Alternative Regimens |
|---|---|---|---|
| **Epididymitis**[7] | Likely due to gonorrhea or chlamydia | | |
| | • Ceftriaxone **plus** | 250 mg IM | |
| | Doxycycline | 100 mg po bid × 10 d | |
| | Likely due to enteric organisms | | |
| | • Ofloxacin[9] **or** | 300 mg po bid × 10 d | |
| | • Levofloxacin[9] | 500 mg po qd × 10 d | |
| **Trichomoniasis**[10] | • Metronidazole | 2 g po | • Metronidazole 500 mg po bid × 7 d |
| **Bacterial vaginosis** | | | |
| Adults/Adolescents | • Metronidazole **or** | 500 mg po bid × 7 d | • Metronidazole 2 g po **or** |
| | • Clindamycin cream[11] **or** | 2%, one full applicator (5 g) intravaginally qhs × 7 d | • Clindamycin 300 mg po bid × 7 d **or** |
| | | | • Clindamycin ovules 100 g intravaginally qhs × 3 d |
| | • Metronidazole gel | 0.75%, one full applicator (5 g) intravaginally qd × 5 d | |
| Pregnant Women | • Metronidazole **or** | 250 mg po tid × 7 d | |
| | • Clindamycin | 300 mg po bid × 7 d | |
| **Chancroid** | • Azithromycin **or** | 1 g po | • Erythromycin base 500 mg po tid × 7 d |
| | • Ceftriaxone **or** | 250 mg IM | |
| | • Ciprofloxacin[2] | 500 mg po bid × 3 d | |

| Disease | Recommended Regimens | Dose/route | Alternative Regimens |
|---|---|---|---|
| **Lymphogranuloma venereum** | • Doxycycline[2] | 100 mg po bid × 21 d | • Erythromycin base 500 mg po qid × 21 d **or** |
| | | | • Azithromycin 1 g po qd × 21 d |
| **Human papillomavirus** | | | |
| External Genital/Perianal Warts | **Patient Applied** | | **Alternative Regimen** |
| | • Podofilox[12] 0.5% solution or gel **or** | | • Intralesional interferon **or** |
| | • Imiquimod[13] 5% cream | | • Laser surgery |
| | **Provider Administered** | | |
| | • Cryotherapy **or** | | |
| | • Podophyllin[12] resin 10%–25% in tincture of benzoin **or** | | |
| | • Trichloroacetic acid (TCA) **or** Bichloroacetic acid (BCA) 80%–90% **or** | | |
| | • Surgical removal | | |
| Mucosal Genital Warts | • Cryotherapy **or** | Vaginal, urethral meatus, and anal | |
| | • TCA or BCA 80%–90% **or** | Vaginal and anal | |
| | • Podophyllin[12] resin 10%–25% in tincture of benzoin **or** | Urethral meatus only | |
| | • Surgical removal | Anal warts only | |

(Continued)

**Table 17-2.** (*Continued*)

| Disease | Recommended Regimens | Dose/route | Alternative Regimens |
|---|---|---|---|
| **Herpes simplex virus**[14] | | | |
| First Clinical Episode of Herpes | • Acyclovir **or** | 400 mg po tid × 7–10 d | |
| | • Acyclovir **or** | 200 mg po 5/day × 7–10 d | |
| | • Famciclovir **or** | 250 mg po tid × 7–10 d | |
| | • Valacyclovir | 1 g po bid × 7–10 d | |
| Episodic Therapy for Recurrent Episodes | • Acyclovir **or** | 400 mg po tid × 5 d | |
| | • Acyclovir **or** | 200 mg po 5/day × 5 d | |
| | • Acyclovir **or** | 800 mg po bid × 5 d | |
| | • Famciclovir **or** | 125 mg po bid × 5 d | |
| | • Valacyclovir **or** | 500 mg po bid × 3–5 d | |
| | • Valacyclovir | 1 g po qd × 5 d | |
| Suppressive Therapy | • Acyclovir **or** | 400 mg po bid | |
| | • Famciclovir **or** | 250 mg po bid | |
| | • Valacyclovir **or** | 500 mg po qd | |
| | • Valacyclovir | 1 g po qd | |
| **HIV Infection**[15] | | | |
| Episodic Therapy for Recurrent Episodes | • Acyclovir **or** | 400 mg po tid × 5–10 d | |
| | • Acyclovir **or** | 200 mg po 5/day × 5–10 d | |
| | • Famciclovir **or** | 500 mg po bid × 5–10 d | |
| | • Valacyclovir | 1 g po bid × 5–10 d | |
| Suppressive Therapy | • Acyclovir **or** | 400–800 mg po bid-tid | |
| | • Famciclovir **or** | 500 mg po bid | |
| | • Valacyclovir | 500 mg po bid | |

| Disease | Recommended Regimens | Dose/route | Alternative Regimens |
|---|---|---|---|
| **Syphilis** | | | |
| Primary, Secondary, and Early Latent | • Benzathine penicillin G | 2.4 million units IM | • Doxycycline[2,16] 100 mg po bid × 2 weeks **or**<br>• Tetracycline[2,16] 500 mg po qid × 2 weeks **or**<br>• Ceftriaxone[16] 1 g IM or IV qd × 8–10 d **or**<br>• Azithromycin[16] 2 g po |
| Late Latent and Unknown Duration | • Benzathine penicillin G | 7.2 million units, administered as 3 doses of 2.4 million units IM, at 1-week intervals | • Doxycycline[2] 100 mg po bid × 4 weeks **or**<br>• Tetracycline[2] 500 mg po qid × 4 weeks |
| Neurosyphilis[17] | • Aqueous crystalline penicillin G | 18–24 million units daily, administered as 3–4 million units IV q 4 hrs × 10–14 d | • Procaine penicillin G, 2.4 million units IM qd × 10–14 d **plus** Probenecid 500 mg po qid × 10–14 d **or**<br>• Ceftriaxone[16] 2 g IM or IV qd × 10–14 d |
| **Pregnant Women**[18] | | | |
| Primary, Secondary, and Early Latent | • Benzathine penicillin G | 2.4 million units IM | • None |
| Late Latent and Unknown Duration | • Benzathine penicillin G | 7.2 million units, administered as 3 doses of 2.4 million units IM, at 1-week intervals | • None |

(Continued)

**Table 17-2.** (Continued)

| Disease | Recommended Regimens | Dose/route | Alternative Regimens |
|---|---|---|---|
| Neurosyphilis[17] | • Aqueous crystalline penicillin G | 18–24 million units daily, administered as 3–4 million units IV q 4 hrs × 10–14 d | • Procaine penicillin G, 2.4 million units IM qd × 10–14 d **plus** Probenecid 500 mg po qid × 10–14 d |
| **HIV Infection** | | | |
| Primary, Secondary and Early Latent | • Benzathine penicillin G | 2.4 million units IM | • Doxycycline[2,16] 100 mg po bid × 2 weeks **or** • Tetracycline[2,16] 500 mg po qid × 2 weeks |
| Late Latent, and Unknown Duration[18] **with Normal CSF Exam** | • Benzathine penicillin G | 7.2 million units, administered as 3 doses of 2.4 million units IM, at 1-week intervals | • None |
| Neurosyphilis[17] | • Aqueous crystalline penicillin G | 18–24 million units daily, administered as 3–4 million units IV q 4 hrs × 10–14 d | • Procaine penicillin G, 2.4 million units IM qd × 10–14 d **plus** Probenecid 500 mg po qid × 10–14 d |

[1] Annual screening for women age 25 years or younger. Nucleic Acid Amplification Tests (NAATS) are recommended. Women with chlamydia should be rescreened 3–4 months after treatment.

[2] Contraindicated for pregnant and nursing women.

[3] Test-of-cure follow-up is recommended because the regimens are not highly efficacious (Amoxicillin and Erythromycin) or the data on safety and efficacy are limited (Azithromycin).

[4] Co-treatment for chlamydia infection is indicated unless chlamydia infection has been ruled out using sensitive technology or if 2g Azithromycin dose is used.

[5] Not recommended for pharyngeal gonococcal infection.

[6] Test-of-cure follow-up is recommended to ensure patient does not have an untreated infection from a resistant gonorrhea strain.

[7] Testing for gonorrhea and chlamydia is recommended because a specific diagnosis may improve compliance and partner management and these infections are reportable by California state law.

[8] Discontinue 24 hours after patient improves clinically and continue with oral therapy for a total of 14 days.

[9] If gonorrhea is documented, test-of-cure follow-up is recommended to ensure patient does not have untreated resistance gonorrhea infection.

[10] If reinfection is ruled out and persistance of trichomonas is documented, evaluate for metronidazole-resistant *T. vaginalis*. Referral to CDC at 770-488-4115 or 404-639-1898.

[11] Might weaken latex condoms and diaphragms because oil-based.

[12] Contraindicated during pregnancy.

[13] Safety in pregnancy has not been well established.

[14] Counseling about natural history, asymptomatic shedding, and sexual transmission is an essential component of herpes management.

[15] If lesions persist or recur while receiving antiviral treatment, HSV resistance should be suspected and a viral isolate should be obtained for sensitivity testing.

[16] Because efficacy of these therapies has not been established and compliance of some of these regimens difficult, close follow-up is essential. If compliance or follow-up cannot be ensured, then patient should be desensitized and treated with Benzathine penicillin.

[17] One dose of 2.4 million units of Benzathine penicillin G recommended at completion of neurosyphilis therapy.

[18] Patients allergic to penicillin should be treated with penicillin after desensitization.

stage, signs of androgen effects (hirsutism and acne), and estrogen effects (breast and vulvar development). Complete external and pelvic examinations should be performed. Laboratory tests include urine pregnancy test, LH, FSH, prolactin, and thyroid function tests. Serum testosterone may be checked if there are any signs of androgen excess. A hormonal challenge can also be performed utilizing oral medroxyprogesterone acetate. If there is no bleeding after the challenge, then an ultrasound should be performed to assess the pelvic organs. A karyotype is obtained in the absence of any combination of the uterus, vagina, or ovaries.

## RECOMMENDED READING

Kass EJ, Reitelman C. Adolescent varicocele. *Urol Clin North Am* 1995;22:151.

Moscicki A: Common menstrual problems. In: *Rudolph's Pediatrics,* 21st ed. Norwalk, Conn: Appleton & Lange, 2002:62. Miller WL. The endocrine system. In: Rudolph CD, Rudolph AM, Hostetter MK, et al, eds. *Rudolph's pediatrics,* 21st ed. New York: McGraw-Hill, 2002:2007–2164.

Skoog S, Scherz H: Office pediatric urology. In: Gillenwater JY, Grayhack JT, Howards SS, et al, eds. *Adult and Pediatric urology,* volume 3, 4th ed. Philadelphia: Lippincott Williams and Wilkins, 2002:2671–2718.

# Genitourinary Trauma and Priapism

Hubert S. Swana and James M. Betts

## I. INTRODUCTION

Five percent of all injured children sustain genitourinary trauma; 80% are due to blunt trauma and 20% due to penetrating trauma. A significant number of children also have associated life-threatening injuries to the central nervous system, and thoracic and abdominal organs. Once initial stabilization and resuscitation have occurred, a careful and directed secondary survey can detect genitourinary injuries.

A. **Renal Injury:** The kidney is the most commonly injured genitourinary organ. Blunt trauma represents 80% to 90% of all renal trauma in children. Of all patients with abdominal trauma—blunt and penetrating—8% to 12% have renal injuries. The pediatric kidney is more susceptible to injury because of its large proportional size compared to the adult organ. The underdeveloped abdominal wall muscles and lower ribs, and lack of perirenal fat do not provide as much protection for the pediatric kidney. In addition, congenital anomalies such as hydronephrosis and renal ectopia make a child's kidney more vulnerable to trauma.

1. Evaluation (Fig. 18–1)

   a. Blunt renal trauma: Any child with gross hematuria or microhematuria greater than 50 red blood cells per high-power field (RBCs/HPF) should be suspected of having a renal injury. Flank contusions, lower rib and vertebral fractures, and multisystem injuries after deceleration injuries should raise the suspicion for renal injury, even in the absence of hematuria. Careful attention should be placed on assessing the contralateral kidney.

   b. Penetrating renal trauma: Any child with hematuria and a penetrating injury to the flank, abdomen, or chest should be evaluated for the possibility of genitourinary injury. In stable children, contrast-enhanced computed tomography (CT) can be used. Intravenous pyelogram (IVP) is reserved for the rare intraoperative evaluation in severe trauma.

2. Management: More than 90% of blunt renal injuries can be managed nonoperatively. Patients can be kept on bed rest until the urine clears. The patient's hematocrit is monitored to determine if bleeding has subsided. Prophylactic antibiotics are given in the case of urinary extravasation and the

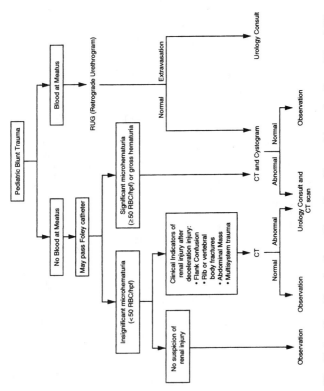

**Fig. 18–1. Algorithm for the systematic radiographic evaluation of the child with suspected urinary tract injury after blunt trauma.**

possibility of infected urine. Light activity is advised for 2 weeks to prevent delayed bleeding. An imaging study is obtained at 3 months to assess function and rule out hydronephrosis. Unstable patients and those with massive urinary extravasation or associated injuries may require additional interventions such as exploration with renal repair or removal, drainage, or angiographic embolization.

**B. Ureter:** Ureteral injuries are rare and most often due to gunshot or stab injuries. Severe blunt injuries can cause tearing and disruption of the ureteropelvic junction (Fig. 18–2).

    **1.** Evaluation: Ureteral injuries are frequently missed. One must maintain a high index of suspicion. Hematuria is present only 23% to 45% of the time.

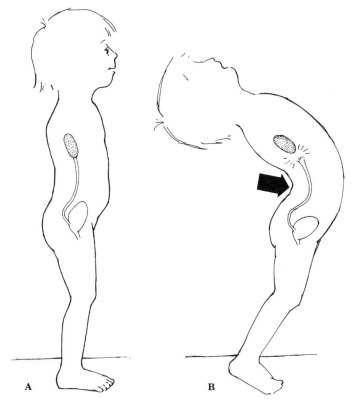

**Fig. 18–2. A:** Normal relation of the urinary tract to the spine in a child. **B:** With a sudden blow to the back, the ureter tenses against the hyperextended vertebral column and avulses at the uteropelvic junction.

Historically, IVP and CT may miss up to 75% of cases. Direct visualization at the time of surgery and retrograde pyelography are more reliable. Delayed imaging studies should be obtained in patients with unexplained abdominal findings after penetrating flank and abdominal trauma.

C.  **Bladder and Urethra:** The vast majority of bladder injuries occur after blunt abdominal trauma sustained in motor vehicle accidents. Of patients with bladder rupture, 89% have a pelvic fracture. Straddle injuries are a common cause of injury to the bulbar urethra. Posterior urethral injuries are associated with pelvic fracture. Blood at the urethral meatus is a harbinger of urethral injury.

1.  Evaluation: If blood is found at the urethral meatus, retrograde urethrography (RUG) should be performed. The patient is carefully placed in an oblique position. Elevation of one hip with a towel and 90 degree abduction of the downside leg is performed. A small catheter is advanced about 2 to 3 cm into the meatus. The balloon is filled with 1 cc of water to secure in place. Films are taken during injection of 20 cc of contrast material.

    If no meatal blood or urethral injury is identified, careful attempt at passing a well-lubricated catheter can be performed. If hematuria is discovered (>5 RBCs/HPF), a cystogram is performed. Complete imaging includes a lower abdominal scout film, a film after bladder distention, and a postdrainage film. Pediatric bladder capacity can be estimated using the following formula (maximum of 300 cc):

    $$[age(y) + 2] \times 30cc$$

2.  Management: If one finds urethral extravasation, immediate urologic consultation should be obtained. Suprapubic cystotomy may be required. Urologic consultation is advised for bladder rupture as well. Extraperitoneal ruptures may be treated with catheter drainage alone, whereas intraperitoneal ruptures require immediate surgical repair.

E.  **Scrotal and Penile Injury:** Scrotal and penile injuries usually occur with blunt injuries sustained in sports activities, straddle injuries, and bicycle falls. Scrotal hematomas can make assessment of testicular integrity difficult. Penile injuries can occur with blunt injuries such as toilet seats. Tourniquet injuries from hair, rubber bands, or entrapment in zippers are not uncommon. Penile lacerations can also be seen.

1.  Evaluation: Scrotal ultrasonography is very helpful in evaluating testicular integrity. The tunica albuginea can be carefully studied. Testicular rupture usually appears as an intratesticular area of

hypoechogenicity and discontinuity of the tunica albuginea.

Evaluation of penile injuries should assess the underlying corpora and urethra (by RUG) as well as the extent of skin defect. Penile fracture can occur after direct trauma to an erect penis, but is extremely rare in prepubertal boys.

2. Treatment: Scrotal hematomas with intact testicles can be managed with scrotal support, bed rest, and pain medications. Patients with testicular rupture should undergo emergent exploration and repair. Nonviable and extruded seminiferous tubules should be excised and closure of the tunica performed. The majority of patients managed emergently can avoid orchiectomy. Patients with tense scrotal wall hematomas may require delayed drainage.

Scrotal lacerations should be closed primarily with chromic catgut sutures after careful debridement and copious irrigation. If injury to the urethral or corpora is discovered, urologic consultation should be obtained.

F. **Vaginal Injuries:** Vaginal injuries may be associated with sexual abuse, foreign body insertion, or the same blunt pelvic forces that cause bladder and pelvic injuries.
   1. Evaluation: If multiple injuries are suspected, stabilization is paramount. Circumstances surrounding the trauma and careful medical historical review are necessary if abuse is suspected.
   2. Management: Vaginal laceration may require repair for hemostasis. Vaginoscopy, cystoscopy, and rectal examinations are necessary to ensure that bladder, vaginal urethral, and anorectal injuries are not overlooked.

II. **PRIAPISM**

*Priapism* is a condition characterized by a prolonged painful erection in the absence of sexual desire. It must be considered a urologic emergency because recurrent episodes can cause fibrosis and subsequent impotence. Prepubertal patients, if treated early, tend to have a better prognosis than adults.

A. **Etiology:** The most common cause of priapism in children is sickle-cell disease. Up to 5% of boys with sickle-cell disease have priapism. Priapism can occur as an isolated event or with other manifestations of sickle-cell crisis. Sludging of sickle cells impairs venous outflow. Leukemia is another important cause of priapism. Here abnormal (leukemic) cells impair penile venous drainage. For these reasons, a complete blood count must be obtained early in the evaluation of the priapism patient.

B. **Treatment:** Initial treatment is usually directed at the underlying cause. For patients with sickle-cell disease, increase the ratio of normal hemoglobin to hemoglobin S with transfusions or exchange pheresis. Additionally, hydration, alkalinization, and analgesia should be used.

When priapism persists despite these measures, surgical intervention may be necessary. Options include corporal aspiration, irrigation, and glans-cavernosal shunting.

## RECOMMENDED READING

Armenakas NA, Duckett CP, McAninch JW. Indications for nonoperative management of renal stab wounds. *J Urol* 1999;161:768–771.

Peterson NE: Genitourinary trauma. In: Feliciano DV, Moore EE, Mattox KL, eds. *Trauma*, 3rd ed. Stamford, Conn: Appleton & Lange; 1996:661–694.

Velmahos GC, Degiannis E. *The management of urinary tract injuries after gunshot wounds of the anterior and posterior abdominal wall injury.* Los Angeles: University of Southern California and Johannesburg, South Africa: University of Witwatersrand, 1997:535–538.

# Hematuria

Robert S. Mathias

*Hematuria* in children is defined as the finding of greater than 5 red blood cells per high-power field (RBCs/HPF) in the urine on microscopic examination. Most children with hematuria have a benign condition that requires no intervention and that has an excellent prognosis. Because the finding of isolated microscopic hematuria is frequently transient, we recommend documentation on at least two of three consecutive urinalyses a few weeks apart before pursuing further workup. Hematuria may be microscopic (typically found in asymptomatic children discovered by routine dipstick screening of urine) or macroscopic, also called *gross* (apparent to the eye as a bright red or brownish discoloration of the urine). When positive, urine dipstick reagents change color and are indicative of the presence of RBCs (at least 5 RBCs/HPF), hemoglobin, or myoglobin. To distinguish them, microscopic examination should be performed on a properly centrifuged, freshly obtained urine specimen (15 mL of urine spun at 2,000 RPM for 5 minutes) to confirm the presence of RBCs, before the diagnosis of hematuria is made. Diagnostic studies should be reserved for those patients who by history, physical examination, and initial laboratory screening tests are deemed to be at high risk for serious renal or urologic disease. Causes of hematuria in children are listed in Table 19–1.

## I. EVALUATION

A. **History** In addition to determining the type, duration, and the pattern of the hematuria, a complete history of previous illnesses and associated genitourinary symptoms, medication use, and activity are essential in the workup of a child. Important historical and familial features, and the possible corresponding diseases are listed in Table 19–2.

B. **Physical Examination** (Distinguishing features on examination and the corresponding diseases are listed in Table 19–3.)

1. Blood pressure should be measured in all children regardless of age, using an appropriately sized cuff.

2. Growth parameters should be plotted on standardized growth charts.

3. Assessment of patient's skin for rash, petechiae, purpura, pallor, or edema.

4. Abdominal examination should evaluate for palpable masses, signs of trauma, and localization of pain or tenderness.

5. Assessment of external genitalia for signs of inflammation, trauma, or the presence of a foreign body.

## Table 19–1.   Causes of hematuria

A. Glomerular disease
   Benign familial hematuria/thin basement membrane disease
   Alport syndrome
   Acute postinfectious or chronic glomerulonephritis
   IgA nephropathy
   Membranoproliferative glomerulonephritis
   Systemic vasculitis: Henoch–Schönlein purpura, systemic lupus
      erythematosus, Wegener granulomatosis, microscopic
      polyangiitis nodosa
   Hemolytic uremic syndrome
B. Interstitial disease
   Interstitial nephritis
   Pyelonephritis
   Acute tubular necrosis
   Polycystic kidney disease: autosomal dominant, autosomal
      recessive
   Wilms tumor
   Hydronephrosis
   Nephrocalcinosis
C. Nonrenal disease
   Vascular thrombosis: renal artery or vein
   Sickle-cell disease/trait
   Vigorous exercise
   Trauma
   Tumors
   Coagulopathy
D. Lower urinary tract
   Urinary tract infection/cystitis
   Hypercalciuria
   Nephrolithiasis
   Perineal irritation
   Hemorrhagic cystitis
   Foreign body (urethra)

**B   Laboratory Investigation**
   1.   Once the diagnosis of hematuria is confirmed on at
        least two separate occasions over a 2- to 3-week
        period, a complete urinalysis should be obtained.
        *Macroscopic* or *gross hematuria* is classically associ-
        ated with hematuria of glomerular origin. In cases
        of brownish, tea-colored, or coca-cola–colored hema-
        turia, glomerular disease is supported by the addi-
        tional findings of proteinuria, hypertension, edema,
        or azotemia. *Macroscopic hematuria of extrarenal
        origin* is bright red and frequently associated with
        pain and blood clots. The examination of urinary
        RBC morphology by microscopy can be helpful in
        determining their site of origin; that is, glomerular
        versus nonglomerular. As RBCs pass through small
        disruptions in the glomerular capillary wall due
        to glomerular disease, RBCs become dysmorphic

**Table 19–2.   Historical features and associated diseases**

| Patient History | Associated Disease |
|---|---|
| Urinary frequency, dysuria, suprapubic, costovertebral or flank pain | Urinary tract infection, pyelonephritis, nephrolithiasis |
| Previous illness (respiratory, throat, or skin) | Postinfectious glomerulonephritis IgA nephropathy |
| Gross hematuria | Urinary tract infection Perineal irritation Trauma Nephrolithiasis IgA nephropathy Postinfectious glomerulonephritis Benign urethralgia |
| Medications (penicillin, nonsteroidal antiinflammatory drugs, protease inhibitors) | Interstitial nephritis |
| Cough, hemoptysis | Systemic lupus erythematosus, Wegener granulomatosis, microscopic polyangiitis nodosa |
| Trauma | Kidney contusion |
| **Family History** | |
| Microscopic hematuria | Benign familial hematuria Alport syndrome Hypercalciuria Nephrolithiasis |
| Hearing loss | Alport syndrome |
| Renal disease (insufficiency, dialysis, or transplantation) | Alport syndrome Polycystic kidney disease |
| Urolithiasis | Hypercalciuria |
| Sickle-cell disease | Sickle-cell nephropathy |

with distorted and irregular contours. Although phase-contrast microscopy is the traditional method for examining RBC morphology in urine specimens, many clinicians can evaluate the morphology on routine microscopy. RBCs with normal morphology represent hematuria of nonglomerular origin. The finding of urinary RBC casts is diagnostic of glomerular disease and is not seen with extrarenal bleeding. Mild proteinuria from the release of hemoglobin from RBCs may be found in all types of hematuria.

2. Children with gross or persistent hematuria (urine dipstick with heme 1+ or greater on two separate occasions over a 2- to 3-week period) warrant further diagnostic evaluation; an algorithm for laboratory tests is provided in Fig. 19–1.

**Table 19–3.   Physical findings and associated diseases**

| Physical Examination | Associated Disease |
|---|---|
| Hypertension | Chronic renal insufficiency |
| | Polycystic kidney disease |
| | Reflux nephropathy |
| Failure to thrive | Chronic renal insufficiency |
| Rash (petechiae, purpura, malar) | Henoch–Schönlein purpura |
| | Systemic lupus erythematosus |
| Edema | Proteinuria/nephrotic syndrome |
| | Fluid retention/acute renal failure |
| Abdominal mass | Polycystic kidney disease |
| | Hydronephrosis |
| | Tumor |
| Costovertebral or suprapubic pain | Urinary tract infection |
| | Pyelonephritis |
| Pallor | Hemolytic uremic syndrome |
| | Chronic glomerulonephritis |
| | Chronic renal insufficiency |

3. The remainder of the urinalysis provides information that may be helpful in determining the cause of persistent hematuria (Table 19–4). Of importance are the findings of leukocytes (infection, interstitial nephritis), bacteria (infection), white blood cell (WBC) casts (pyelonephritis), RBC casts (acute glomerulonephritis, other glomerular diseases), proteinuria (quantity; nephrotic versus nonnephrotic amount), and dysmorphic RBCs (renal versus nonrenal origin). If the urine dipstick or microscopic evaluation reveals evidence of an infection, a urine culture is warranted. If glomerulonephritis is suspected, measurements of serum creatinine, serum complement 3 ($C_3$), CBC, antistreptolysin (ASO), and antideoxyribonuclease B (anti-DNAase B) titers should be determined. Other screening tests should also include both the measurement of the ratio of the urine calcium to urine creatinine and the checking of other family members for the presence of hematuria. For patients with persistent hematuria and proteinuria, significant proteinuria (spot protein to creatinine ratio above 0.5 to 1.0 in the urine) or nephrotic syndrome, elevated serum creatinine, hypertension, or a low $C_3$ levels 8 to 10 after presentation should be referred to a pediatric nephrologist for further evaluation and potential renal biopsy. If the initial screening tests are normal in a patient with persistent asymptomatic microscopic hematuria, no further diagnostic evaluation is necessary and the

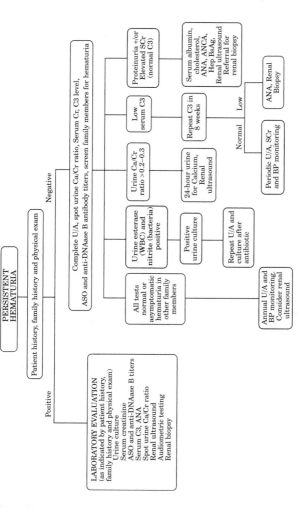

**Fig. 19-1. Treatment algorithm for the child with hematuria.** *Abbreviations:* **ANA**, antinuclear antibody; **ANCA**, antineutrophilic cytoplasmic autoantibody; **ASO**, antistreptolysin; **BP**, blood pressure; **C3**, serum complement 3; **Ca/Cr**, calcium, creatinine; **HBsAg**, hepatitis B surface antigen; **SCr**, serum creatinine; **U/A**, urinalysis.

**Table 19–4.** **Additional laboratory evaluation**

| Laboratory Screen | Further Diagnostic Tests |
| --- | --- |
| Urine dipstick | |
|   Nitrite and Esterase positive | Urine culture |
|   Proteinuria (normal $C_3$) | Serum albumin; hepatitis B surface antigen; cholesterol; 24-h collection for protein; renal ultrasound; consider renal biopsy |
| Urine microscopic examination | |
|   WBCs, bacteria, WBC casts | Urine culture |
|   Dysmorphic RBCs, RBC casts | Serum creatinine, CBC, $C_3$, ASO and anti-DNAase B titers |
| Urine calcium/creatinine ratio $\geq 0.2–0.3$ | 24-h collection for calcium, serum bicarbonate, urine pH, renal ultrasound |
| Persistent low $C_3$ (>8 wk) | ASO and anti-DNAase B titers, ANA |

patient should have an annual urinalysis and blood pressure measurement.

## II. ETIOLOGY

The more common diseases causing hematuria in children are discussed briefly. For each patient, a differential diagnosis can be made based on the knowledge of the likely etiologies and their characteristic features.

### A. Glomerular Basement Disorders

1. Benign familial hematuria (thin basement membrane disease)

    a. In children and young adults, this condition manifests as persistent microscopic hematuria in the absence or presence of mild proteinuria. This condition differs from Alport Syndrome as follows

     (1) Deafness and ocular abnormalities are not seen;

     (2) Deterioration of renal function is rare; and

     (3) thickening and splitting of the glomerular basement membrane are not seen in renal biopsy specimens examined by electron microscopy (although renal biopsy is only rarely indicated in these patients).

    b. In a patient with persistent microscopic hematuria, the diagnosis of benign familial hematuria should be strongly considered when either the screening of family members by urine dipstick is positive for blood or the family history reveals microscopic hematuria without deafness or progressive renal insufficiency. No particular mode of inheritance has been elucidated in this disease even though it is known to cluster in families. This diagnosis is usually made on clinical grounds; however, definitive diagnosis requires examination of renal tissue for electron microscopy obtained by biopsy (peripheral glomerular capillary basement membrane shows decreased thickness of 265 nmole or less). Despite the persistence of microscopic hematuria for many years, this condition is benign and nonprogressive, and therefore requires no therapy.

2. Alport syndrome

  a. Alport syndrome (hereditary nephritis) is characterized by renal disease that initially includes hematuria and proteinuria, and later, progressive renal insufficiency. Alport syndrome is caused by a mutation in the type IV collagen gene that leads to an abnormal basement membrane. Other involvement includes sensorineural deafness and ocular abnormalities. Boys are more severely affected than girls. Because there are no specific laboratory findings in this disease, the definitive diagnosis requires a renal biopsy. In most cases, however, Alport syndrome can be diagnosed clinically in a child with microscopic hematuria in whom a positive family history of either Alport syndrome or sensorineural deafness with progressive renal insufficiency is obtained. Such children should undergo audiologic evaluation.

  b. Because there is no known therapy that alters the progressive course of Alport nephritis, the management of these patients requires close attention to those abnormalities associated with renal insufficiency. For those patients whose disease progresses to end-stage renal failure, renal replacement therapy includes dialysis or kidney transplantation.

B. **Glomerulonephritis**

1. Glomerulonephritis is defined histologically as inflammation of the glomeruli and can be acute, subacute, or chronic. Clinical features of acute glomerulonephritis include both macroscopic and microscopic hematuria, including the presence of red blood cell casts, proteinuria, edema, oliguria, hypertension, and increased serum levels of both urea nitrogen and creatinine (azotemia). Although the classic form of glomerulonephritis, acute poststreptococcal glomerulonephritis (APSGN), often presents as a serious illness with many of these features; glomerulonephritis may also be detected incidentally by the findings of microscopic hematuria or proteinuria on a routine urinalysis.

2. The glomerulonephritides have been classified histologically, with the different types defined by characteristic patterns observed on renal biopsy. These

types can exist as primary renal diseases or as renal manifestations of systemic diseases. The causes of most forms of glomerulonephritis, whether intrinsic to the kidney or as part of a systemic disease, are unknown, but their pathogenesis often involves immune-mediated mechanisms, such as the glomerular deposition of antigen–antibody complexes. Although the prognosis of most of the glomerulonephritides is better in children than in adults, chronic glomerulonephritis is nevertheless one of the most common causes of end-stage renal disease in older children and adolescents. The two most common forms of glomerulonephritis in children, APSGN and IgA nephropathy, are discussed below. For those cases of glomerulonephritis with significant renal involvement, see Chapters 22 and 23 for the management of acute or chronic renal failure.

  **a.** APSGN

    **(1)** After throat or skin infections with certain strains of group A streptococci, glomerulonephritis may develop after a latent period of 1 to 3 weeks. APSGN is primarily a disease of children, with a peak incidence at age 7 years; it is rare in infants. Boys are affected twice as commonly as girls. The disease can present in both sporadic and epidemic forms. The pathogenesis is incompletely understood, but appears to involve the deposition of a streptococcal antigen in the glomeruli with subsequent inflammatory reaction. APSGN is a diffuse, proliferative glomerulonephritis and is the classic example of this pathologic form, although the same pathology also can be observed in glomerulonephritis that follows other bacterial and viral infections. There is marked variability in the clinical presentation and course of the disease, although the majority of patients present acutely with hematuria (more often tea-colored gross, rather than microscopic), hypertension, oliguria with edema, and azotemia. The signs and symptoms of nephritis usually subside within 1 to 2 weeks, although microscopic hematuria and, especially, low-grade proteinuria may persist for months or even years. Complete recovery occurs in more than 95% of children.

    **(2)** In addition to nonspecific laboratory findings that include mild anemia and increased serum levels of creatinine and urea nitrogen, the diagnosis of APSGN depends on the demonstration of elevated serum titers of antibodies against streptococcal antigens (pharyngitis, ASO; impetigo, anti-DNAase B titers) and decreased $C_3$ levels. $C_3$ levels return to normal within 8 to 12 weeks of onset; however, antibody titers to streptococcal antigens remain elevated for 4 to 6 months. If the $C_3$ level remains persistently low after 8 to 12 weeks from onset, this would suggest that the glomerulonephritis is associated with systemic lupus erythematosus (SLE) or membranoproliferative glomerulonephritis (MPGN). Because the majority of patients with PSAGN recover completely, a renal biopsy is not necessary. However, a renal biopsy should be considered when the $C_3$ level remains decreased for longer than 8 to 12 weeks or if there is persistent azotemia, significant proteinuria, or hypertension.

(3) Most patients receive symptomatic treatment for fluid retention, which includes salt and fluid restriction, and for hypertension, which includes the use of diuretics, such as furosemide, and antihypertensive drugs, such as hydralazine and nifedipine. If a streptococcal infection is still present, antibiotics are indicated but they do not shorten the duration of the nephritis.

**b.** IgA nephropathy

(1) IgA nephropathy is the most common cause of glomerulonephritis and is primarily a disease of children and young adults; it is rare in infants. Boys are affected twice as frequently as girls. The etiology and pathogenesis are unknown. The typical presentation features intermittent and recurrent episodes of macroscopic hematuria, or the finding of microscopic hematuria with or without proteinuria on routine urinalysis; the former usually occurs during or shortly after an upper respiratory tract infection and spontaneously resolves after several days. In most children with IgA nephropathy, blood pressure and renal function are normal at the time of diagnosis. However, a small percentage of affected children can present with acute glomerulonephritis or nephrotic syndrome and are at risk of progression to complete renal failure after the onset of disease.

(2) Although the definitive diagnosis by renal biopsy reveals deposition of IgA in

glomeruli on immunofluorescence, the pattern of gross hematuria occurring in association with upper respiratory infection is so characteristic of IgA nephropathy that a presumptive diagnosis can be made without a renal biopsy. However, this pattern also occurs in children with hereditary nephritis (Alport syndrome), Henoch–Schönlein nephritis and, rarely, in benign familial hematuria. Patients who present with gross hematuria characteristic of IgA nephropathy and nephrotic range proteinuria (greater than 3.5 g or 50 mg/kg per 24 hours), azotemia, or hypertension are at risk for a poorer outcome and may require a renal biopsy for prognosis and guidance of therapy. Unfortunately, there are no controlled studies demonstrating a beneficial effect of treatment on either the acute or long-term course of patients with IgA nephropathy. Nonetheless, corticosteroids in patients with poor prognostic features are often used. Patients with IgA nephropathy require close, long-term follow-up.

c. MPGN

   (1) MPGN is one of the less common causes of glomerulonephritides and it affects both children and young adults. Renal involvement is variable in this disease and includes asymptomatic microscopic hematuria, proteinuria, nephrotic syndrome, and acute and chronic glomerulonephritis. Diagnosis is made by renal biopsy and further classified into subtypes (types 1, 2, and 3) by histologic, immunofluorescence, and electron microscopy findings. Renal biopsy is typically performed in any patient with persistent renal involvement and a blood $C_3$ level that remains low for more than 8 weeks.

   (2) The pathogenesis of this disease is unknown. However, there is a significant proportion of cases with MPGN type I associated with hepatitis C infection. Although there is some suggestion that children may respond to alternate-day corticosteroids, the majority of cases fail to respond to any therapy. In most children, the renal disease is usually chronic and there is progression to renal failure.

d. Systemic vasculitis

   (1) Henoch–Schönlein purpura is a multisystem vasculitis seen commonly in children and rarely in adults. It typically involves

the skin (palpable purpura most commonly affecting the lower limbs), kidney (hematuria, proteinuria, or glomerulonephritis), musculoskeletal system (joint pain or swelling), and gastrointestinal tract (vomiting or abdominal pain). The testes may also be affected. This disease is often preceded by an intercurrent illness. Because both the renal manifestations and the renal biopsy findings are similar to those found in IgA nephropathy (see above), the diagnosis is often made on clinical evidence of extrarenal involvement. Therapy is supportive and in severe cases corticosteroids may be an effective treatment, similar to IgA nephropathy.

(2) SLE: Renal involvement in SLE can present with asymptomatic microscopic hematuria, proteinuria, nephrotic syndrome, or acute glomerulonephritis. Although SLE is most common in adult women, it can present in adolescence. If SLE is suspected by history (rash, joint complaints, etc.), physical examination, and laboratory tests (persistently low $C_3$ level), additional blood tests should include an antinuclear antibody and an anti-dsDNA antibody. In any patient with SLE and an abnormal urinalysis, including isolated microscopic hematuria, renal biopsy is warranted. The histologic classification on renal biopsy, in addition to clinical symptomatology and laboratory findings, is used as a guide in determining the treatment (corticosteroids, cyclophosphamide, mycophenolate mofetil) for SLE.

(3) Wegener granulomatosis/microscopic polyangiitis nodosa: These disorders are caused by small vessel vasculitides and account for a large percentage of rapidly progressive glomerulonephritis found in children. Similar to postinfectious glomerulonephritis, these disorders can present with microscopic hematuria, proteinuria, nephrotic syndrome, or acute glomerulonephritis. Extrarenal involvement in Wegener granulomatosis usually involves upper respiratory tract (sinusitis) and lower respiratory tract (cough with pulmonary hemorrhage often associated with granulomatous lesions) and arthralgias. In contrast, microscopic polyangiitis nodosa involves the skin (palpable purpura),

neurologic (mononeuritis multiplex), and arthralgias; in some cases, lower respiratory tract (pulmonary hemorrhage) can be involved. Renal biopsy often shows focal or diffuse proliferative glomerulonephritis with extensive crescent formation. Serologically, these disorders are linked with the presence of antineutrophil cytoplasmic antibodies (ANCA). In Wegener granulomatosis, the antibody staining is directed against the neutrophil cytoplasm (termed C-ANCA) with antigen specificity for proteinase 3 on enzyme-linked immunosorbent assay. For microscopic polyangitis nodosa, the antibody staining is perinuclear (termed P-ANCA) with antigen specificity for myeloperoxidase. For severe disease, treatment involves corticosteroids, cyclophosphamide, and, in some cases, plasmapheresis.

**C. Urinary Tract Infection** (see Chapter 6)
**D. Hypercalciuria or Nephrolithiasis**

   **a.** *Hypercalciuria* is urinary calcium excretion of greater than 4 mg/kg per day. Idiopathic hypercalciuria can result from either excessive gastrointestinal absorption of dietary calcium or from a renal leak of calcium due to decreased tubular reabsorption. The hematuria associated with hypercalciuria is painless and can be either microscopic or macroscopic; the bleeding is thought to result from mechanical trauma to renal cells caused by calcium crystals. Typically, red blood cell casts and proteinuria are absent. On the other hand, nephrolithiasis is rare in children and its presentation is quite varied. Similar to hypercalciuria, the patient may have asymptomatic microscopic hematuria but more often presents with renal colic, abdominal pain, or gross hematuria. The child's medical history may provide significant clues to an underlying condition that predisposes stone formation.

   **b.** To screen for hypercalciuria, a random urine sample is obtained for the calculation of the ratio of urine calcium concentration to that of urine creatinine concentration. A ratio of greater than 0.2 to 0.5 (age dependent) in a fasting morning specimen suggests excessive urinary calcium excretion. To confirm the positive screening test, a more accurate assessment is a 24-hour urine collection that should be obtained in an age-appropriate patient to determine the calcium excretion rate. A calcium excretion of greater than 4 mg/kg per day is considered abnormal. Additional tests to rule out other causes of hypercalciuria should include the serum level of calcium, phosphorus, vitamin D, and parathyroid hormone. A medication history is important to look for the administration of diuretics (furosemide). For example, furosemide therapy in infants with bronchopulmonary dysplasia can cause long-term hypercalciuria and lead to significant rickets of the long bones. A renal ultrasound should be performed at baseline to determine whether nephrocalcinosis or medullary sponge kidney is present. If nephrocalcinosis is found, a serum bicarbonate level and serum pH should be also measured to rule out renal tubular acidosis. Renal ultrasound can detect some stones not visualized on plain radiography; however, the study of choice is a noncontrast spiral CT scan of the abdomen.

  **c.** In isolated hypercalciuria, therapy is generally conservative and includes dietary salt restriction, which by decreasing urinary sodium excretion decreases calcium excretion. Intake of large volumes of oral fluids is recommended because this will dilute urinary calcium and avoid supersaturation, a condition necessary for stone formation. In particular, water or fresh lemonade (to increase urinary citrate levels because citrate is an inhibitor of stone formation) are the best fluids. Hypercalciuric children with nephrocalcinosis or a history of passage of renal stones may require thiazide diuretics, if limitation of sodium does not result in resolution of the hypercalciuria. Thiazide diuretics increase calcium reabsorption in the distal tubule resulting in reduced calcium excretion by the kidney. Large ureteral stones that do not pass require further evaluation by pediatric urologists with experience in endosurgical or lithotripsy intervention.

**D. Other Causes**

  **a.** A history of strenuous exercise, blunt trauma to the abdomen, or a bleeding disorder should be apparent as potential etiologies of isolated hematuria. The occurrence of macroscopic hematuria following minimal trauma to the kidney should raise the possibility of hydronephrosis or a cystic kidney. Blacks or any patient at risk for carrying the sickle cell trait should be tested for the presence of hemoglobin S. Heterozygotes as well as homozygotes for hemoglobin S can develop hematuria due to decreased medullary blood flow as a result of hypoxia and hypertonicity that induces sickling of RBCs within the renal medulla. This results in dilated capillaries in the pelvic mucosa, that can become congested and rupture, the presumed origin of the hematuria.

  **b.** Isolated hematuria, or in rare instances, associated with proteinuria and reduced renal function, can be caused by interstitial nephritis secondary to medications. Medications associated with this condition include nonsteroidal antiinflammatory agents, protease inhibitors, penicillin, cephalosporins, phenytoin, cimetidine, furosemide, and thiazide diuretics.

A history of recent or current use of one of these medications in a patient with hematuria should strongly support this diagnosis. In the majority of patients, withdrawal of the medication results in resolution of the urinary abnormalities.

## RECOMMENDED READING

Diven SC, Travis BT. A practical primary care approach to hematuria in children. *Pediatr Nephrol* 2000;14:65–72.

Patel HP, Bissler JJ. Hematuria in children. *Pediatr Clin North Am* 2001;48:1519–1537.

Trompeter R, Barratt T. Clinical evaluation. In: Holliday M, Barratt T, Avner E, eds. *Pediatric nephrology.* Baltimore: Williams & Wilkins; 1994:366–377.

West C. Asymptomatic hematuria and proteinuria in children: causes and appropriate diagnostic studies. *J Pediatr* 1976;89:173–182.

# Urolithiasis in Children: Medical Management

Anthony A. Portale

Urolithiasis in children is a relatively uncommon problem as compared with that in adult patients. In the northeastern United States, urolithiasis accounts for about 1 in 1,300 pediatric hospital admissions, a rate approximately one-tenth that noted among American adult patients. In parts of North America, notably the southeastern United States, stone disease is endemic. In the majority of children in the United States, urolithiasis is associated with an underlying metabolic disorder or urinary tract malformation, whereas in the majority of European children, urolithiasis is associated with urinary tract infection. This chapter reviews the presentation, causes, evaluation, and treatment of urolithiasis in children.

I. **PATHOPHYSIOLOGY**
  The following factors are known to affect the formation of stones in the urinary tract:
  A. **Supersaturation of urinary solutes:** When the concentration of certain solutes in the urine exceeds its equilibrium solubility product, spontaneous formation of stone crystals can occur. The following metabolic abnormalities are associated with increased urinary solute concentration and thus a predisposition to supersaturation and thereby stone formation.
     1. Hypercalciuria
     2. Hyperoxaluria
     3. Hypocitraturia
     4. Hyperuricuria
     5. Cystinuria
     6. Low urine volume
  B. **Decreased urinary inhibitors of crystallization:** At any given level of urinary supersaturation, spontaneous nucleation or further growth of preexisting crystals depends on the presence in the urine of substances that inhibit crystal growth. Inhibitors of urinary crystallization are listed below.
     1. Ions: magnesium, citrate, pyrophosphate
     2. Macromolecules: nephrocalcin, Tamm-Horsfall glycoprotein
     3. Glycosaminoglycans
  C. **Urinary pH:** Urine pH influences saturation by either increasing or decreasing the solubility of potential stone-forming solutes. Solubility of the following substances is *enhanced* at the indicated pH ranges.

    **1.** Calcium phosphate: pH above 6.0
    **2.** Uric acid: pH 6.0 to 7.0
    **3.** Cystine: pH above 7.4
    **4.** Calcium oxalate: no effect of pH within physiologic range

**D. Other Predisposing Factors**
    **1.** Developmental anomalies of the urinary tract can predispose to stone formation by promoting urinary stasis and thereby infection.
    **2.** Urinary tract infection, or the presence of foreign body, can cause uroepithelial damage and thereby predispose to stone formation by acting as a nidus on which crystal formation can occur.
    **3.** Positive family history.

## II. INITIAL MANIFESTATIONS

Urolithiasis in children can present with the following clinical features, with their approximate incidence.

**A. Pain:** 45% to 50%
**B. Hematuria:** 35% to 40%
**C. Incidental x-ray findings:** 15%
**D. Symptoms of infection:** 10% to 15%
**E. Positive family history:** 35% to 40%

The frequency of these findings varies with age, with pain being three times more common in adolescents than young children. Classic flank pain is not commonly seen in children, particularly those under 5 years of age. Symptoms of infection are fever, dysuria, frequency, or urgency.

## III. LOCATION OF GENITOURINARY STONES AND APPROXIMATE FREQUENCY

**A. Kidney:** unilateral or bilateral, 78%
**B. Ureter:** 5%
**C. Kidney and ureter:** 4%
**D. Bladder:** 9%
**E. Urethra:** 2%
**F. Ileal conduit:** 2%

## IV. CHEMICAL COMPOSITION OF URINARY STONES

**A. Calcium oxalate:** 45%
**B. Calcium phosphate:** 24%
**C. Magnesium ammonium nitrate** (struvite): 17%
**D. Cystine:** 8%
**E. Uric acid:** 2%
**F. Mixed:** 3%
**G. Other:** 1%

The incidence of struvite stones is approximately twofold higher in children 0 to 5 years of age than in adolescent patients. This reflects a higher association of urinary tract infection with stones in infants than in older children.

## V. CLINICAL DISORDERS ASSOCIATED WITH UROLITHIASIS

**A. Metabolic Disorders**
    **1.** Hypercalciuric states
        **a.** Idiopathic hypercalciuria
        **b.** Primary hyperparathyroidism
        **c.** Renal tubular acidosis

       **d.** Corticosteroid excess
       **e.** Immobilization
       **f.** Medullary sponge kidney
       **g.** Phosphorus depletion
       **h.** Vitamin D intoxication
       **i.** Idiopathic hypercalcemia of infancy
       **j.** Hyperthyroidism
       **k.** Hypothyroidism
       **l.** Malignancy
       **m.** Bartter syndrome
       **n.** Furosemide use in infants
       **o.** Sarcoidosis
    **2.** Hyperoxaluria
       **a.** Primary hereditary hyperoxaluria
       **b.** Enteric hyperoxaluria
    **3.** Cystinuria
    **4.** Hyperuricuria
       **a.** Leukemia, lymphoma
       **b.** Idiopathic, familial
       **c.** Inborn error of metabolism: hypoxanthine-guanine phosphoribosyltransferase deficiency
       **d.** Glycogen storage disease, type 1
    **5.** Hypocitraturia
       **a.** Renal tubular acidosis
       **b.** Medullary sponge kidney
       **c.** Malabsorption syndromes
    **6.** Xanthinuria
    **7.** Orotic aciduria
  **B.** **Abnormalities of the Urinary Tract**
    **1.** Ureteropelvic junction obstruction
    **2.** Vesicoureteral reflux
    **3.** Neurogenic bladder
    **4.** Hydronephrosis
    **5.** Ileal conduit, ureterosigmoidostomy
    **6.** Bladder exstrophy
    **7.** Other: duplication of the collecting system, bladder diverticula, multiple anomalies

**VI. EVALUATION OF THE CHILD WITH UROLITHIASIS**
  **A.** Initial evaluation focuses on a search for an underlying metabolic disorder or structural anomaly of the urinary tract because these predisposing conditions are present in the majority of children.
  **B.** A positive family history, present in approximately one-third of children with stones, can give clues to the underlying cause.
  **C.** Children with stones should undergo the following evaluation.
    **1.** History and family history: The following historical features are important.
       **a.** Recurrent urinary tract infection
       **b.** Infection with urea-splitting organisms (proteus)
       **c.** Recurrent abdominal pain

   **d.** Dysuria without infection
   **e.** Recurrent macroscopic or persistent microscopic hematuria
   **f.** Documented passage of calculus or gravel
   **g.** Heavy crystaluria
   **h.** Positive family history
   **i.** Also important are a history of chronic disease, prior urologic surgery, recent immobilization, diuretic use, or vitamin D intake.
**2.** Physical examination, including blood pressure, height, weight
**3.** Biochemical evaluation of blood and urine (Table 20–1)

**Table 20–1. Initial laboratory evaluation of the child with urolithiasis**

---

Serum
   CBC, electrolytes, BUN, creatinine, calcium, phosphorus, alkaline phosphatase, uric acid, total protein, albumin, intact PTH
Urine
   Urinalysis
   Urine culture and sensitivity
   Second morning urine sample for calcium:creatinine ratio
   *24-h urine collection for calcium, phosphorus, magnesium, oxalate, uric acid, citrate, cystine, protein, and creatinine

---

***Normal Urinary Solute and Protein Excretion Rates***

---

| | |
|---|---|
| Calcium | <4 mg/kg/24 h |
| Second morning urine calcium:creatinine ratio (mg/mg), 95th percentile | |
| 1–7 mo | 0.80 |
| 8–18 mo | 0.55 |
| 19 mo–6 y | 0.35 |
| 7–18 y | 0.22 |
| Oxalate | <40 mg/1.73 m$^2$/24 h |
| <1 y | <0.21 mg/mg creatinine |
| 1–12 y | <0.12 mg/mg creatinine |
| >12 y | <0.07 mg/mg creatinine |
| Uric acid | <815 mg/1.73 m$^2$/24 h |
| Cystine | <75 mg/g creatinine |
| Citrate* | (a) >180 mg/g creatinine |
| | (b) >300 mg/g creatinine (girls) |
| | >125 mg/g creatinine (boys) |
| Magnesium | >88 mg/1.73 m$^2$/24 h |
| Protein | >4 mg/h/m$^2$ |
| Creatinine clearance | ≥80 mL/min/1.73 m$^2$ |

---

*Just after completion of collection and prior to analysis, urine for determination of calcium, phosphorus, magnesium, oxalate, and cystine should be acidified to a pH ≤1.5; and for determination of uric acid to a pH >7.5.

4. Imaging: All children presenting with urinary tract infection should have a renal ultrasound to detect the presence of anomalies of the urinary tract, nephrolithiasis, or nephrocalcinosis. An ultrasound is more sensitive than conventional radiology for the detection of nephrocalcinosis. Cysteine stones are weakly radiopaque and uric acid stones radiolucent by conventional radiography, whereas both are strongly echogenic by ultrasound or computed tomography. In a patient with flank pain and a history of urolithiasis, an intravenous pyelogram (IVP) should be considered to better evaluate the ureter and the possibility of obstruction. A voiding cystourethrogram should be performed in all patients with urolithiasis and urinary tract infection.

5. Stone analysis: Chemical analysis of urinary stones should be performed as part of the initial evaluation whenever stone material is available for analysis. Depending on the composition of the stone, subsequent metabolic evaluation of the patient should proceed accordingly.

## VII.  MANAGEMENT OF UROLITHIASIS IN CHILDREN
### A.  Acute Complications

1. Pain: Children with urolithiasis may have severe pain, which should be treated promptly and may require administration of narcotic analgesics.

2. Diagnosis and relief of obstruction: If obstruction is suspected, an abdominal plain film and IVP should be performed to determine the site of obstruction. Consultation with a pediatric urologist should be obtained.

3. Hydration: A relatively high urine flow should be maintained. If the patient cannot take fluids by mouth, intravenous fluids should be administered at a rate of approximately 1.5 to 2.0 times the maintenance rate, in the absence of renal insufficiency.

4. Infection: After obtaining urine for culture, antibiotics should be administered to patients in whom urinary tract infection is suspected. The combination of infection and an obstructing stone requires emergency treatment.

### B.  Spontaneous passage of urinary stones occurs in 8% to 50% of patients within approximately 2 weeks of the onset of symptoms. Urine should be strained in an attempt to recover a calculus or gravel for chemical analysis.

### C.  Chronic Therapy

1. The long-term goal of therapy is to prevent recurrence of stone formation. Specific therapy should be guided by knowledge of the underlying factors that predispose to stone formation in the individual patient. Thus, a search for such factors should be undertaken in every child with urinary stones.

2. The underlying predisposing condition should be corrected whenever possible.
3. Fluid intake: One of the most important aspects of therapy is to increase fluid intake to lower urinary solute concentration and thus decrease the rate of stone formation. A modest restriction of dietary sodium helps to reduce calcium excretion in patients with hypercalciuria.
4. Dietary calcium: In children with calcium-containing stones, one should avoid restricting dietary calcium to less than the recommended dietary allowance for age, so as to avoid negative calcium balance, which might compromise bone health in growing children.
5. Hypocalciuric agents: Thiazide diuretics can be used to reduce urinary calcium excretion in patients with urolithiasis and hypercalciuria unresponsive to other treatments. This treatment is often necessary in patients with idiopathic hypercalciuria.
6. Urine pH: Manipulation of urine pH is helpful in decreasing the formation of uric acid and cysteine stones, but not of calcium oxalate stones.
7. Inhibitors of crystallization: Oral citrate can be useful in reducing stone formation in patients with idiopathic hypercalciuria. Oral magnesium and phosphate have been used to reduce stone formation in patients with primary hyperoxaluria.
8. Indications for surgical intervention
   a. Intractable pain
   b. Persistent obstruction
   c. Persistent infection

## VIII. PROGNOSIS

In most children, urolithiasis is a recurrent problem. The ultimate prognosis is determined to the greatest extent by the underlying metabolic or other factors that predispose to stone formation.

**RECOMMENDED READING**

Gearhart JP, Herzberg GZ, Jeffs RD. Childhood urolithiasis: experiences and advances. *Pediatrics* 1991;187:445–450.

Harmon EP, Neal DE, Thomas R. Pediatric urolithiasis: review of research and current management. *Pediatr Nephrol* 1994;8:508–512.

Milliner DS, Murphy RE. Urolithiasis in pediatric patients. *Mayo Clin Proc* 1993;68:241–248.

Moxey-Mims MM, Stapleton FB. Hypercalciuria and nephrocalcinosis in children. *Curr Opin Pediatr* 1993;5:186–190.

Polinsky MS, Kaiser BA, Baluarte HJ. Urolithiasis in children. *Pediatr Clin North Am* 1987;34:683–710.

So NP, Osorio AV, Simon SD, et al. Normal urinary calcium/creatinine ratios in African-American and Caucasian children. *Pediatr Nephrol* 2001;16:133–139.

# Urolithiasis in Children: Surgical Management

Hubert S. Swana

In developed countries, the incidence of nephrolithiasis in children has remained stable over the last 20 years. In Europe the incidence of stone disease ranges from 0.13 to 0.95 cases per 1,000 hospital admissions while in the United States it is between to 1 per 7,600 hospital admissions, although regional variation is considerable. The incidence tends to be higher in warm climates and in areas with immigrants from countries with endemic stone disease. Boys and girls appear to be equally affected. Currently 75% to 80% of these children have upper tract stones. Metabolic disorders are responsible for 50% of stones.

Multiple factors must be considered when planning pediatric stone surgery. Patient age and size often require special instruments. Stone size and location may limit access to the stone. Stone composition is also important. Knowledge of anatomic abnormalities such as calyceal diverticula or ureteropelvic junction obstructions is important as well. Extracorporeal shock wave lithotripsy (ESWL), ureteroscopy, and percutaneous nephrolithotomy, alone or in combination, are the main surgical modalities in contemporary stone management. Open surgery or laparoscopy is rarely necessary.

## I. SURGICAL MANAGEMENT

The initial management of children presenting acutely with symptoms of stone disease is no different than that of adults. Children should receive ample pain medications and hydration, usually 1.5 to 2.0 times maintenance fluids. Infection should be treated with antibiotics and, when present, concomitant obstruction should be relieved quickly with either ureteral stent placement or percutaneous nephrostomy. In all cases, renal imaging guides treatment (Fig. 21–1).

In afebrile children with a stone less then 4 mm and no associated anatomic abnormalities, observation is appropriate. Uncontrolled pain, nausea, and emesis, even in the presence of a relatively small stone, are indications for intervention.

### A. SWL

1. SWL is a noninvasive method of stone fragmentation. Children have decreased shock wave attenuation, because of their small size, which limits trauma to surrounding organs. Long-term studies indicate that after SWL children do not develop renal scarring. Renal function and linear growth are not affected and there is no increased risk of hypertension or other medical renal disease.

2. In children with small to moderate upper tract calculi and no anatomic defect, SWL is the preferred

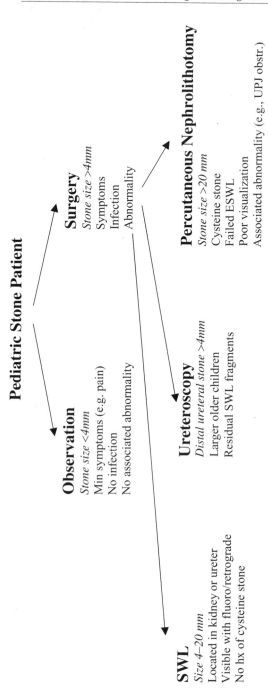

**Pediatric Stone Patient**

**Observation**
*Stone size <4mm*
Min symptoms (e.g. pain)
No infection
No associated abnormality

**Surgery**
*Stone size >4mm*
Symptoms
Infection
Abnormality

**SWL**
*Size 4–20 mm*
Located in kidney or ureter
Visible with fluoro/retrograde
No hx of cysteine stone

**Ureteroscopy**
*Distal ureteral stone >4mm*
Larger older children
Residual SWL fragments

**Percutaneous Nephrolithotomy**
*Stone size >20 mm*
Cysteine stone
Failed ESWL
Poor visualization
Associated abnormality (e.g., UPJ obstr.)

**Open/Laparoscopic Surgery**
Very rarely needed

**Fig. 21-1.** **Surgical treatment of kidney stones.** *Abbreviations:* **SWL,** extracorporeal shock wave lithotripsy; **hx,** history; **Min, minimal;** **UPJ obstr,** ureteropelvic junction obstruction.

first-line therapy. Success with stones up to 1.5 cm has been reported. Most centers report a stone-free rate between 70% and 86% for medium-size stones. Use of SWL in staghorn calculi is possible with reports of stone-free rates in excess of 70%; however, a significant number of these patients required one or more retreatments. Older machines require fluoroscopy for stone localization. Reported complications include the accumulation of obstructing stone fragments in the distal ureter (*steinstrasse*), hematuria, flank pain, and urosepsis. In addition, the type of lithotripsy machine affects results greatly, with newer machines that are generally less powerful having lower stone-free rates.

B. **Percutaneous Nephrolithotomy**

   1. Percutaneous nephrolithotomy (PCNL) is useful in children with large upper tract calculi or very hard (cysteine or calcium monohydrate) stones. It is also useful for failed SWL and allows visualization of radiolucent stones (e.g., uric acid stones). PCNL has been performed successfully in children of all ages. Depending on the child's size, smaller instruments may be required. PCNL allows the use of ultrasound, electrohydraulic, pneumatic, or laser energy for stone fragmentation and suction, baskets, or graspers for extraction.

   2. Stone-free rates of 83% to 100% have been reported. Hematuria (sometimes requiring transfusion), urine leak, sepsis, and hypothermia have been reported. Bowel and pleural injury are also possible.

C. **Ureteroscopy**

   1. Distal ureteral stones can be managed in a similar fashion to adults; however, in children, stones that are 4 mm or larger are unlikely to pass spontaneously. For this reason, children with a distal ureteral stone of 4 mm or larger should be considered for ureteroscopic stone extraction. Either prior placement of a ureteral stent for passive dilation or acute dilation of the ureterovesical junction may be necessary. Ureteral access sheaths can help to minimize trauma associated with repeated scope passage. Small rigid or flexible ureteroscopes can be used in conjunction with laser lithotripsy. Postoperative stenting is prudent in most cases.

   2. Stone-free rates of between 77% and 100% have been reported. Reported complications include stone migration, bleeding, pyelonephritis, ureteral stricture, and ureteral avulsion. Ureteral injuries can be caused by the lithotripsy energy or mechanical injury associated with scope passage and stone manipulation. The incidence of vesicoureteral reflux after ureterovesical junction dilation is less than 1%.

## RECOMMENDED READING

Al-Shammari A, Al-Otaibi K, Leonard M, et al. Percutaneous nephrolithotomy in the pediatric population. *J Urol* 1999;162:1721.

Gschwend JE, Haag U, Hollmer S, et al. Impact of extracorporeal shock wave lithotripsy in pediatric patients: complications and long-term follow-up. *Urol Int* 1996;56:241.

Minevich E. Pediatric urolithiasis. *Pediatr Clin North Am* 2001;48:1571–1585.

# Acute Renal Failure

Paul R. Brakeman

*Acute renal failure* (ARF) is an abrupt reduction in renal function leading to an inability to excrete metabolic wastes and maintain proper fluid and electrolyte balance. ARF results in increased serum levels of creatinine, urea nitrogen, potassium, and phosphorus and frequently is accompanied by oliguria and an increase in extracellular fluid volume.

I. **CAUSES**
   The etiology of renal failure is typically divided into three categories: prerenal, renal, and postrenal (Table 22–1).
   A. **Prerenal Azotemia:** Prerenal azotemia describes any condition in which blood flow to the kidneys is decreased. Causes of reduced renal blood flow include intravascular volume depletion, shock, sepsis, and heart failure. If the reduction of renal blood flow persists long enough, renal tubular cell death occurs (acute tubular necrosis [ATN]). Prerenal azotemia is a common cause of ARF in intensive care units, often related to sepsis or poor renal perfusion during complex surgery, especially cardiac procedures with bypass.
   B. **Renal Causes:** The most common renal cause of ARF is ATN, usually induced by ischemia or toxins. Other renal causes of ARF include glomerular disease such as acute glomerulonephritis (GN), renal vascular diseases such as hemolytic-uremic syndrome (HUS), acute interstitial nephritis, and, in newborns, congenital anomalies of the kidneys. Pyelonephritis is an uncommon cause of ARF because it usually affects only one kidney.
   C. **Postrenal ARF:** Postrenal ARF is caused by obstruction of the flow of urine at any level of the urinary tract.
II. **CLINICAL FEATURES AND DIAGNOSIS**
   A. **History:** Many patients with ARF are asymptomatic and present only with alterations in laboratory findings. The patient and his or her medical record should be evaluated for recent fluid intake, last void, hematuria, stooling pattern, recent blood pressures (including intraoperative blood pressures), heart rate, flank pain, malaise, rash, joint pain, fever, and recent medication exposures. A history of dehydration, sepsis, or previous complex surgery suggests prerenal azotemia or ATN. Exposure to tubular toxins such as amphotericin, IV contrast agents, aminoglycosides, or drugs such as indomethacin that reduce renal blood flow suggest toxin-induced ARF. Bloody diarrhea with malaise suggests hemolytic uremic syndrome. Gross hematuria or bilateral flank pain suggests acute GN.

**Table 22–1.  Causes of acute renal failure**

| Prerenal | Renal | Postrenal |
| --- | --- | --- |
| Hypovolemia | ATN | Calculi |
|   Diarrheal | GN | Posterior |
|     dehydration | HUS |   urethral valves |
|   Third-space losses | Interstitial nephritis | UPJ obstruction |
|   Hemorrhage | Vasculitis | Uretrocele |
|   Burns |   Lupus erythematosus | |
|   Nephrotic syndrome |   Henoch–Schönlein | |
| Shock (septic/ |     purpura | |
|   cardiogenic) | Nephrotoxins (tubular | |
| CHF |   injury) | |
| Hepatorenal syndrome |   Aminoglycosides, | |
| |     amphotericin, radio | |
| |     contrast agents, | |
| |     myoglobulin | |
| | Nephrotoxins | |
| |   (vasoconstriction) | |
| |   NSAIDs | |
| | Pyelonephritis | |
| | Renal artery or vein | |
| |   thrombosis | |
| | Polycystic kidneys | |
| |   (newborn) | |

Abbreviations: ATN, acute tubular necrosis; CHF, congestive heart failure; GN, glomerulonephritis; HUS, hemolytic-uremic syndrome; NSAIDs, nonsteroidal antiinflammatory drugs; UPJ, uretropelvic junction.

  **B.  Physical Examination:** Patients should be examined for mental status; hyper- or hypotension; tachycardia; facial, presacral (especially in the supine critically ill patient) or extremity edema; skin turgor; mucous membrane dryness; flank pain; abdominal mass; a palpable bladder; and rash. Poor skin turgor, tachycardia, and hypotension suggest prerenal azotemia or ATN. Commonly, children with ARF present with oliguria and signs of fluid overload, such as edema and hypertension. Bilateral flank tenderness suggests GN or interstitial nephritis. An enlarged bladder in a newborn suggests urinary obstruction such as posterior urethral valves.

  **C.  Laboratory and Imaging:** A complete blood count, urinalysis, and serum electrolytes, blood urea nitrogen (BUN), creatinine, calcium (including ionized calcium if the total calcium is low), phosphorus, and albumin should be obtained in all cases. If pyuria is present, a urine culture should be obtained. A renal ultrasound is frequently useful and should be obtained if there is any chance that urine obstruction is the cause. Table 22–2 describes test results that can be used to differentiate causes of ARF.

**Table 22–2. Evaluation of causes of acute renal failure**

| | Prerenal | Acute Tubular Necrosis | Glomerulonephritis and Hemolytic Uremic Syndrome | Obstruction |
|---|---|---|---|---|
| Urine output | Low | Low-normal or high | Low | Variable |
| Urine osmolality (mOsm/kg) | >500 | <350 | NA | <350 |
| Urine sodium (mEq/L) | <20 | >40 | NA | >40 |
| Fractional excretion of sodium (%) | <1 | >2 | NA | >2 |
| Serum BUN/creatinine | >20 | <20 | NA | NA |
| Urinalysis | Minimal findings | Proteinuria ± Tubular epithelial cells Brown granular casts | Proteinuria Hematuria RBC casts | Proteinuria ± |
| Ultrasound | Normal | ↑Renal size and echogenicity | ↑Renal size and echogenicity | Dilatation of urinary proximal to obstruction, e.g., hydronephrosis |

1. Urinalysis is the most important test in evaluating ARF. Mild proteinuria (1+ or less) is a nonspecific finding that occurs in many types of ARF. Severe proteinuria with or without hematuria and RBC casts is associated with intrarenal processes such as GN, vasculitis, HUS, or nephrotic syndrome. Pyuria is suggestive of pyelonephritis or interstitial nephritis.

2. The fractional excretion of sodium {(urine [Na]/urine[Cr]) / (serum [Na]/serum[Cr])} is useful to distinguish prerenal azotemia from ATN. Prerenal azotemia is characterized by oliguria and concentrated urine with a low sodium concentration (<20 mEq/L) and a low fractional excretion of sodium, whereas ATN is characterized by low or normal urine volume and a dilute urine with a high sodium concentration (>40 mEq/L). This measurement is not applicable to newborns who are unable to generate very concentrated urine.

3. Blood tests that can be used to diagnose various forms of GN or vasculitis include complement levels, antinuclear antibody titer, antinuclear cytoplasmic antibody titer, and antistreptolysin O titer (to detect previous strep infection in cases of poststreptococcal GN).

4. Ultrasound is the most important test for the diagnosis of congenital abnormalities or obstructive ARF (indicated by the finding of hydronephrosis). However, in the oliguric patient or very early after obstruction, no hydronephrosis may be detected despite the presence of postrenal obstruction. The finding of enlarged kidneys with bilateral increased echogenicity is most consistent with medical renal disease such a ATN, GN, interstitial nephritis, HUS, or renal vein thrombosis.

## III. TREATMENT

Many causes of ARF such as ATN, most types of GN, and HUS have no specific treatment and are self-limiting diseases. Steps should be taken to maintain or correct fluid and electrolyte abnormalities. Finally, the kidneys should be protected from further toxic or ischemic insults during recovery from ARF. In cases of drug-induced ATN, the offending agent should be removed. In the case of obstructive renal failure, catheter drainage should be initiated and, if necessary, urgent surgical correction. In the oliguric patient with presumed prerenal ARF, hydration with saline should be started with 10 to 20 mL/kg over 30 to 60 minutes and continued until volume repletion is attained as indicated by the normalization of blood pressure, heart rate, skin turgor, and central venous pressure. To prevent further renal damage in ARF, drugs that detrimentally affect renal function such as ACE inhibitors, nonsteroidal antiinflammatory drugs, and nephrotoxic antibiotics should be discontinued if possible.

A.  **Fluids:** Children who are oliguric require salt and water restriction. Fluids should be restricted to calculated insensible water losses (35 mL/100 kcal/24 h), adjusted for fever and measured urine output, usually given as $D_5$/0.25% saline. Furosemide, 1 to 2 mg/kg IV may be tried to increase urine output, but in many cases it is ineffectual due to severely reduced glomerular filtration rate. There is no evidence that furosemide decreases the duration of ATN or changes other outcome measures of hospitalized patients with ATN. Fluid overload resulting in pulmonary edema that occurs despite fluid restriction is one of the indications for acute dialysis.

B.  **Hyperkalemia:** Intake of potassium should be restricted in most patients with ARF and potassium should be removed from IV fluids, particularly total parental nutrition. Mild hyperkalemia (serum $K^+$ <6 mEq/L) is treated with IV furosemide (if the patient is furosemide responsive), IV sodium bicarbonate (1 mEq/kg) if the patient is acidotic, or with sodium polystyrene sulfonate (Kayexelate), 0.5 to 1.0 g/kg PO or 1.5 to 2.0 g/kg PR. More severe hyperkalemia is treated with IV calcium gluconate, 100 mg/kg (maximum 2 g) over 10 minutes; sodium bicarbonate, 1 to 2 mEq/kg over 15 to 30 minutes; 50% dextrose in water 1 mL/kg; and insulin, 0.15 U/kg over 15 to 30 minutes for short-term reduction and with sodium polystyrene sulfonate as above for more long-term treatment. The patient with severely elevated potassium should be assessed for the presence of peaked T waves on the electrocardiograph.

C.  **Hypocalcemia:** In ARF, reduction of renal excretion of phosphorus results in hyperphosphatemia that, in turn, causes hypocalcemia. Hypocalcemia is exacerbated by a reduced ability to hydroxylate vitamin D in ARF. Hypocalcemia severe enough to result in a positive Chvostek sign, Trousseau sign, or tetany (usually <6.0 mg/dL) is treated with IV calcium gluconate 100 mg/kg (maximum 1 g) every 6 hours. Serum phosphorus should be reduced by treating with a phosphorus-binding agent such as calcium carbonate, 50 mg/kg PO with meals and snacks. Hemodialysis is only minimally effective in reducing serum phosphorus levels.

D.  **Acidosis:** Severe acidosis (serum pH <7.2 or serum bicarbonate level <16 mEq/L) is initially treated with sodium bicarbonate, 2 to 3 mEq/kg, IV over 30 to 60 minutes followed by slow correction with IV or PO sodium bicarbonate over 24 hours with a goal of a serum level of 20 mEq/L. Maintenance therapy with sodium bicarbonate is 1 to 3 mEq/kg/day IV or PO; correction of acidosis requires providing 1 to 3 mEq/kg per day of sodium bicarbonate in addition to the amount required to achieve correction. Correction of acidosis exacerbates hypocalcemia, thus treatment of hypocalcemia should precede or accompany treatment of acidosis.

E. **Anemia:** Severe anemia (hematocrit <20%) is treated with packed red blood cells. Transfusion can exacerbate hypocalcemia, hypervolemia, and hypertension and should be given slowly.

F. **Azotemia:** In ARF increased catabolism due to fever, fasting, and stress aggravates elevated BUN levels. Adequate calories [75% to 100% of the recommended daily allowance (RDA)] and restriction of protein intake to RDA levels can decrease the accumulation of BUN. Severe azotemia (usually >100) can lead to symptoms of uremia including bleeding, malaise, encephalopathy (in severe azotemia), nausea, and vomiting, which are indications to initiate acute dialysis. In the absence of these uremic symptoms, dialysis in the setting of ARF can be delayed until BUN exceeds 120 to 150 mg/dL.

G. **Hypertension:** Hypertension in ARF is usually caused by fluid retention and can be treated with salt and water restriction, diuresis with furosemide (1 to 2 mg/kg in the diuretic responsive patient), or both. Inability to respond to these therapies suggests the presence of increased plasma renin levels that can result from ARF. Though not specifically approved by the FDA for use in children, those unresponsive to fluid restriction or diuresis can be treated with amlodipine, 0.1 to 0.5 mg/kg per day PO every 12 or 24 hours, or acutely with nifedipine, 1 to 5 mg PO every 4 to 6 hours. Severe hypertension associated with end-organ damage such as seizure, pulmonary edema, or stroke constitutes a hypertensive emergency and merits transfer to a pediatric intensive care unit for aggressive IV blood pressure control.

## RECOMMENDED READING

Flynn JT. Causes, management approaches, and outcomes of acute renal failure in children. *Curr Opin in Pediatr* 1988;10;184–189.

Phillips AS. Management of acute renal failure. In: Holliday MA, Barratt TM, Avner ED, eds. *Pediatric nephrology*. Baltimore: Lippincott Williams and Wilkins; 1998:1109–1118.

# Chronic Renal Failure

Paul R. Brakeman

I. **DEFINITION**
Chronic renal failure (CRF) is a permanent and progressive reduction in renal function that results in a variety of clinical signs and symptoms and multiple metabolic, hormonal, and organ system abnormalities.

II. **PREVALENCE**
The prevalence of CRF varies significantly between studies and is in the range of 25 to 50 per million children.

III. **CAUSES**
The most common causes of end-stage renal disease (ESRD) in North America are listed in Table 23–1. The most common cause of ESRD in children in North America is glomerulonephritis; however, urologic tract abnormalities combined (reflux nephropathy, obstructive uropathy, and hypoplasia/dysplasia) represent almost 40% of all cases of ESRD in children. In younger patients, congenital anomalies represent the most common causes of ESRD, while in adolescent patients the various forms of glomerulonephritis are the most common cause of ESRD.

IV. **PATHOGENESIS**
As CRF progresses, individual nephrons are lost and the total glomerular filtration rate (GFR) decreases. To compensate, the remaining nephrons increase the fraction of filtrate that is excreted as urine. Thus, substances that depend on glomerular filtration for excretion such as urea nitrogen accumulate, and substances such as salt, potassium, and water may remain in homeostasis until the final stages of CRF. This is specifically true in the case of CRF resulting from congenital obstructive uropathy or hypoplastic/dysplastic kidneys, in which a patient may reach ESRD with a normal urine output and near-normal excretion of sodium and potassium.

V. **CLINICAL MANIFESTATIONS**
The major clinical manifestations of CRF are listed in Table 23–2. Many of the same biochemical abnormalities occur in CRF and ARF; however, in CRF persistence of these abnormalities results in organ system pathology such as renal osteodystrophy.

VI. **DIAGNOSIS**
   A. **History** A patient with CRF should be evaluated thoroughly for a family history of cystic kidney disease; family members receiving dialysis or renal transplantation, indicating other heritable causes of CRF; or a family history of renal failure and hearing loss, suggestive of Alport syndrome. A CRF patient should be questioned for a history of dysfunctional voiding,

**Table 23–1.   Most common causes of ESRD in North America**

| Causes | Percentage of Total |
|---|---|
| Glomerulonephritis | 21.4 |
| Obstructive uropathy | 18.8 |
| Dysplasia/hypoplasia | 15.9 |
| Reflux nephropathy | 5.3 |
| Cystic diseases | 5.6 |
| Hemolytic uremic syndrome | 2.7 |
| Congenital nephrotic syndrome | 2.5 |
| Familial nephritis | 2.4 |
| Cystinosis | 2.1 |
| Chronic pyelonephritis/interstitial nephritis | 2.0 |
| SLE | 1.6 |
| Renal infarct | 1.6 |
| Henoch-Schönlein purpura | 1.3 |

Adapted from the North American Pediatric Renal Transplant Cooperative Study, *Annual Report*, 2002.

**Table 23–2.   Clinical manifestations of chronic renal failure**

**Cardiovascular**

Fluid retention, hypertension, pulmonary edema, pericarditis, cardiomyopathy

**Biochemical and metabolic**

Hyperkalemia, hyperphosphatemia, hypocalcemia, acidosis, hyperlipidemia, glucose intolerance

**Gastrointestinal**

Anorexia, nausea and vomiting, gastritis, colitis, malnutrition → growth retardation

**Neurologic**

Drowsiness, obtundation, seizures, peripheral neuropathy

**Musculoskeletal**

Renal osteodystrophy, metastatic calcification, myopathy

**Hematopoietic**

Anemia, platelet dysfunction

**Hormonal**

Increased parathyroid hormone, increased renin–angiotensin, decreased 1.25 dihydroxyvitamin D, decreased erythropoietin, decreased insulin-like growth factor activity → growth retardation recurrent urinary tract infection, vesicoureteral reflux, or meningomyelocele, any of which would suggest obstructive uropathy, infection, or both as a cause for CRF. The patient should be evaluated for a history of proteinuria, hematuria, flank pain, or edema consistent with chronic glomerulonephritis (GN) and for previous episodes of skin rashes, fever, adenopathy, or arthralgias consistent with systemic lupus erythematosus (SLE) or a vasculitis. Many times the absence of a previous history of symptoms or renal disease is indicative of congenital anomalies of the kidneys such as hypoplasia/dysplasia or medullary cystic disease as the cause of CRF.

**B.** **Physical Examination** The infant with CRF should be examined for enlarged kidneys indicative of hydronephrosis or autosomal recessive polycystic kidney disease; enlarged bladder indicative of obstructive uropathy; and abnormal bony structure of the lumbar spine indicative of meningomyelocele associated with neurogenic bladder. Older patients should be evaluated for short stature indicating long-standing renal failure; blood pressure control; fever, rash, or arthralgia indicative of SLE; and hearing loss consistent with Alport syndrome.

**C.** **Laboratory and Imaging Studies**

1.  **Urinalysis:** Hematuria with moderate to severe proteinuria is suggestive of chronic GN or Alport syndrome. Milder proteinuria with or without mild hematuria is more typical of congenital dysplasia or obstructive uropathy.

2.  **Blood:** Complete blood count, iron studies, serum electrolytes, blood urea nitrogen (BUN), creatinine, calcium (including ionized calcium if the total calcium is low), phosphorus, serum alkaline phosphatase, parathyroid hormone level, and albumin should be obtained initially and monitored in patients with CRF.

3.  **Imaging:** Renal ultrasound is the most important imaging modality in diagnosing congenital anomalies of the kidneys, obstruction, and scarring due to chronic pyelonephritis. In children who present with advanced renal failure and no previous history of renal disease, the kidneys are often small and echogenic on ultrasound. This appearance is nondiagnostic, and a voiding cystogram should be considered to rule out the diagnosis of vesicoureteral reflux as the etiology of renal failure. The absence of reflux in such a patient is also nondiagnostic, because reflux may have resolved after scarring occurred.

**D.** **Biopsy** Renal biopsy is used to diagnose the many forms of glomerulonephritis, interstitial nephritis, and Alport syndrome. Rarely, it establishes a diagnosis of medullary cystic disease. In children with small kidneys by ultrasound, biopsy is not usually performed because small kidneys generally exhibit only nonspecific scarring on pathologic examination.

**VII. MANAGEMENT**

Most of the signs, symptoms, and biochemical abnormalities occurring in CRF are the same as those occurring in ARF. Usually in CRF the biochemical abnormalities are detected at early stages and the goal of management is to prevent or slow their progression. The most important clinical manifestations of CRF are listed below. Intractable hyperkalemia, persistently elevated BUN (>100), and pulmonary edema are late findings in CRF and indicate the need to initiate dialysis.

**A. Fluid Retention:** Children with CRF who are oliguric require sodium restriction to 2 to 3 g of sodium per day for older children. Furosemide, 1 to 2 mg/kg per dose PO one to two times per day, may also limit edema in the furosemide responsive patient.

**B. Hypertension:** Many patients with CRF are hypertensive and hypertension can accelerate the progression of CRF. Common treatments for hypertension include the following.

1. Salt restriction, as above.

2. Angiotensin-converting enzyme (ACE) inhibition: Captopril suspension (1 mg/mL), 0.1 to 0.5 mg/kg per day in two divided doses, or benazepril, 2.5 to 20 mg per day in one to two divided doses, for older children. *In vitro* data in animals and extrapolation of data from patients with diabetes mellitus and SLE indicate that the use of ACE inhibitors in patients with proteinuria, renal insufficiency, or both may provide some renoprotection and slow the progression of CRF. Because of the side effects of hyperkalemia and reduced GFR, serum electrolytes, BUN, and creatinine must be monitored in patients receiving ACE inhibitors.

3. Calcium channel blockers: Amlodipine 0.1 to 0.5 mg/kg per day in one to two divided doses.

4. Diuretics: Chlorthiazide suspension 5 to 10 mg/kg twice a day in infants and young children or hydrochlorothiazide; or 12.5 or 25.0 mg once daily in older children; or furosemide, 0.5 to 1.0 mg/kg twice a day.

**C. Renal Osteodystrophy**

1. Restrict phosphorus to 15 mg per gram of protein per day.

2. Calcium carbonate, 500 to 5,000 mg with meals and snacks, to bind phosphorus in the gut and maintain a normal serum phosphorus level.

3. Active vitamin D: dihydrotachysterol, 0.1 to 0.2 mg per day, in infants and young children or calcitriol, 0.25 to 1.00 $\mu$g/kg per day, in older children. Vitamin D should be used with caution in children whose calcium $\times$ phosphorus product exceeds 60 mg/dL$^2$ because of the danger of metastatic calcification.

**D. Anemia:** When the hematocrit is below 25%, synthetic erythropoietin is started, 100 U/kg three times per week. When the hematocrit increases to 30%, the dose is reduced with a goal of a hematocrit of 30% to 35%. Iron is almost always given as adjunctive therapy with erythropoietin. Transfusions are avoided when possible to prevent sensitization to antigens that might complicate transplantation and are given only if the child is symptomatic or has a hematocrit below 18% to 20%.

**E. Acidosis:** Sodium citrate solution, 1 to 3 mEq/kg per day in three divided doses is given to infants and young children and sodium bicarbonate; 1 to 2 mEq/kg per day in three divided doses is given to older children.

**F. Azotemia:** High levels of BUN (>80 mg/dL) can cause anorexia, fatigue, and other uremic symptoms. Protein restriction to the RDA minimum can help to prevent the development of azotemia. Protein restriction below the RDA interferes with growth in children. In humans, protein restriction has proven to be of only marginal benefit in delaying the progression of CRF.

**G. Nutrition and Growth:** Anorexia probably related to uremia frequently causes inadequate calorie intake in CRF. Inadequate calorie intake is treated with supplementation with carbohydrates and fats while maintaining the protein restriction as described. In younger children and infants, inadequate calorie intake can detrimentally affect brain growth and development causing decreased head circumference and delayed developmental milestones. Frequently gastrostomy feedings are necessary in younger patients to achieve adequate growth. Acidosis, anemia, and renal osteodystrophy can also limit growth. Patients who do not achieve normal linear growth despite adequate calorie intake, correction of acidosis, and the absence of renal osteodystrophy are treated with recombinant growth hormone, 0.5 mg/kg per day.

**H. Imaging With Intravenous Radiocontrast Dye:** There is significant risk of contrast-induced ARF in patients with preexisting renal insufficiency. There have been several recent studies in adults indicating that the administration of oral *N*-acetylcysteine and IV hydration before and after the procedure can reduce the number of patients that have a rise in creatinine following computed tomography scans and coronary angiography. A typical protocol for adults is to hydrate with 1 cc/kg per hour of 0.45% normal saline for 12 hours before the procedure and for 12 hours after the procedure and to give *N*-acetylcysteine, 600 mg PO every 12 hours starting 1 day prior to the procedure for a total of four doses, two before and two after the procedure. Given the data in adults, it is reasonable to use this protocol for adolescents or older children receiving IV contrast with a creatinine below 1.5 mg/dL or creatinine clearance below 50 mL/min. In the outpatient setting, IV hydration can be given the day of the procedure, 5 to 10 cc/kg of 0.9% normal saline over 1 to 2 hours with careful monitoring for signs of hypertension or pulmonary edema. This may be contraindicated in patients with oliguria. Alternatively, consideration should be given to magnetic resonance imaging because contrast may not be needed and if so, gadolinium is not nephrotoxic.

I. **Dialysis and Transplantation:** The indications for initiating chronic dialysis in a patient with CRF are lethargy; nausea, or vomiting due to uremia; BUN persistently below 100; GFR below 8 to 10 mL/min/ 1.73 $m^2$; persistent hyperkalemia; or pulmonary edema. Dialysis can be undertaken either as hemodialysis, typically three times per week, or daily peritoneal dialysis that can be administered at home either manually throughout the day (continuous ambulatory peritoneal dialysis) or continuously during the night using a cycling machine (continuous cycling peritoneal dialysis). Both forms of dialysis provide only approximately 15% of normal renal function; therefore, dialysis patients still experience many of the complications of CRF.

The optimum treatment for children with ESRD is transplantation. The child with CRF should be evaluated for transplantation before reaching ESRD. If a suitable living donor can be identified, the transplant can be performed before the child develops significant symptoms of CRF. When there is no living donor, the child is placed on a waiting list to receive a cadaveric kidney. Because of the shortage of cadaveric organs, most children on the cadaver waiting list require some type of dialysis before receiving their transplant. The current 5-year renal graft survival for children in North America is higher than 80% for living-donor kidneys and above 70% for cadaveric kidneys.

## RECOMMENDED READING

Warady B, Watkins SL. Current advances in the therapy of chronic renal failure and end stage renal disease. *Semin Nephrol* 1998;18:341–354.

Wassner SJ, Baum M. Chronic renal failure: physiology and management. In: Holliday MA, Barratt TM, Avner ED, eds. *Pediatric nephrology*. Baltimore: Lippincott Williams and Wilkins, 1998:1155–1182.

# Pediatric Renal Transplantation

Martin A. Koyle and Gerald C. Mingin

In children with end-stage renal disease (ESRD), renal transplantation represents the current optimal standard of care for renal replacement. Despite the effectiveness of hemodialysis and peritoneal dialysis, even with the addition of recombinant erythropoietin and growth hormone for the prevention of anemia and lack of growth to the armamentarium, neither of these options have proven more effective than renal transplantation. The success rate of renal transplantation in children has steadily improved over the past 20 years.

The North American Pediatric Renal Transplant Cooperative Study (NAPRTCS) was established in 1987 to collect and distribute clinical data regarding pediatric transplantation in North America. One-year graft survival from living-related donors (LRD) has risen from 91% (1987 to 1995) to 94% (1996 to 2000), and cadaver donor survival has increased from 81% to 93% during the same interval. In fact, most recent data show equal 1-year allograft survival rates, regardless of whether the donor source of the allograft was living or cadaveric. This is of importance because allograft half-lives—that is, long-term transplant kidney survival—directly correlate with 1-year survival rates.

Unfortunately, the number of children with ESRD is increasing exponentially. The number of transplants performed (530), as well as the number of cadaveric donors, has not changed over the last several decades. Fortunately, LRD allografts as donor sources have increased dramatically in the pediatric subgroup (from 42% in 1987 to 60% currently). This is partially due to a more invested potential donor pool, including the use of unrelated living donors. The advent of laparoscopic donor nephrectomy and minimally invasive techniques with their perceived reduction in donor morbidity and more rapid convalescence also have had an impact in stimulating the potential use of LRD allografts.

It has been recognized that preemptive transplantation decreases the morbidity associated with chronic dialysis, thus potentially improving physical health, statural growth, and mental well-being. In recognition of the overt benefits of transplantation, pediatric patients with ESRD are given special consideration in the allocation of organs; despite this, waiting times remain long for the fixed source of cadaveric organs and this problem is not likely to be solved in the near future.

Currently, increased graft survival depends on identifying the most appropriate donor and recipient characteristics and employing ongoing improvements in immunosuppressive therapy. Some of the recent and important changes in pediatric renal transplantation are discussed.

## I. ETIOLOGY AND DEMOGRAPHICS

A. The etiologies of renal failure in pediatric patients differ significantly from that of adult patients (those over 18 years of age) in that urologic etiologies, comorbidities, or both can be found in 30% to 40% of children compared to less than 10% of adults.

B. The major urologic conditions associated with ESRD in pediatric patients requiring renal replacement include obstructive uropathy (16%), hypoplastic/dysplastic kidney disease (15%), and reflux nephropathy (5%). The most common medical causes of ESRD include focal glomerular sclerosis, membranous nephropathies, autoimmune disease, metabolic defects, and tumor.

C. Although these etiologies have remained relatively constant, the demographics have shifted significantly. This is most pronounced in the ethnic mix, where white recipients have decreased. In turn, the number of black and Hispanic patients has increased from 28% in 1987 to almost 40% currently.

## II. SELECTION OF RENAL DONORS

A. Although the short-term survival of cadaveric allografts has been shown to be nearly equal to that of LRD allografts, the use of a LRD is still preferable in children. Families are better able to plan and prepare for the surgery; in addition, there is a potential psychological benefit to the recipient knowing the source of the organ and to the donor by virtue of being a Good Samaritan. However, this must be weighed against the knowledge that if the graft is lost, there can be considerable anguish, grief, and guilt from both the donor and recipient.

B. Donor–recipient compatibility is based on several immunologic factors. The cytotoxic cross-match, where donor lymphocytes are mixed with recent recipient sera, is performed prior to any transplant. A positive cross-match, where recipient preformed reactive antibodies (PRA) attack specific antigens on recipient cells, is a contraindication to transplantation because it will lead to hyperacute (immediate) rejection.

C. The two primary antigen systems associated with graft rejection are the ABH and HLA systems. Similar to blood transfusions, type O represents the universal blood donor and type AB represents the universal recipient. Hence an appropriate match should be assured to avoid hyperacute rejection. The Rh status appears to be a minor antigen system that does not influence the risk of rejection. The short- and long-term survivals of a transplanted kidney appear to be primarily related with HLA compatibility at the -A, -B, and -D (DR) loci. Ideally a perfect six-antigen match is desired. In an LRD from parent to child there is at worst a one haplotype or three HLA match (there is also a one haplotype or three HLA mismatch). An identical twin should be a two haplotype (same maternal and paternal alleles)/six antigen match/zero mismatch donor. In a sibling group, there is a 50% chance of sharing one haplotype (one maternal or one paternal) and a 25% chance of being either identical or totally mismatched. Clearly, with cadaveric donors, the chances of obtaining a perfect match is far less because of the HLA distributions in various populations and ethnic/cultural groups.

**D.** All donors must be free of systemic infection such as acquired immunodeficiency syndrome and viral hepatitis as well as malignancy (with the exception of some primary brain tumors). In selected individual cases, the criteria have been expanded to include kidneys from non–heartbeating donors; donors younger than 5 or older than 60 years; as well as selected kidneys from donors with diabetes and hypertension. Any living donor should be healthy, free of systemic illness, malignancy, and willing to donate. The perioperative donor risk is small, with a mortality rate between 0.03% and 0.06%. Long-term data have substantiated that there is no evidence of significant long-term morbidity or mortality from becoming uninephric.

## III. PRETRANSPLANT RECIPIENT PREPARATION

### A. Metabolic Diseases

1. The activity of systemic diseases such as systemic lupus erythematosus and vasculitis require a stable and quiescent state prior to transplantation. Often, the autoimmune responses in these diseases can be controlled with the same immunosuppression required for antirejection therapy and maintenance.

2. Metabolic disease such as cystinoses and primary hyperoxalosis require adequate medical therapy prior to transplantation. Recurrence of the disease is 100% for primary hyperoxalosis without simultaneous liver transplantation; thus, combined hepatic and renal transplantation must be considered the current treatment of choice for these patients.

### B. Upper Urinary Tract

1. Clinical conditions requiring pretransplant nephrectomy are limited. However, consideration to nephrectomy(ies) include those children who have severe polyuria with electrolyte wasting and for those with significant proteinuria. Polyuria, dehydration, electrolyte disturbances, and, importantly, a reduced circulating volume can lead to a hypercoagulable state. It should be emphasized that the child often receives a larger donor kidney that requires a significant cardiac output and perfusion pressure. Thus, a low recipient volume status can precipitate thrombosis, a surgical complication more prevalent among pediatric patients than adults, and often thought to be technical in etiology.

2. As opposed to years gone by when routine nephrectomies were performed in patients with a history

of obstructive uropathy and vesicoureteral reflux, this is rarely an indication today, unless the patient is prone to relapsing recurrent infections that can be attributed to the kidney. Renal hypertension that cannot be controlled with medication may be considered a rare indication for nephrectomy to improve blood pressure control. In children who have an associated predisposition to the development of malignant renal neoplasms, such as those with Denys–Drash syndrome, nephrectomy(ies) should be performed because these tumors tend to occur early in life.

C. **Lower Urinary Tract**
   1. As discussed earlier, a substantial minority of children with ESRD have associated urologic anomalies that may have contributed to native kidney loss and potentially might negatively impact an allograft. Investigation must be individualized to ensure that the lower tract is hospitable to a new kidney. The goal in all cases is to ensure that the bladder serves its two primary functions: storage of urine (at an adequate capacity with pressures below 35 cm $H_2O$) and emptying (completely and reliably). Patients with a history of posterior urethral valves, neurogenic bladder, urethral strictures, and anatomic anomalies such as bladder exstrophy should be scrutinized closely. Depending on age and other parameters, urologic investigation may range from none, to uroflow with pre- and postvoid bladder scans, all the way to multichannel videourodynamics.
   2. Clean intermittent catheterization (CIC) can be performed safely via the urethra or using the Mitrofanoff technique when spontaneous voiding is not possible. In addition, if anticholinergic medications are insufficient in controlling the inhospitable bladder, augmentation cystoplasty will be required. Occasionally the anuric patient has a defunctionalized bladder. If the bladder was normal prior to the onset of anuria, then the majority of these bladders stretch and contract normally after successful transplantation. If there is a doubt, bladder cycling using CIC or suprapubic catheter installation of saline can be used to test the distensibility and emptying parameters of the bladder. In patients with preexisting continent cutaneous diversions, reimplantation of the transplant ureter can be performed into these systems. In the case of the incontinent diversion, conversion to a continent catheterizable system can be performed electively either pre- or posttransplant, provided the child exhibits stable renal function and is on maintenance immunosuppression.

D. **Blood Transfusions:** It is well known that renal failure leads to a decrease in the production of erythropoietin and subsequent anemia in patients with ESRD. Early on it was noted that patients who received red cell transfusions had fewer episodes of rejection and as a result in many centers it became routine for potential recipients to receive multiple transfusions. In the case of the LRD, multiple donor-specific transfusions were performed. However, a number of these patients went on to develop unacceptably high levels of cytotoxic antibodies and a high PRA level in their serum, which delayed or even precluded subsequent transplantation. Because of the use of recombinant erythropoietin the need for transfusion has decreased dramatically from a high of 83% in 1987 to 45% in 1999. Most recent data suggest that, with current immunosuppressive protocols, the risk of transfusions and their associated hypersensitivity outweigh their potential immunologic benefits and transfusion for this purpose should be abandoned.

## IV.  IMMUNOSUPPRESSIVE AGENTS

With the improvement in graft survival over the last several years due to advances in immunosuppressive protocols, focus is now on optimizing immunotherapy to decrease potential recipient side effects while maintaining or even improving graft survival. It should be understood that immunosuppression is used to prevent acute rejection and treat that form of rejection should it develop. Hyperacute rejection is preventable in virtually all cases by ensuring a negative cross-match; regardless, it cannot be reversed. Acute rejection, a cell-mediated event, can occur anytime after the graft is placed. The most common cause of graft loss, however, is chronic rejection, an antibody-mediated process that also cannot be prevented or reversed with current therapeutic agents. The optimal immunosuppressive agent or combination of agents still eludes the transplant surgeon and thus their use is often dictated by a center-by-center preference or even patient-by-patient protocol. Immunosuppressive agents can be grouped broadly into those used for induction, those used for maintenance, and those used for anti–acute rejection therapy.

A.  **Corticosteroids:** Corticosteroids have a wide range of nonspecific and specific antiinflammatory effects on cell-mediated immunity and have been a mainstay in the immunosuppression armamentarium for almost 50 years. They are employed for induction, maintenance, and when administered in high doses (pulses), in anti–acute rejection protocols as well. Although it has been standard practice to use steroids in children, their side effects can be severe. Some of the more common problems seen with steroid use include Cushingoid habitus, susceptibility to infection, impaired wound healing, and growth suppression. In recognition of these deleterious effects, lower steroid dose protocols or alternative-day dosing or even replacement with daclizumab appear to have no deleterious effect on the acute rate of rejection.

B. **Interleukin-2 Inhibitors/Blockers:** Cyclosporine and Tacrolimus are sister peptides of fungal origin that are utilized in induction and maintenance.

1. Cyclosporine inhibits T-cell response by binding to cellular proteins called cyclophilins. This complex then blocks the movement into the nucleus of those transcription factors required for interleukin (IL)-2 production. The introduction of cyclosporine or cyclosporin A in the 1980s, when it failed in its initial development as an antibiotic but demonstrated unique immunosuppressive properties, essentially ushered in the modern era of transplantation and indeed has been responsible for the explosive expansion in multiorgan transplantation.

2. Tacrolimus is produced from the fungal species *Streptomyces tsukubaensis*; however, its binding site is distinctly different from that of cyclosporine. Tacrolimus complexes with FK-binding protein inhibit T-cell–derived lymphokines such as IL-2. The use of cyclosporine is associated with nephrotoxicity, hepatotoxicity, hypertension, hirsutism, gingival hyperplasia, susceptibility to infection, and increased risk of malignancy. Tacrolimus is associated with a slightly better side effect profile when compared to cyclosporine, with less hypertension seen. Tacrolimus, in addition to being effective in inducing graft tolerance, appears to be just as successful in the absence of steroids when used as monotherapy. The most serious side effect of tacrolimus is an increased incidence of lymphoproliferative disease. Because both of these drugs are metabolized by the cytochrome P-450 system, it is important to be aware of those drugs that can induce or inhibit cytochrome P-450 will alter serum levels. These should be monitored closely.

3. A second group of drugs used for induction are antibodies directed to the IL-2 receptor. Basiliximab blocks the alpha chain of the IL-2 receptor, and daclizumab acts at the alpha chain of that receptor. Both of these antibodies have been shown to significantly reduce the incidence of biopsy-proven acute rejection. They also have the added benefit of being well-tolerated despite significant side effects.

C. **Antimetabolites**

1. Azathioprine is an antiproliferative agent, a prodrug of 6-mercaptopurine. Once metabolized, its derivatives inhibit purine synthesis, which prevents gene replication and in turn inhibits antibody formation. Myelosuppression is a major side effect of this drug and its use has diminished over recent years with the introduction of more specific agents.

2. Mycophenolate mofetil also interrupts purine metabolism in B and T lymphocytes and is now

replacing azathioprine in many protocols. Recent studies report that mycophenolate mofetil in combination with cyclosporine and prednisone provides early graft survival rates of 98% with a low rate of acute rejection. Side effects are limited to hematologic and gastric problems, in particular neutropenia, thrombocytopenia, diarrhea, nausea, and vomiting.

3. The newest of these drugs is sirolimus, which was just approved for use by the U.S. Food and Drug Administration. Although the mechanism is not fully understood, it blocks cytokine mediated proliferation of T and B lymphocytes. Again, sirolimus in combination with cyclosporine and corticosteroids results in a very low acute rejection rates. An added benefit is the apparent synergistic effect of sirolimus and cyclosporine, allowing for a decrease in the dose of the latter.

**D. T-Cell Antibody Therapy**

1. Two antibodies currently in common use are OKT3, a monoclonal antibody that binds to the lymphocyte–CD3 complex, and antithymocyte globulin (Atgam), a polyclonal horse-derived antilymphocyte globulin. An alternative agent, antithymocyte globin (Thymoglobin), has also been shown to be effective in the depletion of T lymphocytes. These parentally administered anti-antibody preparations are associated with infusion-related side effects that include fever, chills, nausea, and hypotension. Premedication with acetaminophen, corticosteroids, and diphenhydramine is therefore recommended. Because of the morbidity as well as the significant reduction in circulating active lymphocytes, with resultant risk of infection, associated with these preparations, they are utilized primarily for the treatment of rejection and occasionally for induction in selected protocols. They are never utilized for long-term maintenance.

2. Although many new agents continue to target the activation or the proliferation of lymphocytes, such as everolimus, an agent similar to sirolimus, even newer immunosuppressive drugs will have radically different mechanisms of action. One of these drugs, FTY720, prevents lymphocytes from reaching the transplanted kidney. It impairs activated T cells from traveling through the blood stream into the grafted tissue without affecting cellular or humoral immunity to systemic infection.

**E. Typical Immunosuppressive Regimens:** Although protocols differ depending on the institution, the following is fairly representative. Induction takes place using either T-cell antibody therapy or an antibody directed at the IL-2 receptor. The choice depends on the individual patient. In those who are highly sensitized or have had a previous transplant, T-cell antibody therapy is the better choice. For all others, an antibody to the IL-2 receptor is acceptable. Maintenance therapy is accomplished in most cases using a steroid either every day or when growth is a concern on an alternate-day schedule, with the addition of cyclosporine and an antiproliferative agent such as mycophenolate mofetil. In the future the latter may be replaced by sirolimus to decrease the dose of cyclosporine. Acute rejection is treated with pulse steroids and antibody preparation such OKT3, antilymphocyte globin, or antithymocyte globulin. The morbidity of repeated treatments must be evaluated with the philosophy that the patient is more valuable than graft survival and that there is the fall back of dialysis if an allograft is lost.

## V. GRAFT LOSS

A. Graft loss may be due to hyperacute rejection, acute rejection, chronic rejection, vascular thrombosis, technical mishaps or recurrence of the primary disease. Acute rejection is the second leading cause of allograft loss as well as being the biggest contributor to chronic rejection. Acute rejection is increased among blacks, in HLA mismatch, and in those patients who did not have induction therapy. Silent rejection has become an important issue in children, where it is postulated that because of the larger adult kidney acute rejection requires a greater amount of time to become clinically apparent.

B. Chronic rejection is still the primary cause of graft failure, accounting for 30% to 40% of allograft loss. Even so, more recent analysis of the NAPRTCS database has shown that the incidence of chronic rejection has fallen significantly since 1987. This is most likely due to improvements in immunosuppression leading to a decrease in acute rejection. This improvement may also be related to improved renal storage methods that promote early graft function.

C. Vascular thrombosis is the third leading cause of graft failure and according to the NAPRTCS registry is responsible for graft loss in 11.6% of children. Some patients have an increased risk for thrombosis: peritoneal dialysis patients, donor kidneys less than 5 years of age, recipients less than 2 years of age, patients previously transplanted, and cadaveric donors with a cold ischemia time of more than 24 hours. As mentioned, recipient hydration and oxygen-carrying capacity must be optimal at the time of engraftment to ensure appropriate allograft perfusion. Engraftment of an organ can be a challenge in smaller patients and those who have undergone multiple prior transplants. Thus, it requires ingenuity at times by the transplant surgeon to find appropriate vasculature and recipient lower urinary tract into which the donor renal artery and vein and ureter can be implanted to prevent technical complications and graft loss.

## VI. COMPLICATIONS AND GROWTH

### A. Complications

1. Infections, both bacterial and viral, account for a majority of hospital admissions posttransplantation. Viral infections, especially those due to herpes virus and cytomegalovirus, can lead to systemic morbidity in this immunosuppressed population and often mimic acute rejection. Even more worrisome is Epstein–Barr virus exposure. The virus may cause posttransplant lymphoproliferative disease and lymphoma. The incidence of this disease has been reported at 1.6%; however, recent NAPRTCS data suggest the prevalence to be as high as 10%. Pneumocystis, an opportunistic infection, is preventable in most recipients by administering prophylactic sulfonamide and trimethoprim (Sulfatrim) in the early posttransplant period. The same antibiotics also minimize the risk of lower and upper urinary tract infections.

2. As opposed to infection, cardiovascular disease is a leading cause of death in children posttransplantation. Hypertension, often with decreased allograft function, is common in children after transplantation. NAPRTCS reports that 58% of children 5 years posttransplant require antihypertensive therapy. What is still unknown is if hypertension results in allograft damage, or if previous allograft damage causes hypertension. In any event, cardiovascular disease leads to almost 25% of the deaths in this population.

### B. Growth and Development:

Growth failure continues to be a serious concern in children posttransplantation; many experience no improvement in growth. Subsequent growth correlates with patient age and amount of growth failure at the time of transplantation. Those children who undergo transplantation when younger than 5 years have the greatest degree of catch-up growth. However, these children never reach normal adult size. The cause of continued decreased growth after transplantation is due to several factors, including an inherent abnormality of the growth hormone axis, steroid use, renal tubular acidosis, and failing allograft function. Although the use of alternate-day dosing of steroids can lead to improved growth, only 30% of patients are currently on this regimen. Finally, the use of recombinant growth hormone leads to improvement in growth, but recent data suggest that its use may lead to increased acute and chronic rejection.

## VII. CONCLUSION

In reviewing the status of renal transplantation in children, we have seen that graft survival has improved tremendously over the past two decades. In spite of this, these patients are still plagued by complications such as infection and growth failure. The present challenge is to find ways to decrease the morbidity attendant with current immunosuppression and continue to discover new and superior medications. Until tissue engineering becomes a reality, providing a better source of organs, the limited cadaveric donor pool means that LRD will continue to provide the principal source of kidneys for pediatric renal transplantation.

## RECOMMENDED READING

Barnett CC, Partrick DA, May DJ, et al. Update in pediatric transplantation. *Curr Opin Urol* 1997;7:103–108.

Barocci S, Valente V, Gumano R, et al. HLA matching in pediatric recipients of a first kidney graft. *Transplantation* 1996;61:151–154.

Benfield MR, McDonald RA, Bartosh SM, et al. Changing trends in pediatric transplantation: 2001 annual report of the North American Pediatric Renal Transplant Cooperative Study. *Pediatr Transplant* 2003;7:321–335.

Furness III PD, Hostan JB, Grampsas SA, et al. Extraperitoneal placement of renal allografts in children weighing less than 15kg. *J Urol* 2001;166:1042–1045.

Hatch DA, Koyle MA, Baskin LS, et al. Kidney transplantation in children with urinary diversion or bladder augmentation. *J Urol* 2001;165:2265–2268.

Koyle MA, Woo HH, Kam I, et al. Management of the lower urinary tract in pediatric transplantation. *Semin Urol* 1994;2:74–83.

Rosenthal JT, Miserantino DP, Mendez R, et al. Extending the criteria for cadaver kidney donors. *Transplant Proc* 1990;22:338.

Smith JM, Nemath TL, McDonald RM. Current immunosuppressive agents: efficacy, side effects, and utilization. *Pediatr Clin North Am* 2003;50:1283–1300.

Wood EG, Hand M, Briscoe DM, et al. Risk factors for mortality in infants and young children on dialysis. *Am J Kidney Dis* 2001;37:573–579.

# Pediatric Urologic Oncology

Michael Ritchey

I. **NEUROBLASTOMA**
   A. **Epidemiology:** Neuroblastoma is the most common extracranial solid tumor in children, accounting for 8% to 10% of all childhood tumors. It is the most common malignant tumor in infancy and 75% of the cases are noted by the fourth year of life.
   B. **Genetics:** Neuroblastoma can be familial with an autosomal dominant mode of inheritance. Most cases are sporadic, however. Numerous chromosomal abnormalities occur in neuroblastoma and are of prognostic significance. Deletion of the short arm of chromosome 1 is found in 70% to 80% of cases and is an adverse prognostic factor.
   C. **Clinical Presentation**
      1. Most primary tumors arise within the abdomen. Many children present with a palpable abdominal mass. Extrinsic compression of the bowel can produce symptoms.
      2. Metastasis is present in 70% of patients at diagnosis and can be responsible for a variety of symptoms. Some children present with rather unique paraneoplastic syndromes. One of these is acute myoclonic encephalopathy that results in myoclonic activity and ataxia. It is thought to result from antibodies produced against the neuroblastoma.
   D. **Diagnosis**
      1. Increased levels of urinary metabolites of catecholamines, vanillylmandelic acid, and homovanillic acid are found in 90% of patients.
      2. Bone marrow involvement from metastatic tumor can produce anemia. Bone marrow biopsies are performed to detect metastatic tumor.
      3. Screening for metabolites of catecholamines has been employed widely in Japan. The goal is to detect disease at an earlier stage. To date, screening has not had an impact on survival.
      4. Plain radiographs may demonstrate a calcified abdominal or posterior mediastinal mass. Skeletal metastasis can be detected with skeletal survey and bone scans. Imaging of both the primary tumor and metastatic sites can be performed with radiolabeled metaiodobenzylguanadine (MIBG). Magnetic resonance imaging (MRI) has advantages in the evaluation of intraspinal tumor extension.

**E. Pathology and Staging**

    **1. Pathology**

        **a.** Autopsy examination in infants has found neuroblastoma in situ in 1 out of 224 infants. Most of these small tumors regress spontaneously as the incidence of neuroblastoma is lower. It has been suggested that overt neuroblastomas can regress spontaneously. Neuroblastoma, ganglioneuroblastoma, and ganglioneuroma display a histologic spectrum of maturation and differentiation. Ganglioneuroma may arise *de novo* or result from maturation of preexisting neuroblastoma.

        **b.** The Shimada classification is used to stratify patients according to tumor prognosis. The classification determines whether the tumor is stromal poor or stromal rich. Stromal-poor tumors have a poor prognosis.

    **2.** Prognostic variables: Children age 1 year or younger have an improved survival when compared with older children. This is attributed to more favorable biologic parameters in this age group.

        **a.** Site of origin has been correlated with survival. Thoracic tumors have a better prognosis.

        **b.** Stage of disease is one of the most important prognostic indicators. More advanced tumors—stages III and IV—require much more aggressive treatment.

        **c.** A special category is stage IV-S. These tumors primarily occur in infants. They often have small primaries associated with the liver, as well as skin and bone marrow metastases. These patients have a very good prognosis with many tumors undergoing spontaneous regression.

        **d.** $n$-myc amplification is associated with rapid tumor progression and a poor prognosis. $n$-myc amplification is found in 30% to 40% of advanced-stage tumors. This is an adverse prognostic factor, independent of the patient's age or stage of disease.

        **e.** Stage of the disease is a significant prognostic variable. It is used to determine postoperative adjuvant therapy.

**F. International Neuroblastoma Staging System**

    **1.** Stage 1: Localized tumor with complete gross excision, with or without microscopic residual disease.

    **2.** Stage 2A: Localized tumor with incomplete gross excision; representative ipsilateral nonadherent lymph nodes negative for tumor microscopically.

    **3.** Stage 2B: Localized tumor with or without complete gross excision, with ipsilateral nonadherent lymph nodes positive for tumor.

4. Stage 3: Unresectable unilateral tumor infiltrating across the midline, with or without regional lymph node involvement; or localized unilateral tumor with contralateral regional lymph node involvement; or midline tumor with bilateral extension by infiltration (unresectable) or by lymph node involvement.

5. Stage 4: Any primary tumor with dissemination to distant lymph nodes, bone, bone marrow, liver, skin, or other organs.

6. Stage 4S: Localized primary tumor with dissemination limited to skin, liver, or bone marrow (less than 10% tumor) in infants younger than 1 year.

G. **Surgical Management**

1. Low-risk disease (stage I, II, IVS): Children with low-stage disease have an excellent survival with surgical excision alone.

2. High-risk disease (stage III, IV): There is some controversy regarding aggressive surgical resection at diagnosis. Many centers defer surgery until after completion of chemotherapy. Timing of surgery is generally after 13 to 18 weeks of therapy.

H. **Postoperative Treatment**

1. Chemotherapy: A variety of multiagent treatments have been developed to treat high-risk patients. Despite marked treatment intensification, relapse continues to be a problem with 4-year overall survival for patients with stage IV disease of only 20%. The use of marrow ablative chemoradiotherapy followed by autologous marrow transplant has resulted in higher survival rates. Other modalities are being developed to target the tumor using biologic therapy.

2. Radiation therapy: Radiation therapy is primarily used for treatment for unresectable disease. Intraoperative radiation can deliver higher radiation doses while sparing local tissues.

## II. RHABDOMYOSARCOMA

A. **Epidemiology:** Rhabdomyosarcoma (RMS) accounts for 15% of all pediatric solid tumors with 20% of RMS arising in the genitourinary (GU) tract. The most common GU sites are prostate, bladder, and paratesticular. There is a bimodal age distribution with a peak incidence in the first 2 years of life and again in adolescence.

B. **Genetics**

1. The Li-Fraumeni syndrome associates childhood sarcomas with those mothers who have an increased risk of breast cancer. Mutation of the P53 tumor suppressor gene was found in patients with this syndrome.

2. A number of cytogenetic abnormalities have been noted in RMS. Correlation of these abnormalities with clinical behavior has not yet been proven.

C. **Clinical Presentation**
   1. Presentation varies by tumor site. Bladder and prostate tumors often have a clinical presentation of urinary obstruction. This can be stranguria or urinary retention. Hematuria is common. Physical examination often reveals a palpable abdominal mass.
   2. Paratesticular RMS presents as a painless scrotal mass. It is usually detected at an earlier stage because of its superficial location.
   3. Vaginal and vulvar RMS present with a vaginal mass and/or bleeding. Prolapse of the mass from the vaginal introitus can be quite striking. This is a typical finding with the sarcoma botryoides variant.
D. **Diagnosis:** Computed tomography (CT) or MRI is used to stage the extent of disease. It can be difficult to determine the site of origin of pelvic tumors. This is particularly true for distinguishing bladder and prostate tumors. In paratesticular RMS, it is important to assess the lymph node status. Lymph nodes are the primary site of initial extension.
E. **Pathology and Staging**
   1. Pathology: There are three main pathologic variants of RMS. Embryonal RMS is the most common subtype and accounts for most GU tumors. This type can present as sarcoma botryoides, a polypoid variety that occurs in hollow organs or body cavities such as the bladder or vagina. The botryoides variants have excellent survival. The second most common type is alveolar, and has a worse prognosis.
   2. Staging: Intergroup Rhabdomyosarcoma Study (IRS) Clinical Staging Classification
      a. Stage 1: Favorable site, nonmetastatic
      b. Stage 2: Unfavorable, small, negative nodes, nonmetastatic
      c. Stage 3: Unfavorable, big or positive nodes, nonmetastatic
      d. Stage 4: Any site, metastatic
F. **Surgical Treatment:** The role of surgery varies by site.
   1. Paratesticular tumor: Initial intervention is radical orchiectomy. The tumor arises in the distal spermatic cord and may invade the testis or surrounding tissues. Retroperitoneal sampling is not recommended in children younger than 10. Children older than 10 should undergo ipsilateral retroperitoneal lymph node dissection prior to chemotherapy.
   2. Bladder or prostate: Surgical management of a bladder/prostate primary has become more conservative. Most patients receive chemotherapy, radiation, or both prior to surgery. The goal is to shrink the tumor to allow bladder preservation. With intensification of treatment, 60% of the patients now retain a functional bladder with an overall survival of 85%. Tumors that are in the periphery of the bladder can be managed with partial cystectomy. If chemotherapy does not result in adequate shrinkage to allow partial resection, a radical cystectomy

may be necessary. Radical prostatectomy has been used for selective primaries confined to the prostate gland.

G. **Postoperative Treatment:** Multimodality therapy is used in the treatment of RMS. The primary chemotherapy is vincristine, dactinomycin, and cyclophosphamide. For higher-risk tumors, more intensive regimens have been utilized. Radiation therapy is given if the tumor fails to regress on chemotherapy. Survival rates vary by site.

1. Paratesticular: Survival of stage 1 and 2 is excellent with a greater than 90% 3-year survival.

2. Vagina or uterus: These tumors respond very well to preoperative therapy. Less than 15% require surgical resection. Survival exceeds 90%.

3. Bladder or prostate: A major goal in treatment of patients with these tumors is bladder preservation. Survival has improved, although relapse continues to be a problem.

H. **Late Effects:** A primary concern is the late risk of bladder dysfunction in patients treated with pelvic irradiation. This can result in decreased compliance leading to renal problems. Cyclophosphamide can cause hemorrhagic cystitis. The use of mesna in conjunction with drug administration has decreased the incidence of cystitis.

III. **WILMS TUMOR**

A. **Epidemiology:** The incidence of Wilms tumor in children age less than 15 years is 7 to 10 cases per million. Median age at presentation is 3 years with 80% of the cases presenting under age 5. Children with bilateral tumors present at a younger age.

B. **Genetics**

1. A number of recognizable syndromes are associated with increased incidence of Wilms tumor. These are divided into overgrowth and non-overgrowth syndromes. The non-overgrowth syndromes include aniridia and the Denys–Drash syndrome. Aniridia is found in 1% of Wilms tumor patients. It is associated with WAGR syndrome (Wilms tumor, aniridia, genital anomalies, mental retardation). A deletion of chromosome 11 was first detected in these patients. Approximately 50% of the patients with the WAGR syndrome and chromosome 11 deletion will develop Wilms tumor.

2. An example of an overgrowth syndrome is the Beckwith–Wiedemann syndrome. This is characterized by organomegaly such as nephromegaly and liver enlargement. Children with isolated hemihypertrophy also are at increased risk for Wilms tumor. The risk of Wilms tumor in Beckwith–Wiedemann syndrome and hemihypertrophy is approximately 10%.

3. A study of children with these syndromes has led to the identification of two genes responsible for the development of Wilms tumor. WT-1 is located

on chromosome 11p13 and is associated with patients with aniridia and Denys–Drash syndrome. WT-2 has been identified on chromosome 11p15. It has been linked to the Beckwith–Wiedemann syndrome.

4. Other chromosomal abnormalities have been found in Wilms tumor patients. The loss of heterozygosity for chromosome 16q and 1p has been found to be associated with an adverse prognosis. This is currently under study by the National Wilms Tumor Study Group.

C. **Clinical Presentation:** A palpable abdominal mass is present in over 90% of children. Tumor rupture can occur leading to the signs and symptoms of an acute abdomen. Hematuria is a less common presentation, but microscopic hematuria is common. Extension of the tumor into the venous drainage from the kidney can produce varicocele, ascites, and even congestive heart failure due to extension into the right atrium.

D. **Diagnosis**
   1. Ultrasound confirms a solid tumor and may identify the site of origin. Either CT or MRI are next performed in all children, but cannot distinguish Wilms tumor from other renal tumors of childhood.
   2. Preoperative imaging should exclude intracaval extension. Ultrasound is useful in this regard. MRI is the study of choice if ultrasound is inconclusive.
   3. Diagnosis of extrarenal extension of the tumor is important in staging. Imaging studies may suspect regional extension to surrounding organs but it is not that reliable. The contralateral kidney should be evaluated to exclude bilateral disease. Very few lesions are missed by imaging.

E. **Pathology and Staging**
   1. Pathology: Most tumors are categorized as favorable histology. Wilms tumor typically has three components: blastema, epithelial, and stroma. Anaplasia of the tumor is found in approximately 5% of children. It is associated with resistance to therapy. Complete excision of these tumors is mandatory. Other variants once thought to be Wilms tumor are now considered to be separate entities (see below).
   2. Staging
      a. Stage I: Tumor limited to the kidney and completely excised. The renal capsule is intact and the tumor was not ruptured prior to removal. There is no residual tumor.
      b. Stage II: Tumor extends through the perirenal capsule, but is completely excised. There may be local spillage of tumor confined to the flank or the tumor may have been biopsied. Extrarenal vessels may contain tumor thrombus or be infiltrated by tumor.

    **c.** Stage III: Residual nonhematogenous tumor confined to the abdomen: lymph node involvement, diffuse peritoneal spillage, peritoneal implants, tumor beyond surgical margin either grossly or microscopically, or tumor not completely removed.

    **d.** Stage IV: Hematogenous metastases to lung, liver, bone, brain, or other sites.

    **e.** Stage V: Bilateral renal involvement at diagnosis.

**F. Surgical Treatment**

  **1.** Nephrectomy should be done via a transperitoneal approach. The surgeon is responsible for staging of the tumor. Sampling lymph nodes is imperative. Surgeons should look for evidence of extension to the other organs and ruptured tumor within the peritoneal cavity.

  **2.** The surgeon is responsible for removing the tumor intact. Tumor spillage results in a sixfold increase in local abdominal relapse. Local relapse is associated with a significant reduction in survival. Surgical complications remain common occurring in 11% of patients.

**G. Postoperative Treatment:** In North America, most patients with Wilms tumor are treated with primary surgery followed by postoperative regimen therapy. In Europe and other countries, preoperative chemotherapy is the initial treatment. Results of these studies are reviewed.

  **1.** National Wilms Tumor Study Group

    **a.** The overall survival for patients with favorable histology now exceeds 90%. Stage I and II patients are treated with dactinomycin and vincristine for 18 weeks. Survival is 94%. Stage III and IV tumors also receive doxorubicin. Radiation therapy is given for residual tumor, diffuse tumor spill, and distant metastasis. The 4-year overall survival in stage III patients is 90% and for stage IV is 80%.

    **b.** Children with anaplastic tumors continue to do poorly. More intensive chemotherapy regimens have been employed without any survival advantage. The 4-year relapse-free survival remains poor. Current trials are utilizing biologic factors to stratify patients for therapy. In particular, chromosome 16q and 1p are evaluated in all patients.

  **2.** International Society of Pediatric Oncology (SIOP): SIOP has adopted the approach of preoperative therapy. Chemotherapy, consisting of dactinomycin and vincristine, is given for 4 weeks followed by surgery. Preoperative therapy can produce a fairly dramatic response with shrinkage of the tumor. This will result in more postchemotherapy stage I patients. More recently, the SIOP group has used the response of the tumor on histologic examination to determine chemotherapy treatment. Low-risk patients are those with marked necrosis of the tumor with chemotherapy. One concern regarding preoperative therapy is less precise staging due to eradication of extrarenal tumor deposits that could result in increased local relapse if these patients are undertreated.

3. Bilateral tumors: Five percent of patients present with bilateral tumors at diagnosis. These tumors often arise from precursor lesions known as *nephrogenic rests*. Preservation of renal tissue is necessary in this group of children who are at increased risk of renal failure. Preoperative chemotherapy is used in all patients with bilateral tumors. Using this approach, nephrectomy can be avoided entirely in almost 50% of the patients.

**H. Late Effects of Treatment**

1. Numerous organ systems are subject to late sequelae of anticancer therapy. Early reports found that irradiation could result in scoliosis. The radiation dose has been decreased and the radiation portals were changed. Musculoskeletal problems are now much less common.

2. Gonadal radiation can produce infertility in both boys and girls. A 12% incidence of ovarian failure has been noted after abdominal radiation therapy. This abdominal radiation can also lead to adverse pregnancy outcomes.

3. Doxorubicin is associated with an increased risk of congestive heart failure. Cardiomyopathy can develop many years after treatment. The incidence of congestive heart failure is 4.4% among Wilms tumor patients receiving doxorubicin as their initial chemotherapy regimen.

4. An increased risk of renal failure has been found in patients with bilateral tumors. Patients with Wilms tumor in association with aniridia and GU anomalies also have an increased risk of renal failure, occurring more than 10 years after initial treatment. Children with the Denys–Drash syndrome have an increased risk of renal failure due to co-existent glomerulopathy.

**IV. OTHER RENAL TUMORS**

**A. Congenital Mesoblastic Nephroma (CMN):** CMN is the most common renal tumor in infants. These tumors are predominately composed of bundles of spindle cells resembling smooth muscle cells. Most of these patients are cured with nephrectomy alone. Some tumors with increased cellularity have been noted to develop local recurrence. The risk is greatest in children under 3 months of age.

**B. Cystic Partially Differentiated Nephroblastoma:** The majority of these tumors occur in the first year of life. Some authorities consider multilocular cystic

nephroma to be the same entity. They are indistinguishable radiographically. The CT shows varying size cysts
sometimes with a prominent septa. Surgery is curative in almost all patients if the tumor is completely
removed. For those with incomplete resection, postoperative dactinomycin and vincristine are administered.
Partial nephrectomy can be performed if the tumor is
confined to the pole of the kidney.

C. **Clear Cell Sarcoma of the Kidney (CCSK):** CCSK
accounts for 3% of renal tumors. The age at diagnosis is similar to nephroblastoma. Prognosis is improved
in those with lower stage. Doxorubicin has greatly improved survival of these children. They all require radiation therapy. Patients with stage I tumor have a 98%
survival rate. Late recurrences can occur. These tumors
are unique in that they are prone to bone, as well as
brain metastasis.

D. **Rhabdoid Tumor of the Kidney (RTK):** RTK is the
most aggressive and lethal renal tumor. It accounts for
2% of renal tumors. It typically occurs at a very young
age with a median age at diagnosis of 16 months. It is
very unresponsive to chemotherapy and most patients
with metastatic disease do not survive.

E. **Renal Cell Carcinoma:** Renal cell carcinoma is the
most common renal tumor in the second decade of life.
Complete tumor resection is the most important determinant of outcome. Patients with stage I tumors usually survive. No studies have been conducted to identify
effective adjuvant treatment for higher stage patients.

F. **Angiomyolipoma:** Angiomyolipoma develops in 80%
of patients with tuberous sclerosis. The incidence of angiomyolipoma increases with age in these patients. Annual ultrasounds are recommended to detect growth
of tumors. Less commonly, renal cell carcinoma occurs in these children. The risk of bleeding increases
with lesions greater than 4 cm in diameter. Selective angiographic embolization has been used for treatment.

V. **TESTICULAR TUMORS**

A. **Epidemiology:** Testicular tumors represent 1% to 2%
of all solid pediatric tumors. Benign lesions occur more
commonly in children than adults. Recent reports have
noted benign testicular lesions such as teratoma occur
more often than germ cell malignancy. The incidence
of childhood testicular tumor peaks at age 2 years, but
rises again after puberty.

B. **Genetic:** A variety of chromosomal abnormalities have
been found in both adolescent and adult germ cell tumors. It is not yet clear what association these have
with development of testicular tumor. Nor have they
been found to be of prognostic importance. There is a
clear increased risk of germ cell tumors in children with
a history of cryptorchidism. Intratubular germ cell neo-
plasia has been found with increased incidence in adults
with a history of undescended testes.

C. **Clinical Presentation:** Painless testicular mass is the most common clinical finding. Unfortunately, many patients can be misdiagnosed with other benign conditions such as epididymitis, hydrocele, or hernia. Testicular ultrasound is invaluable in assessing scrotal pathology. Ultrasound is particularly helpful to identify cystic components of testicular teratoma as well as epidermoid cysts. Recognition of these lesions preoperatively can provide for a testis-sparing procedure.

D. **Diagnosis**

1. CT of the retroperitoneum and chest are necessary to exclude metastatic lesions in germ cell tumors. Most retroperitoneal lymph node metastasis can be identified but 15% to 20% are missed.

2. Tumor markers are important in germ cell tumors. $\alpha$-Fetoprotein (AFP) is produced by tumors that contain yolk sac elements. Assessment of AFP after removal of tumor is essential. Persistently high levels reflect metastatic disease. The exception is that, in infants, normal adult levels are not reached. $\beta$-hCG is produced by embryonal and mixed germ cell tumors. It is not commonly elevated in prepubertal patients.

E. **Pathology and Staging**

1. **Staging**

   a. Stage I: Tumor is limited to the testis. Tumor markers are negative after appropriate half-life decline.

   b. Stage II: Microscopic residual disease is present in the scrotum or spermatic cord. Tumor markers remain elevated after appropriate half-life interval. Tumor rupture or scrotal biopsy occurred prior to complete orchiectomy.

   c. Stage III: Retroperitoneal lymph node metastases.

   d. Stage IV: Distant metastases.

2. **Pathology**

   a. Teratoma is the most common germ cell tumor in prepubertal children. The tumor may have elements from more than one germ cell layer. The microscopic appearance varies with the degree of maturation and the amount of tissue from each germ cell layer.

   b. Yolk sac tumor is also known as endodermal sinus tumor. A characteristic finding in yolk sac tumors is Schiller–Duval bodies. Special staining will demonstrate the presence of AFP.

   c. Leydig cell, Sertoli cell, and granulosa cell tumors have a common embryologic origin. The pathologic feature characteristic of Leydig cell tumors is Reinke crystals present in 40% of the tumors.

   d. Gonadoblastomas are the most common tumors found in patients with intersex disorders.

The germ cell component of gonadoblastoma is prone to malignant degeneration. The tumors occur in dysplastic or streak gonads.

**F.  Surgical Treatment:** Malignant tumors are managed by radical inguinal orchiectomy. Scrotal approach to a testicular mass is avoided. This leads to an increase in stage of the tumor and requires more intensive therapy. Benign tumors such as teratoma and epidermoid cysts are amenable to a testis-sparing approach in some cases. With complete excision of the lesion, no cases of recurrence have been noted.

**G.  Postoperative Treatment**

1.  Mature teratoma: Radical or partial orchiectomy is curative in prepubertal patients. After puberty assessment of retroperitoneal lymph nodes is mandatory. Immature teratoma is less common. It occurs more often in the ovary than the testis. Recurrence of an immature teratoma may occur in patients with elevated AFP or evidence of yolk sac tumor in the specimen.

2.  Yolk Sac Tumors

    a.  Initial treatment for yolk sac tumors is radical orchiectomy. This is curative in most children. Clinical stage I patients do not receive adjuvant therapy after radical orchiectomy. Careful surveillance is performed. If elevation of AFP is noted, chemotherapy is begun.

    b.  Patients with stage II to IV tumors are treated with three cycles of compressed PEB (cisplatin, etoposide, and bleomycin). If a patient has only a partial response then six cycles of chemotherapy are given. Persistent retroperitoneal masses after chemotherapy are uncommon.

3.  Gonadal stromal tumors: Inguinal orchiectomy is curative for Leydig cell tumors in prepubertal children. The patient with a Sertoli cell tumor should undergo retroperitoneal lymph node sampling after orchiectomy.

# VI.  MISCELLANEOUS TUMORS

**A.  Adrenal Tumors**

1.  Pheochromocytoma

    a.  These tumors originate either in the adrenal gland or in extraadrenal sites along the paraaortic sympathetic chain. These tumors can occur in association with syndromes such as neurofibromatosis, tuberous sclerosis, or von Hippel–Lindau syndrome.

    b.  Pheochromocytomas secrete catecholamines and can produce symptoms of catecholamine excess, which can include headache, hypertension, tachycardia, and arrhythmia. Laboratory studies demonstrate increased levels of urinary metanephrines and plasma levels of epinephrine and norepinephrine. MRI shows hyperdense lesions on T2 images. MIBG scans can also localize the tumor. The primary treatment is surgical removal.

2. Cushing syndrome

   a. Adrenal tumors can produce elevated levels of corticosteroids leading to the diagnosis of Cushing syndrome. The features of corticosteroid excess include increased weight gain with moon facies and truncal obesity. Hypertension can also result.

   b. Evaluation of the patient should include biochemistry studies to demonstrate the excess corticosteroid production. Urinary steroids will demonstrate markedly elevated 17-ketosteroid levels. Plasma cortisol is also elevated due to the excess secretion of steroids. Adrenocorticotropic hormone is decreased.

B. **Bladder Tumors**

   1. Nephrogenic adenoma: Nephrogenic adenoma is a benign tumor that can occur both in children and adults. It is typically seen in patients with prior bladder surgeries and recurrent infections. It has also been reported after renal transplantation in immunosuppressed patients. It is felt to be a metaplastic lesion. Endoscopically the lesions are typically small and consistent with papillary transitional cell carcinoma. A biopsy is necessary to make the initial diagnosis. Treatment consists of excision and fulguration. These tumors can recur and surveillance is required although at less frequent intervals than for transitional cell carcinoma of the bladder.

   2. Transitional cell carcinoma: Transitional cell carcinoma of the bladder rarely occurs in children. Most cases are found in isolated case reports. There is some suggestion that there is a lower risk for recurrence for transitional cell carcinoma that occurs in younger children. These tumors can also occur as a second malignant neoplasm after prior treatment with cyclophosphamide.

**RECOMMENDED READING**

Andrassy RA, Corpron C, Ritchey ML. Testicular tumors. In: O'Neill J, Rowe M, Grosfeld JL, et al, eds. *Pediatric surgery*, 5th ed. Chicago: Mosby Year Book, 1998:541–545.

Grundy PE, Green DM, Coppes MJ, et al. Renal tumors. In: Pizzo PA, Poplack DG, eds. *Principles and practice of pediatric oncology,* 4th ed. Philadelphia: Lippincott Williams & Wilkins, 2001;865–894.

Ritchey ML. Nephroblastoma. In: Belman DB, King LR, Kramer SA, eds. *Clinical pediatric urology.* Oxford: Isis Medical, 2002:1269–1290.

Ritchey ML, Coppes M, Raney RB, et al. Pediatric urologic oncology. In: Walsh PC, Retik AB, Vaughan ED, et al, eds. *Campbell's urology,* 8th ed. Philadelphia: Saunders, 2002:2469–2507.

# Laparoscopy in Pediatric Urology

Eric A. Kurzrock

Laparoscopy has been used for the diagnosis of abdominal testicles, hernias, and intersex for over 20 years. Only in the last decade has laparoscopy been applied therapeutically. Newer, less-invasive techniques have had a profound impact on the practice of urology. Laparoscopic surgery has the advantages of smaller incisions, less pain, shorter hospitalization, and reduced convalescence. For adults, the laparoscopic approach to nephrectomy is quickly becoming the standard. For children, who rarely require nephrectomy, laparoscopy is most commonly used for the management of abdominal testicles.

Infants and children may also benefit from laparoscopic kidney and bladder surgery, but the advantages are arguably less. Because a child's bladder and kidneys are much closer to the surface and smaller, they can be repaired or removed through small (3- to 5-cm) open incisions with less division of muscle. Most children can be discharged home within 24 hours of a standard nephrectomy, pyeloplasty, or ureteral reimplantation.

Laparoscopy does have a substantial role in pediatric urology. There are a number of surgical procedures for which laparoscopy has utility and others that are controversial. In some instances, laparoscopy can be combined with open surgery. With the development of smaller robotic instruments and increasing experience, laparoscopy is certain to become a major component of pediatric urologic surgery.

## I. INSTRUMENTATION AND TECHNNIQUE

Telescopes are available in 2- to 10-mm sizes. The initial port placement can be done blindly with a Veress needle, through an open incision, or with newer trocars that allow direct vision. Other ports are then placed under direct laparoscopic vision. Most pediatric procedures are performed with 3.5- or 5-mm working instruments. A full array of instruments is available including dissectors, graspers, needle drivers, and cautery and suction devices. Morcellators and bags may be used for specimen removal. The laparoscope provides magnification, but the instruments and port angles limit the surgeon's dexterity and movement. Robotics should obviate these problems in the future.

Most laparoscopic procedures are performed within the peritoneum. However, retroperitoneoscopy is becoming popular for kidney procedures. Operating within the peritoneal space has the advantage of more working space, but there is also a risk of injuring the bowel or inducing bowel adhesions. Retroperitoneoscopy provides a smaller working area, but the kidney is closer and there is no bowel, liver, or spleen obstructing the view.

## II. DIAGNOSTIC USES

### A. Inguinal Hernia:
A metachronous, contralateral hernia will develop in 5% to 10% of children. Age, sex, and side affect the risk. Prior to laparoscopy, contralateral, open, inguinal exploration was the standard for young children. Laparoscopy obviates a contralateral incision in most children. During hernia repair, a 70- or 120-degree telescope is passed through the ipsilateral hernia sac. The contralateral, internal ring is easily visualized from within the peritoneal cavity. If patent, contralateral hernia repair is typically performed. What remains to be determined is the correlation between a patent contralateral internal ring detected by laparoscopic inspection and the incidence of a clinical hernia in the future. Diagnostic laparoscopy via the umbilicus may be valuable in the patient with a persistent hydrocele after ligation of a patent processus vaginalis. It will determine whether or not the hydrocele is due to persistence of the communication.

### B. Nonpalpable Undescended Testis:
There is no imaging modality that is 100% sensitive in identifying an intraabdominal testis. Laparoscopy can easily determine the presence and location of a testicle. Findings include the following.

1.  Intraabdominal testis
    Usually near the internal ring
    Occasionally the testis is in the pelvis or near the kidney.
2.  Vas deferens and gonadal vessels pass through internal ring
    a.  Robust vessel suggests an inguinal testis.
    b.  Thin vessel suggests an atrophic testis in the scrotum or inguinal canal.
        Inguinal exploration is required in either case.
3.  Gonadal vessels fade away before entering the internal ring
    If a blind-ending vessel is absolutely evident, inguinal exploration is unnecessary. Some would recommend fixation of the contralateral testis to prevent a torsion.

### C. Intersex:
Laparoscopy allows delineation of internal genital structures and possible biopsy of internal gonads.

## III. THERAPEUTIC USES

### A. Abdominal Testis:
For the intraabdominal testis, laparoscopic orchiopexy appears to be comparable to open techniques. Outcome measures include testicular scrotal position and atrophy. Laparoscopy is particularly advantageous for older boys or boys with high, abdominal testicles. For a two-stage Fowler-Stephens orchiopexy, clipping of the gonadal artery during the first stage is simplified by laparoscopy. The second stage can be completed using either an open or a laparoscopic technique.

**B.  Nephrectomy and Nephroureterectomy**
1.  Indications
   a.  Nonfunctional kidney secondary to
      (1)  Cystic disease
      (2)  Reflux nephropathy
      (3)  Hydronephrosis
   b.  Donor transplant
   c.  Pretransplant nephrectomy
2.  Contraindications
   a.  Tumor
   b.  Trauma
   c.  Infection
**C.  Partial Nephrectomy**
   Primary indication is a duplex kidney
      (1)  Poorly functioning upper pole associated with ureterocele or ectopia
      (2)  Poorly functioning lower pole associated with reflux
**D.  Pyeloplasty and Ureteral Reimplantation:** Although slowly becoming common for adults, laparoscopic pyeloplasty is performed by very few pediatric urologists. Most consider this application to be in the investigational stage. Standard open pyeloplasty and ureteral reimplantation are over 95% successful and can be performed through very small, muscle-splitting incisions. Hospitalization is less than 24 hours in experienced hands. Both procedures require significant suturing. With the popularization of robotics, the laparoscopic approach may one day equal or better open techniques. It is important to remember that, as noted, the morbidity of these procedures in children is comparable in the open and laparoscopic approaches, so that the advantages of laparoscopy are minimal. The exception may be nephroureterectomy, in which a much larger incision is needed for laparoscopic nephrectomy.
**E.  Uncommon Laparoscopic Procedures**
1.  Renal biopsy
2.  Urachal abnormality
3.  Enterocystoplasty
4.  Vaginoplasty
5.  Continent urinary diversion
6.  Appendicocecostomy

## RECOMMENDED READING

Docimo SG, Peters CA. Pediatric endourology and laparoscopy. In: Walsh PC, Retik AB, Vaughan ED, et al, eds. *Campbell's urology,* 8th ed. Philadelphia: WB Saunders, 2002:2564.

Franks M, Schneck FX, Docimo SG. Retroperitoneoscopy in children. In: Caione P, Kavoussi LR, Micali F, eds. *Retroperitoneoscopy and extraperitoneal laparoscopy in pediatric and adult urology.* Milan: Springer, 2003:103.

# Anesthesia for Pediatric Urologic Procedures

## Melissa A. Ehlers

Surgery is a stressful event for everyone, and even more so for children who may not understand the reason for their surgery. Coupled with potential feelings of embarrassment or shame involved with examinations of the genitalia, the presurgical time is a high-anxiety state that the knowledgeable practitioner should anticipate and work to alleviate. A plan can be fashioned that reduces anxiety for the patient, parents, and everyone involved, as well as providing a safe anesthetic and assisting in postoperative pain control.

## I. PREOPERATIVE PREPARATION

A. **Allay Fears Early!** Preparation of a pediatric patient for urologic surgery begins in the surgeon's office or clinic. Besides discussing the risks and benefits of a certain procedure with the parents (and the patient if age appropriate), it is usually helpful to describe to the child what to expect when he or she arrives for the operation. Many hospitals give tours or Perioperative Ambulatory Care Unit (PACU) parties for prospective patients and their families where they can see the check-in area, surgical holding area (hopefully an area separate from the adult presurgical area, and stocked with toys!), PACU area, and possibly one of the rooms in the pediatric ward or intensive care unit (ICU) if admission is planned. Alternatively (or in addition), many anesthesia groups provide their own handout or pamphlet to be passed out to the patient and their family that delineates NPO guidelines as well as discussing some of the rudiments of anesthesia for their child and methods of postoperative pain control.

B. **Who Needs the Prescreening Clinic?** Many institutions are allowing healthy pediatric patients to bypass the prescreening clinic and instead do the screening on the day of surgery, thus preventing extra lost days from school and work, as well as probably helping to keep the child's anxiety level at a minimum. Of course, this is only applicable to healthy children and any child who is by standards of the American Society of Anesthesiologists (ASA) 3 or higher (see section IIC) or who has a systemic disease that is not stable should be prescreened to avoid a possible delay or cancellation on the day of surgery. Patients with some syndromes warrant a very close look because they frequently have physiologic abnormalities with specific implications during anesthesia (see section IID). In addition, any history of problems with anesthesia in the past, or even more significantly a family history of malignant hyperthermia, warrants referral to the prescreening clinic.

C. **ASA Classification of Physical Status**

   a. Class 1: There is no organic, physiologic, biochemical, or psychiatric disturbance. The pathologic process for which the operation is to be performed is localized and is not a systemic disturbance.

   b. Class 2: Mild to moderate systemic disturbance caused either by the condition to be treated surgically or by other pathophysiologic processes.

   c. Class 3: Severe systemic disturbance or disease from whatever cause, even though it may not be possible to define the degree of disability with finality.

   d. Class 4: Indicative of the subject with a severe systemic disorder already life threatening, not always correctable by the operative procedure.

   e. Class 5: The moribund subject has little chance of survival, but is submitted to an operation in desperation.

D. Common syndromes with specific implications for anesthetic management (not meant to be an all-inclusive list)

   1. Beckwith (Wiedemann) syndrome: Difficult airway, neonatal hypoglycemia

   2. Down syndrome (trisomy 21): Difficult airway, sleep apnea, atlantoaxial instability, congenital heart disease

   3. Goldenhaar syndrome: Difficult airway, congenital heart disease

   4. Hemolytic uremic syndrome: Renal failure, hepatic dysfunction, seizures, coagulopathy

   5. Pierre Robin syndrome: Difficult airway, congenital heart disease

   6. Prune-belly syndrome: Difficult airway, congenital heart disease

   7. VATER (or VACTERL) syndrome: Congenital heart disease, gastrointestinal atresias, tracheoesophageal fistula, renal issues

E. **NPO Guidelines:** Guidelines for *nulla per os* vary from hospital to hospital, but in general are starting to become more liberalized for pediatric patients. A recent ASA publication evaluated the evidence supporting current NPO practices and came up with the following recommendations for fasting prior to anesthesia.

   1. No clear liquids for 2 or more hours.

   2. No breast milk for 4 or more hours.

   3. No meals or nonhuman milk for 6 hours. High-fat foods may prolong gastric emptying time.

II. **DAY OF SURGERY**

A. **Parental Reassurance:** Studies have shown that one of the major factors in determining a child's anxiety level is the anxiety level of his or her parents. Calm parents keep the young child from being unduly alarmed about their trip to the hospital, and likewise provide a model for the older child or adolescent who is undergoing an operation. Needless to say, it is difficult for a child to control his or her own fears when the child has parents who are struggling to control their own fears!

**B. Premedication:** Depending on the child's level of anxiety and anticipated cooperation, an oral premedication is frequently given. Midazolam is the most frequently used drug because it has a relatively fast onset, ease of administration (works as well orally as it does intranasal or PR), and a low side effect profile. Studies have shown that children who receive a premedication show less anxiety at induction, are more cooperative, and have fewer regressive behaviors postoperatively (e.g., bedwetting, temper tantrums), all of which contribute to a significant decrease in parental anxiety as well.

**C. Parents in the OR:** Many institutions allow the presence of parents during anesthesia induction for pediatric patients. For hospitals with induction rooms this is accomplished quite easily, but at other institutions this may involve extensive preparation, including dressing the parents up in some type of cover suit as well as hat and mask, escorting them through the OR with the child, and then ensuring that personnel are available to escort them back out to the surgical waiting area after induction has been accomplished.

Studies have shown no significant difference in reduction of the child's anxiety between parental presence in the OR versus premedication. Indeed, it may be more stressful for all parties when there are potential difficulties with induction or the airway.

**D. Mode of Anesthesia:** The vast majority of pediatric urologic procedures are performed under general anesthesia, but spinal anesthesia is an option for infants (usually up to around 6 months old) or in the mature adolescent. When a spinal anesthetic is used, it is important to remember not to allow anyone to lift the legs (usually this occurs for electrocautery grounding pad placement) for at least 10 minutes after the spinal is in place as this may allow the local anesthetic to migrate so far cranially as to cause respiratory compromise or even a total spinal.

**E. Pain Control:** Numerous studies have found that children's pain in general is seriously undertreated, so it is important to have assessment tools in place to rapidly diagnose and treat pain in this population. For instance, many institutions use the Wong-Baker faces scale (Fig. 27–1) to evaluate pain in grade-school children. Almost all scales used for pain assessment use a range of 0 to 10 to describe the pain numerically; a score of less than 4 is considered to be mild pain, whereas a score of 4 or greater is classified as moderate to severe pain.

Good postoperative pain control begins during the anesthetic. Pain management may be approached in a

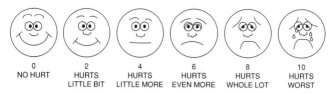

**Fig. 27–1.   Wong-Baker Faces Pain Rating Scale. (From Wong DL, Hockenberry-Eaton M, Wilson D, et al. *Wong's essentials of pediatric nursing*, 6th ed. St. Louis: Mosby, 2001:1301. Copyrighted by Mosby, Inc. Reprinted by permission.)**

variety of different ways, using different routes, and certainly by many different medications. Although adequate pain control is the end-point, ease of use, feasibility, and side effects are important to consider as well.

1. Neural blockade: Regional nerve blocks are useful to reduce intraoperative anesthetic doses as well as to provide postoperative pain control. Blocks can be performed with local anesthetics, narcotics, or both.

   a. Lumbar/thoracic epidural: This is the most invasive regional technique and is used mainly for operations involving large incisions above the umbilicus. Because children would rarely be cooperative with awake placement, epidural catheters are usually performed under very heavy sedation or more commonly under general anesthesia. Although the complication rate is relatively low, many anesthesiologists feel uncomfortable performing this mode of regional anesthesia in children unless they do it on a regular basis. Pain control is usually excellent postoperatively, but it does require the patient to be connected to one more tubing line; urinary retention may be an issue (especially with a lumbar epidural), and occasionally motor block is present to such a degree as to cause difficulty with ambulation (this usually can be resolved by adjustment of the epidural infusion concentration, rate, or both). Narcotics are often added to the local anesthetic solution being used in the epidural; they act synergistically to decrease the total amount of local anesthetic required. Occasionally they will cause pruritus, and rarely nausea and vomiting or respiratory depression. Because of these potential complications, some centers require that the patient be monitored in the ICU. This may cause issues with bed availability and increases the cost considerably.

   b. Caudal epidural: This is probably the most common type of regional anesthesia performed in pediatric urologic patients. It is quickly placed, using just a needle and syringe, has an extremely low incidence of side effects, and provides pain control below the umbilicus for at least 4 hours when bupivicaine is used, longer when other adjuncts such as clonidine, neostigmine, or epinephrine are mixed with it. Alternatively, many institutions use narcotics that when placed in the epidural space can remain efficacious for up to 24 hours postoperatively. Depending on the additives to the local anesthetic mixture, the caudal can be repeated at the end of surgery if at least 2 hours have elapsed since the first caudal dose was placed. Because the sacrococcygeal ligament progressively ossifies, the block becomes more difficult technically and has a significant failure rate after the age of 7. Urinary retention is very rare after this type of block, but has been reported.

c. Spinal narcotics: An alternative to epidural narcotics, this block can usually be placed more quickly than a lumbar or thoracic epidural, and like epidural narcotics may provide analgesia for up to 24 hours. Disadvantages include its ability to produce respiratory depression depending on the narcotic used, as well as pruritus or nausea and vomiting at higher doses (note: this may also be seen with epidural narcotics).

d. Ilioinguinal block: This easily performed technique blocks sensory innervation to the scrotum and inner aspect of the thigh, thus making it popular for herniorrhaphy, orchiopexy, and hydrocoelectomy. It is performed by infiltrating local anesthetic 1 cm medial and 1 cm caudal to the anterior superior iliac spine, immediately below the plane of the external oblique muscle where the ilioinguinal and iliohypogastric nerves are found.

e. Penile block: This block can provide analgesia for circumcision or hypospadias repair. The most common technique involves injection of local anesthetic at the base of the penis deep to Buck's fascia on either side of the suspensory ligament; a potential drawback to this method is that it does not provide blockade of the genitofemoral and ilioinguinal nerves that provide sensation to the base of the penis. Alternatively, the Dalens method involves infiltration of local anesthetic into the subpubic space, blocking the nerves before their entry into the penis. This also theoretically decreases the risk of injury to neurovascular or other penile structures. A third method entails a subcutaneous ring-block at the base of the penis, which also avoids trauma to important structures while still providing analgesia along the entire shaft.

2. Intravenous agents

    **a.** Narcotics: Narcotics are the traditional cornerstone of pain treatment. Their safety and efficacy in children when used in appropriate doses has been well documented. Morphine is the most commonly used opiate in this class. Dosing is usually 0.03 to 0.05 mg/kg IV every 2 to 4 hours for patients older than 6 months, and 0.05 to 0.20 mg/kg IV every 2 to 4 hours for older patients. If frequent dosing is anticipated (or is in fact occurring), consider using a patient-controlled anesthesia with a basal rate. Keep in mind that the metabolites of morphine are also active and may accumulate in patients with renal disease. Side effects include nausea and vomiting, respiratory depression, and decreased bowel motility.

    **b.** Nonsteroidal antiinflammatory drugs (NSAIDs): Ketorolac (Toradol) is a frequent favorite in urologic surgery because it has a strong analgesic effect with minimal side effects. Ketorolac usually allows opiate use to be reduced or eliminated, thereby reducing opiate side effects. In addition, ketorolac is effective in reducing bladder spasms, a common problem in children who have catheters postoperatively. Because NSAIDs inhibit renal prostaglandin synthesis, they should be used cautiously in patients with renal failure or if administered concomitantly with nephrotoxic drugs (e.g., IV gentamicin and ketorolac probably should not be given too close to one another). In addition, the NSAIDs inhibit platelet function that, in theory, can be dangerous in any patient at increased risk for bleeding intra- or postoperatively.

3. Oral agents

    **a.** Acetaminophen (Tylenol): A very widely used drug, especially for pain control at home. Because of its ability to decrease opioid requirements, its ease of administration (PO if appropriate, PR is an alternative, and soon an IV formulation will be available) as well as its low side effect profile, it should probably always be included as part of any analgesia plan, unless significant hepatic disease is present. To get the most advantage possible from this drug, it is important to prescribe it on an around-the-clock basis and not PRN.

    **b.** COX-2 inhibitors: This newest class of NSAIDs claims to have no effect on platelet function while still inhibiting prostaglandin synthesis. Current studies in adults show great promise for overall improvement of pain scores as well as reduction in opiate requirements. Although currently not approved for use in children, multiple studies are underway to prove their efficacy and safety in this age group, and an IV formulation is also being developed. Concerns about cardiovascular side effects in adults are probably not relevant in children but this remains to be investigated.

    **c.** Opiates: Oral opiates are often used for pain control once the patient's gastrointestinal system is working, especially if an IV line is no longer in place. For patients unable to swallow pills, elixirs or syrups are available. Major problems are delayed onset of action and decreased bioavailability, which ranges from 15% to 50%, depending on the patient. Constipation is also common and should be treated aggressively; gas pains may increase the child's discomfort.

   **4.** Nonpharmacologic adjuncts: Never forget the importance of therapeutic maneuvers not found in the PDR—cuddling with a parent may often turn a crying and inconsolable child into a cooperative, sleepy, adorable toddler. Other things to try include gentle heat therapy at the site of discomfort, distraction techniques (with games, toys, etc.), massage therapy, low-stimulation environments (minimal lighting, sounds, and manipulation), and even comfort foods (if medically allowed).

## III. CONCLUSION

A happy and pain-free child with satisfied parents should be the goal after every surgical procedure. To achieve this end, it is important for the surgeon, parents, anesthesiology staff, and nursing staff to work together to optimize their roles and thus optimize patient care.

**RECOMMENDED READING**

Berry FA, Castro BA. Anesthesia for genitourinary surgery. In: Gregory GA, ed. *Pediatric anesthesia*, 4th ed. New York: Churchill Livingstone, 2002:587–616.

Deshpande JK, Tobias JD. *The pediatric pain handbook*. St. Louis: Mosby, 1996.

# Sports Recommendations for Children With Solitary Kidneys and Other Genitourinary Abnormalities

Jack S. Elder

Adequate data on the risks of a particular sport for an athlete with a medical problem are limited or lacking, and an estimate of risk becomes a necessary part of medical decision making. In recent legal decisions, athletes have been permitted to participate in sports despite known medical risks (AAP, 1994). When an athlete's family disregards medical advice against participation, the physician should ask all parents or guardians to sign a written informed consent statement indicating that they have been advised of the potential dangers of participation and that they understand them. The physician should also document, with the child's signature, that the child athlete also understands the risks of participation (AAP, 2001).

I. **CONDITIONS THAT ARE ASSOCIATED WITH IN-CREASED RISK OF INJURY**
   A. **Renal Conditions**
      1. **Solitary Functioning Kidney**
         a. Typically has compensatory hypertrophy, thereby increasing the risk of injuring the kidney, because it is not as well protected by the ribs; the majority of solitary kidneys are right sided, and the right kidney usually is displaced inferiorly by the liver.
         b. Renal agenesis: incidence as high as 1 in 1,000; male:female ratio 1.8:1.0; left side more commonly affected; contralateral vesicoureteral reflux in 20%.
         c. Multicystic dysplastic kidney: nonfunctioning kidney with multiple cysts; incidence 1 in 1,000 to 1,500; contralateral renal abnormality in 20% to 30%, including vesicoureteral reflux and hydronephrosis; may involute and be mistaken for renal agenesis.
         d. S/P nephrectomy for tumor (e.g., congenital mesoblastic nephroma, Wilms tumor, multilocular cystic nephroma, renal cell carcinoma) or nonfunctioning or poorly functioning kidney [ureteropelvic junction (UPJ) obstruction, ureterovesical junction obstruction, vesicoureteral reflux; renal vein thrombosis].

> **2. Hydronephrosis**
> > **a.** UPJ obstruction
> > **b.** Ureterovesical junction obstruction
> > **c.** Vesicoureteral reflux
>
> **3. Anomalies of Renal Position**
> > **a.** Horseshoe kidney: incidence 1 in 400; male: female 2:1; most common renal fusion anomaly; isthmus inferior to inferior mesenteric artery; hydronephrosis common; unilateral multicystic dysplasia more common than in general population.
> > **b.** Other renal fusion anomalies: estimated incidence 1 in 1,000; male:female 2:1; crossed fused ectopia, with or without renal fusion: left crossing to right side accounts for two-thirds; sigmoid kidney, lump kidney, and disc kidney uncommon.
> > **c.** Renal ectopia: pelvic, lumbar; more common on left.
> > **d.** Renal transplant: pelvic position
>
> **4. Abnormal Renal Size**
> > **a.** Autosomal recessive polycystic kidney disease: survival beyond infancy is uncommon, but kidneys are very large.
> > **b.** Autosomal dominant kidney disease: typically diagnosed in adulthood, but affected children typically have hypertension, proteinuria, and renal enlargement.
> > **c.** Angiomyolipoma associated with tuberous sclerosis; both kidneys typically affected.
>
> **5. Reduced Renal Function**
> > **a.** Renal disease: glomerulonephritis, renal cystic disease.
> > **b.** Renal dysplasia: may or may not be associated with vesicoureteral reflux.

**B. Abdominal Conditions**

> **1. Prune-Belly Syndrome:** lax abdominal musculature predisposes to injury of solid abdominal organs as well as fluid-filled organs (e.g., bladder) from blunt trauma.
>
> **2.** S/P augmentation cystoplasty or construction of urinary neobladder with continent diversion, for example, in children with bladder exstrophy, VATER syndrome, and spina bifida.

**C. Testicular Conditions**

> **1.** Solitary functioning testis; typically the solitary testis exhibits compensatory hypertrophy.
> > **a.** Secondary to in utero torsion; left side affected in two-thirds.
> > **b.** Secondary to postnatal testicular torsion; most common in adolescence.
> > **c.** Following removal of testicular tumor.
> > **d.** Following removal of testis from trauma.
> > **e.** Following unsuccessful orchiopexy.

2. **Undescended Testis:** incidence 1 in 60
   a. Unilateral: fertility typically nearly normal, most probably because unaffected testis is functioning normally.
   b. Bilateral: fertility approximately 30% to 60%, in part because of impaired germ cell development, and in some cases because of intraoperative iatrogenic testicular or spermatic cord injury.

## II. DATA ON RENAL TRAUMA

A. Gerstenbluth et al (2002): Reviewed 68 children with blunt renal trauma, mean age 10 years.
   1. Twenty (29%) associated with recreational sports: bicycling ($n = 8$), hockey ($n = 3$), all-terrain vehicle ($n = 2$), sledding ($n = 2$), football ($n = 1$), and jet ski ($n = 1$).
   2. Injury severity score mean 20.6 for bicycle injury and 6.7 for nonbicycle sports-related trauma ($p < 0.05$).
   3. Bicycle injuries: none involved collision with vehicle; grade III ($n = 1$), grade IV ($n = 2$), grade V ($n = 3$) renal injuries; one nephrectomy for life-threatening hemorrhage.
   4. Hockey: grade II ($n = 1$), grade III ($n = 1$), grade IV ($n = 1$); sled grade I and II; football grade I.
   5. Conclusion: Bicycle riding most common sports-related cause of renal injury. Team contact sports uncommon risk factor.

B. McAleer et al (2002): Reviewed 14,763 patients in San Diego trauma registry from 1984 to 2000; identified 193 renal injuries.
   1. Sixty-nine (36%) associated with recreational sports: bicycle ($n = 27$), playground equipment ($n = 8$), all terrain vehicle ($n = 8$), skateboard ($n = 6$), rollerblade ($n = 6$), playing ball ($n = 4$), equestrian ($n = 3$), trampoline ($n = 1$), and team sports ($n = 6$).
   2. Team sports
      a. Football: two contusions, one fracture
      b. Soccer: one contusion with UPJ obstruction
      c. Basketball: one hematoma, one contusion
   3. Team sport injury for overall series 3.40%, vs. 0.04% for renal injury.
   4. Conclusion: Recommendations against team sport participation may not be necessary in patients with a solitary kidney or testis.

C. Wan et al (2003): Reviewed 4,921 children in western New York trauma registry, of whom 15 (0.03%) had genitourinary injury related to sports participation.
   1. Etiology: football ($n = 5$), ice hockey ($n = 2$), skiing ($n = 2$), wrestling ($n = 2$), snowboarding ($n = 1$), sledding ($n = 1$), playground ($n = 1$), and bicycle ($n = 1$).

     **2.** Football: grade I to II ($n = 2$), grade III ($n = 1$), grade IV ($n = 2$)

     **3.** Other grade IV injury from snowboarding.

     **4.** One nephrectomy following skiing injury.

     **5.** Conclusion: snow sports more common risk of renal injury than team sports.

 **D.** Wan et al (2003): Reviewed renal injuries from team sports in the National Pediatric Trauma Registry, 1990 to 1999 (50 reporting centers); 42 (0.05% of total) renal injuries reported.

     **1.** Etiology: football ($n = 26$), baseball ($n = 6$), basketball ($n = 5$), ice hockey ($n = 3$), and soccer ($n = 2$).

     **2.** Did not review bicycle injuries.

     **3.** No injury resulted in functional renal loss or nephrectomy.

     **4.** Conclusion: minimal risk from team sports.

 **E.** **Summary: Renal Trauma from Recreational Sports**

     **1.** Highest risk of renal trauma from bicycling, American football, skiing (including snowboarding and sledding), and ice hockey.

     **2.** No denominator to compute risk of renal injury; however, risk of renal loss is remote.

     **3.** In large series of pediatric trauma, renal injury resulted from motor vehicle injury (child either patient or pedestrian) in 17% to 77% and fall in 6% to 50%. Overall, sports-related causes only 10% of renal trauma.

     **4.** Although the kidney is the most commonly injured organ in blunt abdominal trauma, head injuries are more common. The risk of contact sports includes liver, spleen, and brain. Although only 10% of head injuries are related to sports, head injuries cause 70% of traumatic deaths and 20% of permanent disability in sports.

     **5.** Renal loss from sports activity in child with UPJ obstruction and blunt trauma not reported.

     **6.** No reports in medical literature of loss of solitary kidney from trauma.

**III. DATA ON TESTICULAR TRAUMA FOLLOWING SPORTS INJURY**

 **A.** McAleer et al (2002): Reviewed 14,763 patients in San Diego trauma registry from 1984 to 2000; identified 11 testis injuries from recreational sports; analysis focused on team sports.

     **1.** Cause of testicular injury: team sports ($n = 4$; 2 baseball, 1 basketball, 1 soccer), playing ball ($n = 2$), playing on playground equipment ($n = 2$), rollerblading ($n = 1$), bicycling ($n = 1$), and equestrian sports ($n = 1$).

     **2.** Of four testicular injuries from team sports, there were two fractures and two hematomas.

All were explored and none sustained testicular loss.

**B.** Wan et al (2003): Reviewed testicular injuries from team sports in the National Pediatric Trauma Registry, 1990 to 1999 (50 reporting centers); no injuries reported; limited search to team sports, rollerblading, skateboarding, skiing, sledding, and wrestling.

## IV. AAP RECOMMENDATIONS

From the American Academy of Pediatrics Committee on Sports Medicine and Fitness Regarding Sports Participation (2001).

**A. Classified Sports by Level of Contact**

1. Collision or contact: in collision sport, athletes purposely hit or collide with each other or inanimate objects, including the ground, with great force; in contact sports athletes routinely make contact with each other or inanimate objects, but usually with less force than in collision sports. Contact sports include basketball, boxing, diving, field hockey, tackle football, ice hockey, lacrosse, martial arts, rodeo, rugby, ski jumping, soccer, team handball, water polo, and wrestling.

2. Limited contact: contact with other athletes or inanimate objects is infrequent or inadvertent; includes baseball, bicycling, cheerleading, canoeing or kayaking (white water), fencing, field events (high jump, pole vault), floor hockey, flag football, gymnastics, handball, horseback riding, racquetball, skating (ice, in-line, roller), skiing (cross-country, downhill, water), snowboarding, softball, squash, ultimate Frisbee, volleyball, surfing, and windsurfing.

3. Noncontact sports include all other sporting activities.

**B. Kidney, Absence of One:** "Qualified yes" for participation: "Athlete needs individual assessment for contact, collision, and limited-contact sports."

**C. Testicle, Undescended or Absence of One:** "Yes" for participation: "Certain sports may require a protective cup."

## V. SOLITARY KIDNEY: PEDIATRIC UROLOGISTS RECOMMENDATIONS (2002)

**A.** Sharp et al (2002) surveyed 231 members of the American Academy of Pediatrics, Section on Urology; 182 (79%) responded.

1. Sixty-eight percent strongly advised against participation in contact sports

2. What is advice to patient?
   a. Strongly advise against participation: 26%
   b. Recommend against participation with exception for highly skilled or motivated patient: 30%
   c. No recommendation either way: 14%

    **d.** Recommend allowing participation: 25%

    **e.** Feel strongly that patient should have no restrictions: 4%

Note that recommendations to questions #1 and #2 were inconsistent.

    **3.** Seventy-one percent recommended flank protectors, even if not normally used for that sport.

**VI. SOLITARY KIDNEY: SPORTS MEDICINE SOCIETY RECOMMENDATIONS**

Survey indicated 54% of respondents would allow patients with a solitary kidney to participate fully in sports after discussion of the possible risks; many required signed waiver, use of protective padding, or consultation with a urologist or nephrologist before approving contact sports participation (1995).

**VII. PERSONAL RECOMMENDATIONS FOR CHILDREN AND ADOLESCENT WITH SOLITARY KIDNEY OR RENAL ABNORMALITY**

**A.** Advise patient and family that risk of injury is highest with bicycling, American football, skiing (including snowboarding and sledding), and ice hockey. However, risk of renal injury from sports accounts for approximately 0.05% of pediatric trauma.

**B.** Advise that risk in girls participating in team sports appears extremely low.

**C.** Advise against extreme sports involving bicycles.

**D.** Advise that flank protectors are available.

**E.** Advise against collision sports in children with renal fusion abnormality, prune-belly syndrome, augmentation cystoplasty, or renal transplant.

**F.** Document discussion with patient and family carefully in medical record.

**VIII. PERSONAL RECOMMENDATIONS FOR CHILDREN OR ADOLESCENT WITH SOLITARY TESTIS OR ABNORMAL TESTIS**

**A.** Advise patient and family that reports testicular injury uncommon from sports participation, but that lack of reports probably results from most male athletes wearing protective cup.

**B.** Recommend use of protective cup in boys participating in contact sports.

**C.** Document discussion with patient and family carefully in medical record.

**RECOMMENDED READING**

American Academy of Pediatrics, Committee on Sports Medicine and Fitness. Medical conditions affecting sports participation. *Pediatrics* 1994;94:757–760.

American Academy of Pediatrics, Committee on Sports Medicine and Fitness. Medical conditions affecting sports participation. *Pediatrics* 2001;107:1205–1209.

Anderson CR. Solitary kidney and sports participation. *Arch Fam Med* 1995;4:885–888.

Gerstenbluth RE, Spirnak JP, Elder JS. Sports participation and high grade renal injuries in children. *J Urol* 2002;168:2575–2578.

McAleer IM, Kaplan GW, LoSasso BE. Renal and testis injuries in team sports. *J Urol* 2002;168:1805–1807.

Sharp DS, Ross JH, Kay R. Attitudes of pediatric urologists regarding sports participation by children with a solitary kidney. *J Urol* 2002;168:1811–1815.

Wan J, Corvino TF, Greenfield SP, et al. Kidney and testicle injuries in team and individual sports: data from the National Pediatric Trauma Registry. *J Urol* 2003;170:1528–1532.

Wan J, Corvino TF, Greenfield SP, et al. The incidence of recreational genitourinary and abdominal injuries in the western New York pediatric population. *J Urol* 2003;170:1525–1527.

# Urologic Manifestations
# of Sexual Abuse

Angelique C. Hinds

Because of the large numbers of children who have been or will be sexually abused, it is important for all medical practitioners caring for children to be well informed with regard to child sexual abuse. More specifically, some children who have been sexually abused may manifest this abuse with urologic conditions, such as incontinence. In addition, in the process of examining a child's genitalia for a urologic condition unfamiliar findings may be revealed; therefore, it is important to understand the normal and potentially abnormal findings of the genital examination.

### I. DEFINITION
The American Academy of Pediatrics, Committee on Child Abuse and Neglect defines child sexual abuse as "the engaging of a child in sexual activities that the child cannot comprehend, for which the child is developmentally unprepared and cannot give informed consent, and/or that violate the social and legal taboos of society. The sexual activities may include all forms of oral-genital, genital, or anal contact by or to the child, or nontouching abuses, such as exhibitionism, voyeurism, or using the child in the production of pornography."

### II. EPIDEMIOLOGY
**A.** At least one in four girls and one in ten boys will suffer victimization by the age of 18.

**B.** Incidence of sexual abuse rises in preadolescence with a dramatic increase at age 10, preceded by a small rise at about ages six and seven. Children under six constitute at least 10% of victims.

**C.** Adolescents are perpetrators in at least 20% of reported cases.

**D.** Children are more frequently abused by men or boys; however, women may be perpetrators, especially in day care settings.

**E.** Most perpetrators of sexual abuse are trusted adult acquaintances of the child, who often target children lacking close adult supervision and craving adult attention.

### III. RISK FACTORS
**A.** Increased risk for sexual abuse is not related to socioeconomic (education, income, or occupational) status, race, or ethnicity.

**B.** Girls are at more risk than boys; however, in clinical samples boys appear to be underrepresented.

C. Children living in the presence of a stepfather are more than 7 times more likely to be abused by him than by a natural father.

## IV. PRESENTATION

A. Children who are sexually abused are generally coerced into secrecy; therefore, a high index of suspicion is required to recognize the problem.

B. Children who have been sexually abused may present in a variety of ways.

1. History
   a. Genital or rectal complaints (Table 29–1)
   b. A parent may communicate concerns that the child has been sexually abused.
   c. The child may actually make an initial disclosure of sexual contact at a medical visit (rare).
   d. Behavioral and emotional problems may raise concern, although it is important to keep in mind that these are nonspecific and may be related to many other causes.

2. Physical examination: during examination of the genitalia, suspicious findings may be observed.

## V. HISTORY

A. In legally proven cases of child sexual abuse, the majority of victims have no diagnostic physical findings. Therefore, the unbiased interview of the child becomes the most critical part of the diagnostic evaluation. Investigative interviews should be conducted by the designated agency or individual in the community to minimize repetitive questioning of the child. However, one

**Table 29–1. Possible medical indicators of sexual abuse**

Genital, anal, or urethral trauma
Genital or anal bleeding or itching
Genital infection or discharge
Headaches
Chronic constipation, painful defecation
Vulvitis or vulvovaginitis
Pregnancy
Foreign body in the vagina or rectum
Anal inflammation
Dysuria
Recurrent UTI
Abdominal pain
Chronic genital or anal pain
Bruises to hard or soft palate, torn frenulum
Sexually transmitted disease
Bite marks on nipples/breasts
Scratch marks or bruises on hips/buttocks
Enuresis/encopresis

should not hesitate to ask relevant questions needed for a detailed pediatric history.

**B.** Any spontaneous disclosure by the child during the assessment must be documented carefully and thoroughly using the exact terminology that the child used. Although hearsay evidence is typically inadmissible in court, statements made to a doctor in the course of a medical evaluation are generally recognized as reliable and are an important exception to the hearsay rule.

## VI. PHYSICAL EXAMINATION

### A. General Examination

1. A more general physical examination should be done prior to the genital examination. Always discuss the genital examination prior to initiating. Older children should be given the choice whether they would like their parent present or not. Provide for privacy. Try to use distraction and relaxation during the examination. Note the child's behavior during the examination. No child thought to have been sexually abused should ever be forcibly restrained and examined against his or her will; arrangements should be made for an examination under anesthesia.

2. Examination findings change depending on the position of the child (supine, knee-chest, lateral), degree of relaxation, amount of labial traction (gentle, moderate), and time to perform the examination. All these variables influence the size of the orifice and exposure of the hymen and internal structures. The more relaxed the child is, the more visible the hymenal edges and the more dilated the introitus diameter; therefore, it is very important to view findings using varying traction and varying positions.

3. In girls, the genital examination should include inspection of the medial aspects of the thighs, labia majora, labia minora, clitoris, urethra, periurethral tissue, hymen, hymenal opening, fossa navicularis, and posterior fourchette/posterior commissure (Fig. 30–1). In boys, the urethral meatus, thighs, penis, and scrotum are examined.

4. In prepubertal girls, a pelvic examination with a speculum is unnecessary, unless there is unexplained, active vaginal bleeding.

### B. Examination Positions

1. Supine frog-leg position (Fig. 30–2)
   a. The child lies with legs in full abduction like a frog, with feet in apposition. In younger children, seating the child in the caretakers' lap may facilitate the examination.
   b. Examine first without separation or traction, and then with simple separation (where the labia is separated laterally only).
   c. Labial separation should be done gently and cautiously. Labial separation can be

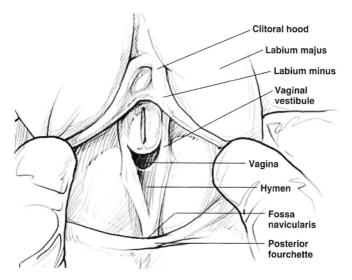

Clitoral hood

Labium majus

Labium minus

Vaginal vestibule

Vagina

Hymen

Fossa navicularis

Posterior fourchette

**Fig. 29–1.** Anatomy of prepubertal female genitalia.

painful, and may cause tears of the posterior fourchette/commissure. If a labial adhesion is present, aggressive labial separation may tear it.

**d.** Gentle traction (Fig. 30–3) should then be applied by placing the thumb and forefinger on the labia majora and pulling laterally and downward. Tension of the other pelvic

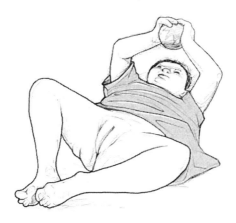

**Fig. 29–2.** Supine frog-leg position.

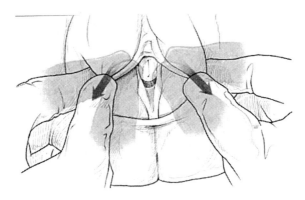

**Fig. 29–3. Labial traction.**

muscles can obscure or change the view of
the vaginal vestibular structures; therefore,
maintain labial traction for a few seconds allowing the child time to relax. This method
is successful in opening the vaginal canal
without causing additional trauma to the
tissues.

2. Knee-chest position (Fig. 30–4)
   a. Instruct the child to lay prone on the examining table. Then assist the child to assume
   a kneeling position while he or she maintains
   head and chest contact with the table and lor-
   dosis of the back. Once the child is positioned
   properly, lift the labia upward and apart gently.
   b. This technique allows excellent noninvasive
   visualization of the posterior hymen, vagina,
   anus, and occasionally the cervix.

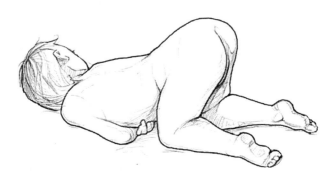

**Fig. 29–4. Knee-chest position.**

      **c.** This position may allow previously adhered and possibly redundant hymenal tissue to drop downward.

      **d.** Use this examination position routinely to clarify questionable examination findings and to verify normal or abnormal findings first noted when the patient is supine.

      **e.** In cases where there is bleeding or suspicion of vaginal foreign body, this position is helpful in that it can provide visualization of the cervix.

**C.** **Examination Techniques**

   **1.** Saline/water

      **a.** Redundancy of estrogenized postpubertal hymen makes close inspection of the hymenal tissues for traumatic injury difficult in adolescents.

      **b.** If the hymenal edges are difficult to visualize, warm normal saline drops or water may be used to float the hymen without any discomfort to the child.

   **2.** Moistened swab

      **a.** A moistened swab may be used to trace the edges of the hymen.

      **b.** The hymenal edge is very sensitive in prepubertal girls; therefore, every effort should be made to visualize the genitalia without using a swab. If a swab is needed to explore the hymenal margin in a prepubertal child, then 2% lidocaine topical gel can facilitate use of the swab. The estrogenized hymen is much more tolerant of the moistened swab.

   **3.** Foley catheter: The catheter is inserted into the vagina, the balloon is then inflated partially, and then the catheter is slowly pulled until the entire hymen can be visualized around the balloon. The balloon should be deflated prior to removal from the vagina.

   **4.** Magnification

      **a.** An otoscope or other handheld magnification can also be used to examine the genitalia and the anus.

      **b.** Colposcopy is the use of magnification and photographic or videographic documentation of physical findings of suspected sexual abuse. It has become routine practice for sexual abuse examinations done by experts; however, it is not a common piece of equipment in most medical practices, and is not recommended.

**D.** **Anal Examination:** The anus can be examined in the supine, lateral, or knee-chest position (Fig. 30–5). As with the vaginal examination, position may influence anatomy. Gluteal folds should be gently separated and assessed for external signs of trauma and to assess if anal dilation will occur. Apply greater traction thereafter in an effort to inspect the anus thoroughly. Only

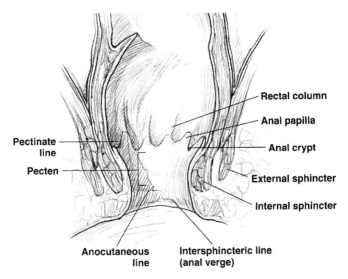

**Fig. 29–5.** Anatomy of the anus.

if there is rectal bleeding is an endoscopic examination indicated. Digital rectal examination is generally not indicated.

**E. Documentation**
1. All physical findings should be clearly documented in the child's medical record.
2. Hymenal or anal findings should be documented using the o'clock designations (i.e., "at 6:00 in the supine, frog-leg position using labial traction").
3. Whenever possible a drawing should be used.
4. For those with limited sexual abuse training it is best to describe the finding in detail and not comment on whether the finding is consistent with abuse or not.
5. Never write "hymen intact," "no signs of penetration," or "no evidence of sexual abuse" because even a normal physical examination does not rule out the possibility of sexual abuse, including penetration.

**F. Examination Findings**
1. Normal hymenal variations
   a. Most common
      (1) Crescentric: Attachments at approximately the 11 o'clock and the 1 o'clock positions without hymenal tissue between the two attachments.
      (2) Annular hymen: The tissue membrane extends completely around the circumference of the entire vaginal orifice.

      **b.** Less common
         **(1)** Cribiform: A hymen with multiple small openings.
         **(2)** Imperforate: The hymenal membrane has no opening.
         **(3)** Septate: The hymenal orifice is bisected by a band of hymenal tissue creating two or more orifices. The septate hymen should be differentiated from a bifid or duplicate vagina.

  **2.** Variations in hymenal appearance
      **a.** Estrogen
         **(1)** The hymenal appearance may vary over time due to the effects of puberty or exogenous estrogen.
         **(2)** Estrogen causes thickening of the hymenal tissue and paleness of the mucosa.
      **b.** The opening size varies according to patient positioning, examination technique, degree of relaxation, patient age, and patient size (generally, an obese child has a larger orifice).
      **c.** There are a range of anatomic variants of normal prepubertal hymens (Table 29–2).
      **d.** Newborn
         **(1)** The normal newborn hymen is generally thickened and redundant and may be described as fimbriated. By 3 years of age the majority of girls have developed a thin crescentric hymen, some with annular hymen.

**G. Physical Findings of Sexual Abuse**
  **1.** Sexual abuse in children will often leave no physical findings for the following reasons.

**Table 29–2.  Genital examination findings in prepubertal girls selected for nonabuse**

| More Common Findings | Less Common Findings |
| --- | --- |
| Erythema of the vestibule | Posterior fourchette friability |
| Periurethral bands | Hymenal clefts |
| Lymphoid follicles on the fossa navicularis | Imperforate hymen |
| Labial adhesions | Hymenal septa |
| Posterior fourchette midline avascular areas | Vaginal discharge |
| Urethral dilation with labial traction | Foreign body |
| Projections: septal remnants, hymenal tags, mounds | |
| Vaginal ridges | |
| Rugae | |

    **a.** Perpetrators will often befriend and avoid physical injury to the child.

    **b.** Digital fondling can occur without tissue damage.

    **c.** The vaginal vestibular tissues are very elastic.

    **d.** Genital tissues heal rapidly and often heal completely.

    **e.** The anus can easily stretch without causing tissue damage.

    **f.** Early pubertal estrogen effects increase hymenal elasticity, hymenal redundancy, and physiologic vaginal secretions, all of which lessen the likelihood of traumatic hymenal tearing.

    **g.** Hymenal defects become less visible following puberty.

    **h.** Some children who have normal genital examinations disclose penile penetration that is verified independently by confession or conviction of the perpetrator.

**2.** Findings consistent but not diagnostic of abuse include

    **a.** Chafing, abrasions, or bruising of inner thighs or genitalia

    **b.** Scarring, tears, or distortion of the hymen

    **c.** Decreased amount of or absent hymenal tissue

    **d.** Scarring, injury, or tears of the fossa navicularis, posterior fourchette, labia minora

    **e.** Enlargement of the hymenal opening

    **f.** Thickened, irregular, or narrowed hymen edges

    **g.** Exposure of the intravaginal contents

**3.** Normal congenital angular concavities or defects may be observed anteriorly, but not posteriorly. The incidence of posterior angular concavities or defects increases with age, suggesting acquired lesions. Physical examination for sexual abuse in girls should focus on the posterior vestibular structures.

**4.** Abnormal findings are rarely noted in sexually abused boys. If present, these findings most often involve the anus and are easily seen with careful inspection. Penile or scrotal injuries are uncommon.

**5.** Acute anal findings in boys or girls can include bruises around the anus, swelling, redness, abrasions, scars, anal tears (especially those that extend into the surrounding anal perianal skin), and occasional fissures extending to the anal verge. If present, laxity of the sphincter should be noted. These superficial injuries heal rapidly. It is unusual to find rectal lacerations from forceful penetration. These deeper injuries occasionally heal as scarring, which may become less visible over time. Anal lacerations often do not leave scars. Anal findings suggestive of chronic, repetitive trauma can include anal deformities or tags outside the midline or dilation greater than 15 mm that occurs within 30 seconds without stool in the ampulla or a marked thickening and irregularity of anal folds after complete dilation. Table 29–3 lists the classification of physical findings.

**H. Differentiation:** Child sexual abuse versus accidental genital injury

1. Conditions most commonly confused with child sexual abuse include vulvovaginitis from poor hygiene, bubble baths, nonsexually transmitted infection (such as strep and shigella), foreign bodies, accidental trauma, and congenital midline structural variations.

2. Female genital trauma caused by accidental straddle injury typically affects the clitoris, clitoral hood, mons pubis, and labial structures.These structures are mostly anterior and are injured when compressed between an object and the pubic bone. Straddle injuries are usually asymmetric and do not involve the hymen.

3. When there is tissue damage resulting from penetrating sexual abuse of girls, the injuries usually involve primarily the posterior commissure, fossa navicularis, and posterior hymen. Injury is considered to have been inflicted in the absence of clear history (witnessed or immediately reported to an adult by the child) of accidental injury consistent with the child's presentation. Even in a child too young to say what happened, if there is tissue injury significant enough to cause tearing, bleeding, or both, it is unlikely a supervising adult would not be aware of the trauma and be able to determine from environmental cues what had occurred (e.g., "I heard her crying and found her straddling the toy box").

**I. Sexually Transmitted Diseases**

1. Routine cultures and screening of all sexually abused children for gonorrhea, syphilis, hepatitis, HIV, or other sexually transmitted diseases (STDs) are not recommended. The yield of positive STDs is very low in asymptomatic prepubertal children, especially those whose histories include fondling only. When epidemiologically indicated, or when the history, physical findings, or both suggest the possibility of oral, genital, or rectal contact, appropriate tests should be obtained.

2. With genital warts there can be vertical transmission that does not manifest itself for up to 2 years or more. In addition, a child still in diapers can have transmission from the hands of a caretaker involved in diapering and hygiene. Older children can autoinnoculate the genital area with warts on their fingers.

**Table 29–3. Classification of physical findings**

**Findings specific/diagnostic for sexual contact** (even in the absence of a history of abuse

- Evidence of ejaculation (semen, sperm, or semen-specific antigens and/or enzymes)
- Pregnancy
- Syphilis, gonorrhea, or HIV infection not acquired perinatally or intravenously
- Fresh genital or anal injuries in the absence of an adequate accidental explanation: laceration, hematoma, ecchymoses, bite mark, abrasion, transection, contusion, petechiae
- Enlarged hymenal opening for age with associated findings of hymenal disruption in absence of an adequate explanation: absent hymen, hymenal remnants, healed transections or scars

**Findings consistent with sexual contact** (history and other investigations may be important)

- Trichomonas, chlamydia, *Condylomata acuminatum*, herpes simplex virus
- Hymenal disruptions: posterolateral angular concavity, transection, decrease amount, scars
- Specific anal changes: anal scars or tags outside the midline, dilation >15 mm without stool in the ampulla, irregularity of the anal orifice after dilation
- Marked dilation of the hymenal opening persisting in different examination positions

**Findings sometimes seen following sexual contact but also following other causes** (history and other investigation is important in diagnosing abuse)

- Bacterial vaginosis
- Extensive labial adhesions in girls several years out of diapers, with no other cause of labial chafing or denudation
- Posterior fourchette friability
- Other anal changes: repeated anal dilation <15 mm, shortening or eversion of the anal canal, perianal fissures, thickened perianal skin and reduction of skin folds
- Penile erection maintained during examination in prepubertal boys

**Findings unlikely to be due to sexual contact**

- Vestibular findings: lymphoid follicles or midline avascular areas of the fossa navicularis
- Urethral findings: periurethral bands, urethral dilation with labial traction
- Hymenal findings: small hymenal mounds/tags, septal remnants, anterior hymenal clefts, smooth, curved, or shallow, imperforate hymen
- Labial findings: small labial adhesions, extensive labial adhesions in girls in diapers, midline avascular areas to posterior fourchette
- Intravaginal ridges or rugae structures behind a normal hymen
- Anal findings: erythema, increased pigmentation, venous engorgement after 2 minutes in knee-chest position, midline skin tags/folds anterior to anus, smooth areas in midline, single episode of anal dilation <15 mm, anal dilation with stool in ampulla, flattening of anal verge and rugae during anal dilation
- *Candida albicans*

3. With herpes, type I must be differentiated by type II; however, both can be found in genital area and both can be transmitted sexually or nonsexually.
4. The presence of vaginal discharge or history of vaginal discharge following sexual abuse increases the likelihood of STDs. Prevalence rates of STDs among sexually abused children are generally less than 4%, but vary among geography and specific STD.
5. If a culture is done, only gold-standard culture systems should be used. Nonculture tests such as direct fluorescent antibody enzyme immunoassay or DNA nucleic acid sequence should not be used; they lack adequate specificity on specimens obtained from the vagina or the anus of children.
6. Of note, the vaginal pool is an acceptable source of culture in the prepubertal child, but a cervical swab must be done for pubertal children.

**J. Acute Sexual Assault:** When the alleged sexual abuse has occurred within 72 hours, the examination should be done immediately by a trained sexual abuse examiner. Rape kit protocols need to be followed to maintain a chain of evidence, and is beyond the scope of routine pediatric practice.

## VII. MANAGEMENT

In all 50 states, physicians are mandated by law to report to child protective services or local law enforcement whenever they suspect that a child has been sexually abused. It is most helpful to have these phone numbers ready in advance, for quick and easy reference. In addition to the numbers of local law enforcement and child protective services, the practitioner should obtain the phone number of the local child sexual abuse medical examiner. This person can be an invaluable resource with questionable examination findings.

## RECOMMENDED READING

Adams J, Harper K, Knudson S, et al. Examination findings in legally confirmed child sexual abuse: it's normal to be normal. *Pediatrics* 1994;94:310–317.

American Academy of Pediatrics Committee on Child Abuse and Neglect. Guidelines for the evaluation of sexual abuse of children. *Pediatrics* 1991;87:254–259.

Chadwick DL, Berkowitz CD, Kerns D, et al. *Color atlas of child sexual abuse.* Chicago: Yearbook Medical Publishers; 1989.

Heger AH. Twenty years in the evaluation of the sexually abused child: has medicine helped or hurt the child and family? *Child Abuse and Neglect* 1996;20:899–906.

Heger A, Emans SJ. *Evaluation of the Sexually Abused Child. A medical textbook and photographic atlas.* New York: Oxford University Press, 1992.

McCann J, Wells R, Simon M, et al. Genital findings in prepubertal girls selected for nonabuse: a descriptive study. *Pediatrics* 1990;86:428–439.

# Pediatric Urology Database

Jeffrey A. Stock and George W. Kaplan

## I. INTRAVENOUS FLUID THERAPY

### A. Maintenance of Normal Kidney Function

1. Fluid requirements
   a. Method to estimate daily maintenance rate of fluid
      (1) First 10 kg body weight: 100 mL/kg per day
      (2) Second 10 kg body weight: 50 mL/kg per day
      (3) Third 10 kg body weight and beyond: 25 mL/kg per day
      (4) Example 1: A 3-kg infant requires 300 mL fluid per day
      (5) Example 2: A 13-kg child requires 1150 mL fluid per day (1000 + 150 mL)
      (6) Example 3: A 40-kg adolescent requires 2000 mL fluid per day (1000 + 500 + 500 mL)
   b. Method to estimate hourly maintenance rate of fluid
      (1) First 10 kg body weight: 4 mL/kg per hour
      (2) Second 10 kg body weight: 2 mL/kg per hour
      (3) Third 10 kg body weight and beyond: 1 mL/kg per hour
      (4) Example 1: A 3-kg infant requires 12 mL per hour (3 kg × 4 mL/kg/h = 12 mL/h)
      (5) Example 2: A 13-kg child requires 46 mL per hour [(10 kg × 4 mL/kg/h) + (3 kg × 2 mL/kg/h) = 46 mL/h]
      (6) Example 3: A 40-kg adolescent requires 80 mL per hour: [(10 kg × 4 mL/kg/h) + (10 kg × 2 mL/kg/h) + (20 kg × 1 mL/kg/h) = 80 mL/h)]
2. Electrolyte requirements
   a. $Na^+$: 50 $mEq/m^2$ per day or 3 to 4 mEq/kg per day
   b. $K^+$: 20 $mEq/m^2$ per day or 2 mEq/kg per day
3. Appropriate solution: The most appropriate solution for routine fluid therapy in postoperative patients is 5% dextrose in 0.2% NaCl, which contains roughly 30 mEq $Na^+$ and 30 mEq $Cl^-$ per liter.
4. Losses: Losses (e.g., nasogastric suction) must be replaced accurately. Children are best followed up for dehydration by monitoring urine output. If the urine output is between 1 and 2 mL/kg per hour,

the appropriate amount of fluid is probably being given.

## II. PEDIATRIC UROLOGY FORMULARY

The information provided is not comprehensive. Please consult a more complete reference before using medications with which you are unfamiliar. (Please note that in the "Supplied As" category, the unit quantity in which a drug is supplied is noted in parentheses after the drug concentration) (Table 30–1.)

## III. DRUG DOSAGES IN RENAL INSUFFICIENCY

**A.** Drug dosage in patients with renal insufficiency (Table 30–2) may be adjusted by

  **1.** Interval extension (IE): Lengthen the interval between doses, keeping the dosage size normal, or

  **2.** Dose reduction (DR): Reduce the amount of individual doses, keeping the interval between doses normal.

**B. Note:** These drug–dosage modifications are approximations. Patients must be followed closely for signs of toxicity.

## IV. BOWEL PREPARATION (TABLE 30–3)

## V. FORMULAS

**A. Ideal Body Weight** (children 1 to 18 years) in kg = [height$^2$ (cm) × 1.65]/1000

**B. Body Surface Area** (Fig. 30–1)

**C. Creatinine Clearance**

  **1.** Estimation of creatinine clearance using body length

  Creatinine clearance (mL/min/1.73 m$^2$)

  $= [K \times \text{length (cm)}]/\text{serum creatinine (mg/dL)}$

  where $K$ = constant that is age specific

   **a.** Low birth weight, 1 year or younger: $K = 0.33$

   **b.** Full-term, 1 year or younger: $K = 0.45$

   **c.** Boys and girls, 7 to 12 years old: $K = 0.55$

   **d.** Girl, 13 to 21 years old: $K = 0.55$

   **e.** Boy, 13 to 21 years old: $K = 0.70$

  **2.** Estimation of creatinine clearance using body surface area (BSA): Children 1 to 18 years old:

  Creatinine clearance (mL/min/1.73 m$^2$)

  $= 0.48 \times \text{height (cm)} \times \text{BSA}$

  serum creatinine level (mg/dL) × 1.73

  **3.** Nomogram (Fig. 30–2)

  **4.** Normal values for glomerular filtration rate in children (Fig. 30–3)

**D. Bladder Capacity**

  **1.** Children younger than 2 years: bladder capacity (mL) = 7.0 × weight (kg)

  **2.** Children 2 to 11 years old: bladder capacity (mL) = [age (years) + 2 × 30]

**E.** Normal stretched penile length (Fig. 30–4)

**F.** Vital signs (Table 30–4)

**Table 30-1.   Pediatric dosages**

| Drug | Dose | Supplied As |
|---|---|---|
| **Analgesics** | | |
| Acetaminophen (Tylenol) | 10–15 mg/kg/dose Q4–6h PO | Tabs: 160, 325, 500, 650 mg<br>Chewable tabs: 80 mg<br>Drops: 80 mg/0.8 mL<br>Elixir: 120, 130, 160, 325 mg/5 mL<br>Caplets: 160, 325, 500 mg<br>Suppositories: 120, 125, 300, 325, 650 mg |
| | NOTE: Contraindicated in patients with glucose-6-phosphate dehydrogenase deficiency.<br>Do not exceed 5 doses per 24 h.<br>Modify dose in patients with renal impairment. | |
| Acetaminophen and codeine<br>(Tylenol with codeine) | Dose based on codeine component: 0.5–1.0 mg/kg/dose Q4–6h PO | Elixir: Acetaminophen, 120 mg, and codeine,<br>12 mg/5 mL, with alcohol 7%<br>Suspension, oral, alcohol-free: Acetaminophen,<br>120 mg, and codeine, 12 mg/5 mL<br>Tabs: Tylenol No. 1: Acetaminophen, 300 mg,<br>+ codeine, 7.5 mg<br>Tylenol No. 2: Acetaminophen, 300 mg, +<br>codeine, 15 mg<br>Tylenol No. 3: Acetaminophen, 300 mg, +<br>codeine, 30 mg<br>Tylenol No. 4: Acetaminophen, 300 mg, +<br>40 mg codeine |
| Ibuprofen (Motrin, Advil) | 4–10 mg/kg/dose Q6–8 h PO | Suspension: 100 mg/5 mL<br>Tabs: 200, 300, 400, 600, 800 mg |
| | NOTE: Use with caution in patients with aspirin hypersensitivity, hepatic/renal insufficiency, or GI disease (bleeding or ulcers). | |

| Drug | Dose | Supplied As |
|---|---|---|
| Meperidine (Demerol) | 1.0–1.5 mg/kg/dose Q3–4 h IV/IM/PO | Injectable<br>Tabs: 50, 100 mg<br>Syrup: 50 mg/5 mL (500 mL) |

NOTE: May cause nausea, vomiting, constipation, and lethargy. Contraindicated in cardiac arrhythmias, asthma, and increased intracranial pressure.

| | | |
|---|---|---|
| Morphine sulfate | Neonate: 0.05–0.2 mg/kg/dose IM/IV Q4h<br>Child: 0.1–0.2 mg/kg/dose IM/IV Q2–4h | Injectable |

NOTE: May cause respiratory and central nervous system depression. Naloxone, 0.01 mg/kg, may be used to reverse effects; repeat every 2–3 min as needed, based on response.

**Local anesthetics**

| Drug | Dose | Supplied As |
|---|---|---|
| Bupivacaine (Marcaine) | Maximum dose:<br>2.5 mg/kg (plain)<br>3.0 mg/kg (with epinephrine 1:200,000) | 0.25% solution = 2.5 mg/mL |
| Lidocaine | Maximum dose—4.5 mg/kg/dose (plain)<br>7 mg/kg/dose (with epinephrine 1:200,000) | 1% solution = 10 mg/mL |

**Antibiotics**

| Drug | Dose | Supplied As |
|---|---|---|
| Amikacin (Amikin) | Neonates: 75 mg/kg/dose IV/IM<br>Dosing interval: | Injectable |

| | Postnatal Age | |
|---|---|---|
| Gestational Age | <7 d | >7 d |
| <28 wk | Q24h | Q18h |
| 28–34 wk | Q18h | Q12h |
| >34 wk | Q12h | Q8h |
| Children: 15–22.5 mg/kg/24 h ÷ Q8–12h IV/IM | | |

NOTE: Therapeutic levels = 20–30 $\mu$g/L (peak); 5–10 $\mu$g/L (trough).
Infusion rate: Infant: 1–2 h; Child: 30–60 min.
Modify dose in patients with renal impairment.

*(Continued)*

**Table 30-1. (Continued)**

| Drug | Dose | Supplied As |
|---|---|---|
| Amoxicillin (Amoxil) | 20–50 mg/kg/24 h ÷ Q8h PO<br>UTI prophylaxis: 25 mg/kg QD | Drops: 50 mg/mL (15, 30 mL)<br>Suspension: 125, 250 mg/5 mL (80, 100, 150, 200 mL)<br>Caps: 250, 500 mg<br>Chewable tabs: 125, 250 mg |
| | NOTE: Modify dose in patients with renal impairment. | |
| Amoxicillin-clavulanic acid (Augmentin) | <40 kg: 20–40 mg/kg/24h ÷ Q8h PO<br>>40 kg: 250–500 mg Q8h PO | Tabs: 250, 500 mg<br>Chewable tabs: 125, 250 mg<br>Suspension: 125, 250 mg/5 mL (75, 150 mL) |
| | NOTE: Incidence of diarrhea is higher than with use of amoxicillin alone.<br>Modify dose in patients with renal impairment. | |
| Ampicillin | Neonates:<br>Postnatal age: <7 d: <2000 g: 50 mg/kg/24 h ÷ Q12h IM/IV<br>>2000 g: 75 mg/kg/24 h ÷ Q8h IM/IV<br>Postnatal age >7 d: <2000 g: 75 mg/kg/24 h ÷ Q8h IM/IV<br>>2000 g: 100 mg/kg/24 h ÷ Q6h IM/IV<br>Infants and children: 50–100 mg/kg/24 h ÷ Q6h IM/IV/PO | Drops: 100 mg/mL (20 mL)<br>Suspension: 125, 250 mg/5 mL (80, 100, 150, 200 mL),<br>500 mg/5 mL (100 mL)<br>Caps: 250, 500 mg<br>Injectable |
| | NOTE: Modify dose is patients with renal impairment. | |
| Aztreonam (Azactam) | Neonates:<br>Postnatal age <7 d:<br><2000 g: 60 mg/kg/24 h ÷ Q12h IM/IV<br>>2000 g: 90 mg/kg/24 h ÷ Q8h IM/IV<br>Postnatal age >7 d:<br><2000 g: 90 mg/kg/24 h ÷ Q8h IM/IV<br>>2000 g: 120 mg/kg/24 h ÷ Q6h IM/IV<br>Children >1 mo:90–120 mg/kg/24 hr ÷ Q6-8h IM/IV | Injectable |
| | NOTE: Reduce dose in patients with cystic fibrosis.<br>Modify dose in patients with renal impairment. | |

| Drug | Dose | Supplied As |
|---|---|---|
| Cefazolin (Ancef) (1st generation) | Neonate: Postnatal age <7 d: 40 mg/kg/24 h ÷ Q12h Postnatal age >7 d: <2000 g 40 mg/kg/d ÷ Q12h >2000 g 60 mg/kg/d ÷ Q8h Infants (>1 mo) and children: 50–100 mg/kg/24 h ÷ Q8h | Injectable |
|  | NOTE: Modify dose in patients with renal impairment. |  |
| Ceftriaxone (Rocephin) (3rd generation) | Infant and child: 50–75 mg/kg/24 h ÷ Q12–24h IM/IV Adult: 1–4 g/24 h ÷ Q12–24h IM/IV | Injectable |
| Cephalexin (Keflex) (1st generation) | Children 25–100 mg/kg/24 h ÷ Q6h PO Adult: 250–500 mg Q6h PO | Caps: 250, 500 mg Drops: 100 mg/mL (10 mL) Suspension: 125 mg/5 mL (50, 60, 100, 200 mL) 250 mg/5 mL (5, 100, 200 mL) Tabs: 250, 500, 1000 mg |
|  | NOTE: Modify doses in patients with renal impairment. |  |
| Ciprofloxacin (Cipro) | 20–30 mg/kg/24 h ÷ Q12h IV/PO | Tabs: 250, 500, 750 mg Injection: 200 mg/20 mL |
|  | NOTE: Not recommended for children <16–18 y. Modify doses in patients with renal impairment. |  |

*(Continued)*

**Table 30-1.**  *(Continued)*

| Drug | Dose | | | Supplied As |
|---|---|---|---|---|
| Gentamicin | Neonates: 2.5 mg/kg/dose IV/IM<br>Dosing interval: | | | Injectable |

| | | Postnatal Age | |
|---|---|---|---|
| | Gestational Age | <7 d | >7 d |
| | <28 wk | Q24h | Q18h |
| | 28–34 wk | Q18h | Q12h |
| | >34 wk | Q12h | Q8h |

Children: 6–7.5 mg/kg/24 h ÷ Q8h IV/IM
Adults: 3–5 mg/kg/d ÷ Q8h IV/IM

NOTE: Therapeutic levels = 6–10 µg/L (peak); <2 µg/L (trough).
Modify dose in patients with renal impairment.

| Drug | Dose | Supplied As |
|---|---|---|
| Metronidazole (Flagyl) | Anaerobic infections: 30 mg/kg/d ÷ Q6h IV/PO<br>*Clostridium difficile* infection: 20 mg/kg/d ÷ Q6h PO | Tabs: 250, 500 mg<br>Injectable |
| Nitrofurantoin (Furadantin, Macrodantin) | Children >1 mo: 5–7 mg/kg/24 h ÷ Q6h PO<br>Prophylaxis: 1–2 mg/kg/QD | Suspension: 25 mg/5 mL<br>Tabs: 50, 100 mg<br>Caps: 25, 50, 100 mg |

NOTE: Contraindicated in infants <1 month of age.
Modify dose in patients with renal impairment.

| Drug | Dose | Supplied As |
|---|---|---|
| Trimethoprim (TMP)-sulfamethoxazole (Septra) | Dose based on TMP component: 8–10 mg/kg/24 h ÷ Q12h PO<br>Prophylaxis: 2 mg/kg/24 h QD | Suspension: 40 mg TMP per 5 mL (20, 100, 150, 200, 480 mL)<br>Tabs: 80 mg TMP (single strength [SS]),<br>160 mg TMP (double strength [DS]) |

NOTE: May cause kernicterus in newborns.
Modify dose in patients with renal impairment.

| Drug | Dose | Supplied As |
|---|---|---|
| Tobramycin (Tobrex) | Neonates: 2.5 mg/kg/dose IV/IM<br>Dosing interval: | Injectable |

| | | Postnatal Age | |
|---|---|---|---|
| | Gestational Age | <7 d | >7 d |
| | <28 wk | Q24h | Q18h |
| | 28–34 wk | Q18h | Q12h |
| | >34 wk | Q12h | Q8h |

Children: 6–7.5 mg/kg/24 h ÷ Q8h IV/IM
Adults: 3–5 mg/kg/24 h ÷ Q8h IV/IM

NOTE: Therapeutic levels = 6–10 $\mu$g/L (peak); <2 $\mu$g/L (trough).
Modify dose in patients with renal impairment.

**Anti-fungal drugs**

| Drug | Dose | Supplied As |
|---|---|---|
| Amphotericin B (Fungizone) | Bladder irrigation: 15–50 mg/d in 1 L sterile water or sorbitol/mannitol irrigation instilled over 24 h<br>Infants and children:<br>  Test dose: 0.1 mg/kg/dose IV to a maximum of 1 mg; infuse over 30–60 min.<br>  Initial therapeutic dose (if test dose is tolerated): 0.25 mg/kg.<br>  The daily dose can then be gradually increased, usually in 0.25-mg/kg increments each subsequent day until the desired dose is reached.<br>  Maintenance dose: 0.25–1 mg/kg/d QD, infuse over 2–6 h. | Injectable |
| | NOTE: Modify dose in patients with renal impairment. | |
| Fluconazole (Diflucan) | Children (3–13 y):<br>  Loading dose: 10 mg/kg IV/PO<br>  Maintenance (begin 24 h after loading dose): 3–6 mg/kg/24 h IV/PO QD | Tabs: 50, 100, 200 mg<br>Injectable |
| | NOTE: PO and IV doses are equivalent.<br>Modify dose in patients with renal impairment. | |

*(Continued)*

**Table 30–1.** *(Continued)*

| Drug | Dose | Supplied As |
|------|------|-------------|
| Flucytosine (5-FC) | Neonates: 20–40 mg/kg/dose Q6h PO<br>Children and adults: 50–150 mg/kg/d ÷ Q6h PO<br>NOTE: Modify dose in patients with renal impairment. | Caps: 250, 500 mg |
| **Anti-emetics** | | |
| Ondansetron (Zofran) | Children >3 y: 0.15 mg/kg/dose IV Q4h<br>NOTE: Decreased effectiveness has been reported when administered for more than 3 doses. | Injectable |
| Prochlorperazine (Compazine) | Oral, rectal: 0.4 mg/kg/24 h ÷ Q6–8h PO/PR<br>IM: 0.1–0.15 mg/kg/dose TID<br><br>NOTE: Safety and efficacy have not been established in children <9 kg or <2 y of age. | Injectable<br>Tabs: 5, 10, 25 mg<br>Syrup: 5 mg/5 mL (120 mL)<br>Suppository: 2.5, 5, 25 mg |
| Trimethobenzamide (Tigan) | Children:<br>Oral, rectal: 15–20 mg/kg/d ÷ 3–4 doses<br>IM: Not recommended<br>Adults:<br>Oral: 250 mg 3–4 times/24 h<br>IM, rectal: 200 mg 3–4 times/24 h<br><br>NOTE: Contraindicated in neonates and premature infants. | Injectable<br>Caps: 100, 250 mg<br>Suppository: 100, 200 mg |
| **Anti-enuresis drugs** | | |
| Desmopressin acetate (DDAVP) | Nocturnal enuresis (>6 y): 20 μg at bedtime intranasally<br>Range 10–40 μg | Spray: 5-mL bottle with spray pump delivering 50 doses of 10 μg |
| Imipramine (Tofranil) | Nocturnal enuresis (>6 yr):<br>Initial: 10–25 mg QHS PO<br>Increment: 10–25 mg/dose at 1–2 wk intervals until maximal dose for age or desired effect achieved<br>NOTE: Maximal dose: 6–12 y: 50 mg/24 h; 12–14 y: 75 mg/24 h or 2 mg/kg/d. | Tabs: 10, 25, 50 mg<br>Caps: 75, 100, 125, 150 mg |

| Drug | Dose | Supplied As |
|---|---|---|
| **Bladder analgesics** | | |
| Phenazopyridine (Pyridium) | Children 6–12 y: 12 mg/kg/24 h ÷ TID | Tabs: 100, 200 mg |
| | NOTE: Colors urine orange, may also stain contact lenses and clothing. | |
| **Histamine₂ blockers** | | |
| Cimetidine (Tagamet) | Neonates: 5–10 mg/kg/d ÷ Q8–12h PO/IV/IM<br>Infants: 10–20 mg/kg/d ÷ Q6–12h PO/IV/IM<br>Children: 20–30 mg/kg/d ÷ Q6h PO/IV/IM<br>Adults: 300 mg/dose Q6h PO/IV/IM<br>400 mg/dose Q12h or 800 mg/dose QHS | Tabs: 200, 300, 400, 800 mg<br>Syrup: 300 mg/5 mL (237 mL)<br>Injectable |
| | NOTE: Modify dose in patients with renal impairment. | |
| Ranitidine (Zantac) | PO: 2–4 mg/kg/24 h ÷ Q12h<br>IV: 1–2 mg/kg/24 h ÷ Q8–8h | Tabs: 150, 300 mg<br>Syrup: 15 mg/mL (7.5% alcohol) |
| | NOTE: Modify dose in patients with renal impairment. | |
| **Drug therapy for neurogenic bladder dysfunction** | | |
| **Anticholinergic** | | |
| Hyoscyamine (Levsin) | SL tabs:<br>Children 2–12 y: 1/2 to 1 tab Q4h<br>Do not exceed 6 tabs in 24 h<br>12 y of age and older: 1–2 tabs Q4h<br>Do not exceed 12 tabs in 24 h or 0.03 mg/kg BID–0.1 mg/kg QID | SL tabs: 0.125 mg |
| Oxybutynin (Ditropan) | Child <5 y: Age in y = mL per dose BID/TID<br>>5 y: 0.2 mg/kg BID-QID | Tabs: 5 mg<br>Syrup: 5 mg/5 mL (473 mL) |
| Propantheline (Pro-Banthine) | 0.5 mg/kg BID-QID | Tab: 7.5, 15 mg |
| **Sympathomimetic** | | |
| Pseudoephedrine (Sudafed) | 0.4 mg/kg BID–0.9 mg/kg TID | Tabs: 30, 60 mg<br>Liquid: 15 mg/5 mL (120 mL), 30 mg/5 mL (120 mL, 240 mL, 473 mL) |
| **Sympatholytic** | | |
| Prazosin (Minipress) | 0.05 mg/kg BID–0.1 mg/kg TID | Caps: 1, 2, 5 mg |

*(Continued)*

**Table 30-1. (Continued)**

| Drug | Dose | Supplied As |
|---|---|---|
| **Hormonal treatment of retractile testes** | | |
| Chorionic gonadotropin (Pregnyl) | 50 USP U/kg IM Q5d × 5 doses<br><br>NOTE: Maximal single dose 2000 USP U.<br>Maximal total dose 10,000 USP U. | Injectable |
| **Cathartics** | | |
| Bisacodyl (Dulcolax) | Oral:<br>Children 3–12 y: 5–10 mg or 0.3 mg/kg/d as a single dose<br>Suppository:<br>Children <2 y: 5 mg/d as a single dose<br>Children 2–11 y: 5–10 mg/d as a single dose | Tabs: 5 mg<br>Suppository: 5, 10 mg |
| Docusate (Colace) | <3 y: 10–40 mg/24 h ÷ QD-QID<br>3–6 y: 20–60 mg/24 h ÷ QD-QID<br>6–12 y: 40–120 mg/24 h ÷ QD-QID<br>>12 y: 50–500 mg/24 h ÷ QD-QID | Caps: 50, 100, 240, 250, 300 mg<br>Tabs: 50, 100 mg<br>Syrup: 20 mg/5 mL (240 mL) |
| Mineral oil | 5–11 y: 5–20 mL QD<br>>12 y: 15–45 mL QD | Emulsion: 1.4 g/5 mL (480 mL)<br>2.5 mL/5 mL (420 mL)<br>2.75 mL/5 mL (480 mL)<br>4.75 mL/5 mL (240 mL)<br>Liquid: 500, 1000, 4000 mL |
| Senna (Senokot) | Oral:<br>Children: 10–20 mg/kg/dose at bedtime<br>Rectal:<br>Children >27 kg: 1/2 suppository at bedtime | Granules: 325 mg/teaspoonful<br>Liquid: 7% (130 mL, 360 mL)<br>6.5% (75 mg, 150 mL)<br>Syrup: 218 mg/5 mL (60 mL, 240 mL)<br>Tab: 187 mg, 217 mg, 600 mg<br>Suppository rectal: 652 mg |

NOTE: Maximal dose = 872 mg.

From Stock JA, Packer MG, Kaplan GW: Pediatric urology facts and figures: Data useful in the management of pediatric urologic patients. *Urol Clin N Am* 22:205–219, 1995.

**Table 30–2. Drug dosages in renal insufficiency**

| Drug | Normal Dose Interval | Method | Creatinine Clearance (mL/min) | | |
| --- | --- | --- | --- | --- | --- |
| | | | >50 | 10–50 | <10 |
| **Antibiotics** | | | | | |
| Amikacin | Q8–12 h | IE | Q12 h | Q12–18h | Q24h |
| | | DR | 60–90% | 30–70% | 20–30% |
| Amoxicillin | Q8 h | IE | Q8 h | Q8–12 h | Q12–16h |
| Amoxicillin and clavulanic acid | Q8 h | IE | Q8 h | Q12–18 h | Q24–36h |
| Ampicillin | Q4–6 h | IE | Q6 h | Q6–12 h | Q12–16 h |
| Aztreonam | Q6–8 h | DR | 100% | 50% | 25% |
| Cefazolin | Q8 h | IE | Q8 h | Q8–12 h | Q24–48 h |
| Cefixime | Q12–24 h | DR | 100% | 75% | 50% |
| Cephalexin | Q6 h | IE | Q6 h | Q6–8 h | Q8–12 h |
| Ciprofloxacin | Q12 h | IE | Q12 h | Q18–24 h | Q18–24 h |
| Gentamicin | Q8 h | IE | Q8–12 h | Q12 h | Q24 h |
| | | DR | 60–90% | 30–70% | 20–30% |
| Nitrofurantoin | Q8 h | IE | Q8 h | Avoid | Avoid |
| Sulfamethoxazole | Q12 h | IE | Q12 h | Q18 h | Q24 h |
| Trimethoprim | Q12 h | IE | Q12 h | Q18 h | Q24 h |
| Tobramycin | Q8h | IE | Q8–12 h | Q12h | Q24 h |
| | | DR | 60–90% | 30–70% | 20–30% |
| **Anti-fungal** | | | | | |
| Amphotericin B | Q24 h | IE | Q24 h | Q24 h | Q24–36 h |
| Fluconazole | QD | DR | 100% | 50% | 25% |
| Flucytosine | Q6 h | IE | Q6 h | Q12–24 h | Q24–48 h |
| | | DR | 50% | 30–50% | 20–30% |
| **Non-antibiotics** | | | | | |
| Acetaminophen | Q4 h | IE | Q4 h | Q6 h | Q8 h |
| Cimetidine | Q12 h | IE | Q6 h | Q8 h | Q12 h |
| | | DR | 100% | 75% | 50% |
| Ranitidine | Q8–12 h | DR | 100% | 75% | 50% |

From Stock JA, Packer MG, Kaplan GW: Pediatric urology facts and figures: Data useful in the management of pediatric urologic patients. *Urol Clin N Am* 22:205–219; 1995.

    **G.**  Blood pressure (Table 30–5)
    **H.**  Renal length versus age (Fig. 30–5A), height (Fig. 30–5B), weight (Fig. 30–5C), and total BSA (Fig. 30–5D)
    **I.**  Physical development (Table 30–6)
    **J.**  Tanner stages (Table 30–7)
    **K.**  Urine Output and Voiding Habits (Tables 30–8 and 30–9)

**Table 30–3.  Bowel preparation**

| Drug | Dose | Supplied As |
|---|---|---|
| Magnesium citrate | 4 mL/kg/dose PO<br>Repeat Q4–6 h until liquid stool results<br>*Note:* Maximal dose = 200 mL. Use with caution in patients with renal insufficiency. | Solution 300 mL |
| Polyethylene glycol electrolyte solution (GoLYTELY) | *Oral:* 25–40 mL/kg/h until rectal effluent is clear<br>*Nasogastric:* 20–30 mL/min to 4 L (1.2–1.8 L/h)<br>*Note:* Monitor electrolyte levels with prolonged administration. Rapid drinking of each portion is preferred to drinking of small amounts continuously. | Powder for oral solution: 2000 mL, 4000 mL, 4800 mL, 6000 mL |
| Neomycin | Preoperative intestinal antisepsis:<br>*Children:* 25 mg/kg PO at 1, 2, and 11 p.m. on day preceding surgery<br>*Adults:* 1 g PO at 1, 2, and 11 p.m. on day preceding surgery | Tab: 500 mg<br>Solution: 125 mg/ 5 mL (480 mL) |
| Erythromycin | Preoperative intestinal antisepsis:<br>*Children:* 20 mg/kg base PO at 1, 2, and 11 p.m. on day preceding surgery<br>*Adults:* 1 g base PO at 1, 2, and 11 p.m. on day preceding surgery | Caps: 125, 250 mg |

From Stock JA, Packer MG, Kaplan GW: Pediatric urology facts and figures: Data useful in the management of pediatric urologic patients. *Urol Clin N Am* 22:205–219; 1995.

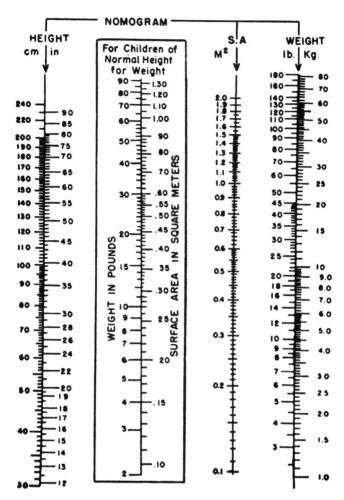

Fig. 30–1.  Nomogram or estimation of surface area. The surface area is indicated when a straight line that connects the height and weight levels intersects the surface area column; or the patient is roughly of average size, from the weight along (enclosed area). (From Behrman RE, Kliegman RM, *Nelson textbook of pediatrics*, 13th ed. Philadelphia: Saunders, 1987:1521.)

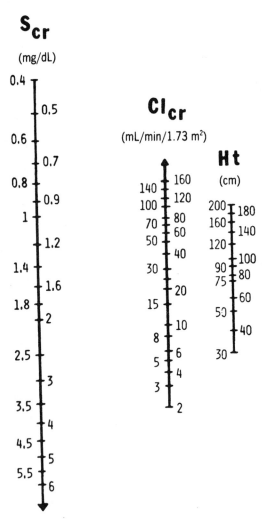

**Fig. 30–2.** Nomogram for rapid evaluation of endogenous creatinine clearance in children (1 to 18 years of age). To predict creatinine clearance, connect the child's serum creatinine concentration and height with a ruler and read the creatinine clearance where the ruler intersects the central line. (From Traub SL, John CE. Comparison of methods of estimating creatinine clearance in children. *Am J Hosp Pharm* 1980;37:195.)

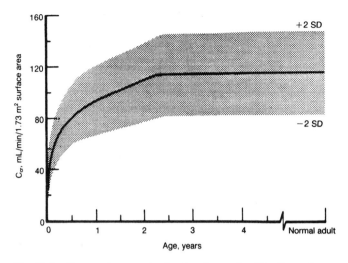

Fig. 30–3. Changes in normal value for glomerular filtration rate (GFR) from birth to later childhood. The GFR was derived by endogenous creatinine clearance. (From McCrory WN. *Developmental Nephrology*. Cambridge, Mass: Harvard University Press, 1972:98. Graph created from data from Winberg J. The 24 hour true endogenous creatinine clearance in infants and children without renal disease. *Acta Pediatr* 1959;48:443–452.)

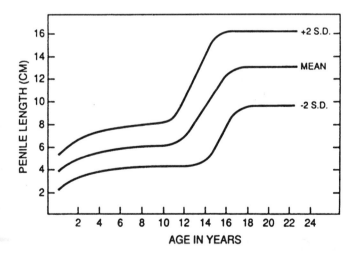

Fig. 30–4. Nomogram of the normal range of stretched penile length in men as a function of age (SD). (From Griffin JE, Wilson JD. Disorders of sexual differentiation. In: Walsh PC, Retik AB, Stamey TA, et al, eds. *Campbell's urology*, 6th ed. Philadelphia: WB Saunders, 1992: 1531.)

**Table 30–4.  Normal values for vital signs in children to 10 years of age**

| Age (y) | Pulse Rate (beats/min) | Blood Pressure (mm Hg) | Respirations (breaths/min) |
|---|---|---|---|
| 0–1 | 120 | 80/40 | 40 |
| 0–5 | 100 | 100/60 | 30 |
| 5–10 | 80 | 120/80 | 20 |

From Coran AG: Perioperative care of the pediatric surgical patient. *Sci Amer Surg* VIII:3, 1994, with permission.

**Table 30–5.  Classification of hypertension by age group**

| Age Group | Significant Hypertension (mm Hg) | Severe Hypertension (mm Hg) |
|---|---|---|
| Newborn (7 d) | | |
| Systolic BP | ≥96 | >106 |
| Newborn (8–30 d) | | |
| Systolic BP | ≥104 | ≥110 |
| Infant (<2 y) | | |
| Systolic BP | ≥112 | ≥118 |
| Diastolic BP | ≥74 | ≥82 |
| Children (3–5 y) | | |
| Systolic BP | ≥116 | ≥124 |
| Diastolic BP | ≥76 | ≥84 |
| Children (6–9 y) | | |
| Systolic BP | ≥122 | ≥130 |
| Diastolic BP | ≥78 | ≥86 |
| Children (10–12 y) | | |
| Systolic BP | ≥126 | ≥134 |
| Diastolic BP | ≥82 | >90 |
| Adolescents (13–15 y) | | |
| Systolic BP | ≥136 | ≥144 |
| Diastolic BP | ≥86 | ≥92 |
| Adolescents (16–18 y) | | |
| Systolic BP | ≥142 | ≥150 |
| Diastolic BP | ≥92 | ≥98 |

BP = Blood pressure. From Task force on Blood Pressure Control in Children: Report on the Second Task Force on Blood Pressure Control in Children. *Pediatrics* 1987;79:1, with permission.

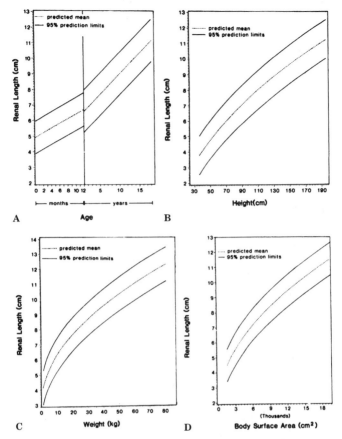

**Fig. 30–5.** Renal length: versus (A) age, (B) height, (C) weight, and (D) total body surface area. Dashed line, predicted mean; solid line, 95% prediction limits. (From Han BK, Babcock DS. Sonographic measurements and appearance of normal kidneys in children. *Am J Roentgenol* 1985;145:611.)

**Table 30–6. Physical development**

| | |
|---|---|
| Weight gain first 6 wk | Head circumference |
| 20 g/d | 35 cm at birth |
| Birth weight | 44 cm by 6 mo |
| Regained by day 14 | 47 cm by 1 y |
| Doubled by age 4 mo | 1 cm/mo in 1st y |
| Tripled by age 12 mo | 0.3 cm/me in 2nd y |
| Quadrupled by age 2 y | |
| Length | Teeth |
| Increases 50% by age 1 y | First tooth: 6–18 mo |
| Doubles by age 4 y | Number of teeth = age (mo) − |
| Triples by age 13 y | 6 (until 30 mo) |

From Taketoma CK, Hodding JH, Kraus DM: *Pediatric dosage handbook*, 2nd ed., Cleveland, Lexi-Comp, 1993; p. 654, with permission.

**Table 30–7.  Tanner stages**

| Stage/Characteristics | Age at Onset (M ± SD) |
|---|---|
| Genital stages: male | |
| 1. Prepubertal | |
| 2. Scrotum and testes enlarge: skin of scrotum reddens and rugations appear | 11.4 ± 1.1 y |
| 3. Penis lengthens: testes enlarge further | 12.9 ± 1 y |
| 4. Penis growth continues in length and width; glans develops adult form | 13.8 ± 1 y |
| 5. Development completed: adult appearance | 14.9 ± 1.1 y |
| Breast development; female | |
| 1. Prepubertal | |
| 2. Breast buds appear; areolae enlarge | 11.2 ± 1.1 y |
| 3. Elevation of breast contour; areolae enlarge | 12.2 ± 1.1 y |
| 4. Areolae and papillae form a secondary mound on breast | 13.1 ± 1.2 y |
| 5. Adult form | 15.3 ± 1.7 y |
| Menarche | 13.5 ± 1 y |
| Pubic hair; both sexes | |
| 1. Prepubertal, no coarse hair | |
| 2. Longer, silky hair appears at base of penis or along labia | M: 12 ± 1 y |
| 3. Hair coarse, kinky, spreads over public bone | F: 12.4 ± 1.1 y M: 13.9 ± 1 y |
| 4. Hair of adult quality but not spread to junction of medial thigh with perineum | F: 13 ± 1 y M: 14.4 ± 1 y |
| 5. Spread to medial thigh | F: 14.4 ± 1 y M: 15.2 ± 1.1 y |
| 6. Male escutcheon | Variable if occurs |
| Maximum growth rate | M: 14.1 ± 0.9 y F: 12.1 ± 0.9 y |

From Taketoma CK, Hodding JH, Kraus DM: *Pediatric dosage handbook,* 2nd ed., Cleveland, Lexi-Comp, 1993; p. 654, with permission.

**Table 30–8.  Urine output per day according to age**

| Age | Output (cc) |
|---|---|
| 0–48 h | 15–60 |
| 3–10 d | 100–300 |
| 10–60 d | 250–450 |
| 2 mo–1 y | 400–500 |
| 1–3 y | 500–600 |
| 3–5 y | 600–700 |
| 5–8 y | 650–1000 |
| 8–14 y | 800–1400 |

From Campbell M: *Clinical pediatric urology.* Philadelphia, WB Saunders, 1951.

**Table 30–9. Percentile information for elimination by age group**

| Age Group (y) | Number of Patients | Voids per Day | | Bowel Movements per Week | |
|---|---|---|---|---|---|
| | | 10th | 90th | 10th | 90th |
| 2 or less | 34 | 4.3 | 9.0 | 5.0 | 10.6 |
| 3 | 137 | 3.5 | 7.5 | 5.0 | 12.0 |
| 4 | 149 | 3.5 | 7.0 | 5.0 | 10.0 |
| 5 | 118 | 3.5 | 7.0 | 4.0 | 9.0 |
| 6 | 100 | 3.2 | 7.5 | 4.0 | 7.3 |
| 7 | 101 | 3.0 | 7.0 | 4.2 | 8.8 |
| 8 | 79 | 3.0 | 7.0 | 4.2 | 7.9 |
| 9 | 78 | 3.0 | 7.0 | 4.0 | 7.9 |
| 10 | 76 | 3.5 | 7.0 | 4.0 | 8.8 |
| 11 | 64 | 3.5 | 7.0 | 4.0 | 8.9 |
| 12 | 56 | 3.0 | 7.6 | 4.0 | 10.2 |
| 13 | 45 | 3.0 | 5.5 | 3.5 | 9.0 |
| 14 | 33 | 3.4 | 9.0 | 3.0 | 10.0 |
| 15 | 33 | 3.0 | 7.0 | 3.6 | 8.7 |
| 16 | 25 | 3.0 | 7.2 | 1.9 | 14.0 |
| 17 | 23 | 3.0 | 5.5 | 3.6 | 9.0 |
| 18 or more | 41 | 3.0 | 8.2 | 4.0 | 8.1 |

From Bloom DA, Seeley WW, Ritchey ML et al.: Toilet habits and continence in children: An opportunity sampling in search of normal parameters, *J Urol* 1993;149:1087, with permission.

## RECOMMENDED READING

Bauer SB. Neuropathology of the lower urinary tract. In: Kelalis PP, King LR, Belman AB, eds. *Clinical pediatric urology,* 3rd ed. Philadelphia: WB Saunders, 1982:399–440.

Fairhurst JJ, Rubin CME, Hyde I, et al. Bladder capacity in infants. *J Pediatr Surg* 1991;26:55.

Filston HC. Fluid and electrolyte management. In: Kelalis PP, King LR, Belman AB, eds. *Clinical pediatric urology,* 3rd ed. Philadelphia: WB Saunders, 1982:272–285.

Forest MG, David M, David L, et al. Undescended testis: comparison of two protocols of treatment with human chorionic gonadotropin. *Horm Res* 1988;30:198.

Johnson KB. *The harriet lane handbook,* 13th ed. St. Louis: Mosby Year Book, 1993.

Koff SA. Estimating bladder capacity in children. *Urology* 1983;21:248.

*Physician's desk reference,* 47th ed. Oradell, NJ: Medical Economics, 1992.

Stock JA, Packer MG, Kaplan GW. Pediatric urology facts and figures: data useful in the management of pediatric urologic patients. *Urol Clin North Am* 1995;22:205–219.

Taketomo CK, Hodding JH, Kraus DM. *Pediatric dosage handbook,* 2nd ed. Cleveland, OH: Lexi-Comp, 1993.

# Online Pediatric Urology Recommendations

Laurence S. Baskin

The Internet is ubiquitous and patients and physicians have easy access to an unlimited amount of unreferenced medical material. The trick is to negotiate the web in a strategic fashion so that reliable, accurate, and up-to-date information can be obtained. Below are monitored web sites that give useful patient information on common pediatric urology problems, including patient handouts in both English and Spanish.

One of the most important pieces of information that can be obtained on the Internet is a physician in your community with expertise in pediatric urology. Urologists who have obtained further training in pediatric urology and confine their practice to children can be found by searching the membership list of the Society of Pediatric Urology at spuonline.edu or http://main.uab.edu/spu/show.asp?durki = 47598.

## RECOMMENDED PEDIATRIC UROLOGY WEBSITES

### Pediatric Urology
http://urology.ucsf.edu/clinicalRes/CRpedUro.html

### Hypospadias
Hypospadias.com
http://urology.ucsf.edu/clinicalRes/CRhypo.html

### General Urology Health Information
http://urologyhealth.org.html

### Pediatric Urology Patient Handouts
http://urology.ucsf.edu/patientGuides/pedUro.html

#### English Version
Bladder Augmentation Surgery
Children's Continence Clinic
Circumcision: Post-Op Instructions for Newborn, Baby & Toddler
Circumcision: Post-Op Instructions for Adolescents
Clean Intermittent Catheterization for Bladder Emptying
Clean Intermittent Catheterization Through an Abdominal Stoma (Appendicovesicostomy)
Enuresis (Bed-wetting)
Hydrocele/Hernia
Hydronephrosis: Prenatal Diagnosis
Hypospadias Overview
Hypospadias Repair, Postoperative Care
Length of Stay for Specialized Pediatric Urologic Care
Pediatric Urinary Continence

Pyeloplasty Surgery for Uretero-Pelvic Junction (UPJ)
    Obstruction
Undescended Testes
Ureteral Reimplant Surgery for Reflux
Urinary Tract Infection (UTI)
VCUG (Voiding cystourethrogram)
Vesicoureteral Reflux

**Spanish Version**
Clínica de Continencia de Niños en Español
Enuresis en Español
Hernia/Hidrocele en Español
Hipospadias en Español
Undescended Testes en Español: El Testiculo Retenido
    (No Ha Decendido)
Ureteral Reimplant Surgery en Español: Cirugia de
    Reimplantacion Ureteral
VCUG en Español: Cistouretrograma de Evacuacion de
    Orina

# Index

NOTE: Italic *f* indicates an illustration; *t* indicates a table.